MAINTAINING THE MIRACLE:

An Owner's Manual for the Human Body

by

Ted D. Adams, Ph.D.
Program Director, The Fitness Institute,
Division of Cardiology, LDS Hospital
Adjunct Associate Professor of Physical Education,
University of Utah
Salt Lake City, Utah

A. Garth Fisher, Ph.D.
Director, Human Performance Research Center,
Professor of Physical Education,
Brigham Young University
Provo, Utah

Frank G. Yanowitz, M.D.
Medical Director, The Fitness Institute,
Division of Cardiology, LDS Hospital
Associate Professor of Medicine (Cardiology),
University of Utah School of Medicine
Salt Lake City, Utah

An up-to-date and personalized owner's manual
for promoting and maintaining
good health.

A user-friendly format that visibly tracks the timetable
of what must be done to prevent disease
and insure optimal health.

Published by VITALITY HOUSE INTERNATIONAL, INC.
Copyright © 1991 by Ted D. Adams, Ph.D., and A. Garth Fisher, Ph.D.

All rights reserved including the right of reproduction in whole or in part in any form by:
VITALITY HOUSE INTERNATIONAL, INC.
1675 North Freedom Boulevard, #11C, Provo, Utah 84604

To order: Call toll-free 1-800-637-0708.
First Printing, August 1991

ISBN #: 0-912547-09-X
Library of Congress #: 91-065532

Cover designed by Jim Knight Design
Text designed by Mark Woodland/Lexicon
Photography by Borge Anderson and Associates

The authors are grateful for permission to reprint the following material: Information from the LDS Hospital's *Total Fitness Workbook*, by Ted D. Adams, Robin L. Lockwood, Timothy G. Butler, Larry S. Carr, Jerry R. Edgington, Mary E. Mahler, Kathleen Nielson, Jill Paxman, Gregory W. Schreeve, Frank G. Yanowitz, and David B. Midget (editor); information and drawings were used from the Cottonwood Hospital Medical Center's *Back School* booklet (authors are Stephen Hunter, Anne Hunter, Kurt Dudley, Laurie Stewart, Doug Green, Bill Tobey, and IHC Publishing Services); condensed information on urinalysis and blood tests from *The Peoples Book of Medical Tests* by Drs. David S. Sobel and Tom Ferguson, published by Summit Books (New York); The Rockport Walking Institute's "The Rockport Fitness Walking Test," and the Rockport Walking Institute's "Exercise Program" charts from *Dr. James M. Rippe's Complete Book of Fitness Walking* by Dr. James M. Rippe and Dr. Ann Ward (Prentice Hall Press, New York); a cartoon by Gary Larsen (Universal Press Syndicate); "Sleep Disorders" list from The Upjohn Company, written by Dr. Peter Hauri; a "Psychological Symptoms Checklist" from Dr. Joan Borysenko's book *Minding the Body, Mending the Mind* (Addison-Wesley Publishing Company, MA); the American Cancer Society's "10-Step Skin Cancer Check" and various figures reproduced from *The American Cancer Society: Cancer Book* (Doubleday and Company, New York); a "Home Safety Checklist" by Dr. Laurence Z. Rubenstein, reproduced from *Practical Care of the Ambulatory Patient* (W.B. Saunders Company, Phil.); condensed material on weight management principles from *How to Lower Your Fat Themostat*, by Drs. Dennis Remington, Garth Fisher, and Edward Parent (Vitality House International, Inc., Provo, UT); norms and percentiles by age and gender for trunk forward flexion and push-ups, developed by Fitness Canada and published in *Exercise in Health and Disease*, by Drs. Michael L. Pollock and Jack H. Wilmore (W.B. Saunders Company, Phil.); a life experience by U.S. Senator Jake Garn; a life experience by former U.S. Senator Wallace Bennett; a modification of "The Relaxation Response" from Dr. Herbert Benson's book *The Relaxation Response* (Avon Books, New York); strength and flexibility standards by the Canadian Standardized Test of Fitness Operations Manual; "Nutrition Goal Sheets" by Martha McMurry and The Cardiovascular Research Clinic, University of Utah Medical Center; excerpts from "Aspirin and Your Heart" (American Heart Association); and medical health questionnaire material from The Cardiovascular Genetics Research Clinic, the University of Utah School of Medicine, The Fitness Institute at LDS Hospital (Salt Lake City, UT), and Dr. Ralph S. Paffenbarger of Stanford University.

To

Suzanne, Joseph, Samuel,
Aubrey, John, Ryan, and Ethel

and

Dr. Webster L. Marxer, a pioneer
in preventive medicine, whose philosophy was:
"The most advanced state of
the art of medicine is dedicated to
the maintenance of function."

CONTENTS

ACKNOWLEDGEMENTS

We acknowledge and give thanks to the following individuals who have assisted the authors in the writing, editing and/or scientific review of this book.

O. Glade Hunsaker, Ph.D.
Professor, English Department,
Brigham Young University,
Provo, Utah

John H. Holbrook, M.D.
Professor, Internal Medicine and
Chief, Div. of General Internal Medicine,
University of Utah School of Medicine,
Salt Lake City, Utah

Charles Smart, M.D.
Chief, Early Detection
Branch, Div. of Cancer
Prevention and Control,
National Cancer Institute,
Bethesda, Maryland

Roger R. Williams, M.D.
Director, Cardiovascular Genetics
Clinic and Professor of Medicine,
University of Utah School of Medicine,
Salt Lake City, Utah

Martha McMurry, M.S., R.D./C.D.
Head Research Nutritionist,
Clinical Research Center,
University of Utah School of Medicine,
Salt Lake City, Utah

Ladd and Nancy Christensen
Technical Reviewers,
Salt Lake City, Utah

Ray W. Squires, Ph.D.
Program Director, Cardiovascular
Health Clinic, Mayo Clinic,
Rochester, Minnesota

Dede B. Lewis, P.T.
Physical Therapist,
The Fitness Institute at LDS Hospital,
Salt Lake City, Utah

George VanKoman, M.D.
Internist, Department of
Internal Medicine, Bryner Clinic,
Salt Lake City, Utah

Stephen Hunter, P.T.
Assistant Director, Back Institute,
Cottonwood Hospital,
Salt Lake City, Utah

Michael J. Wall, M.D.
Internist, Intermountain Clinic,
Salt Lake City, Utah

Timothy G. Butler, M.S.
The Fitness Institute
at LDS Hospital,
Salt Lake City, Utah

Heidi Swinton
Writer
Salt Lake City, Utah

Scott C. Gardner
Research Assistant,
Salt Lake City, Utah

Susan Bellingham
Health Promotion Specialist,
Salt Lake City, Utah

Additionally, we recognize the efforts of many physicians and health-care specialists who have devoted their professional lives to the advancement of health and the prevention of disease. The publications of their experience and research have made this book possible.

We express gratitude to Dr. Glade Hunsaker for his valuable contribution in bringing this important project to its completion. His insight and review of the many manuscript drafts were invaluable. We also acknowledge the contribution of Mark Woodland for his text design.

We express our appreciation to the U.S. Preventive Services Task Force (formed under the direction of The Department of Health and Human Services, Office of Disease Prevention and Health promotion). The outstanding work by this Task Force, which culminated in the *Guide to Clinical Preventive Services: Report of the U.S. Preventive Services Task Force*, was invaluable in the preparation of our book. We used extensively the written text, the recommendations (including the age-specific periodic health examination charts), and the references of the *Prepublication Copy* of this book (1989) to help prepare our manuscript. We anticipate the work of the Task Force will ultimately be viewed as a major contribution towards the advancement of preventive medicine. The U.S. Preventive Services Task Force's report has now been published by Williams and Wilkins Publishing Company, under the same title as the Health and Human Services Prepublication copy.

We also thank the Early Detection Branch of the National Cancer Institute, headed by Dr. Charles Smart, for its booklet, *Working Guidelines for Early Cancer Detection: Rationale and Supporting Evidence to Decrease Mortality*. We have used this booklet extensively in formulating guidelines and in securing pertinent reference material. We understand a second and revised edition of this booklet is soon to be released. We commend the Early Detection Branch for its contribution to preventive medical services.

We specifically commend the untiring efforts of Dr. James O. Mason, U.S. Assistant Secretary for Health and his staff (in particular Dr. Douglas B. Kamerow and Dr. Steven H. Woolf) for helping people take greater responsibility for their own health and for teaching clinicians new skills in the area of health promotion and disease prevention.

We acknowledge the efforts of the American College of Physicians in its careful review of adult health maintenance recommendations. Preventive services guidelines by the American College of Physicians are now published in *Common Screening Tests*, edited by David M. Eddy, M.D., Ph.D., and published by the American College of Physicians (Philadelphia, PA, 1991).

We appreciate and recognize the pioneering efforts of Dr. Paul S. Frame in advancing the understanding of adult health maintenance. His insight has assisted us with this book. We appreciate the data gathered by the National Statistics Division (under the direction of Dr. Harry M. Rosenberg) for use in compiling the leading causes of death. We have departed somewhat from the manner in which the National Statistic Division reports the leading causes of death. We have reported the leading causes of death by decade and we have also included AIDS in the by-decade report. Dr. Rosenberg kindly provided us with the AIDS' statistics for every five years of life.

We also recognize the excellent source book, *The American Cancer Society: Cancer Book*, published by Doubleday and Company, Inc., New York. We made significant use of the information presented in this book, particularly information by Dr. Jerome J. DeCrosse, Dr. Thomas B. Fitzpatrick, and Dr. S. B. Gusberg.

We express also our appreciation to the following individuals: Kent Ririe, Jeffrey Swinton, Gary Felt, Tom Nelson, Robert Clark, Orlan Owen, and Joe Barry for their advice and encouragement; Thomas E. Nelson, Attorney at Law (VanCott, Bagley, Cornwall and McCarthy law firm) for his legal assistance; David Midget for his graphic design assistance; Borge Anderson and Robert Pennington of Borge Anderson and Associates for their photography assistance; Marilyn Garner and Dale Nelson (McCarty Modeling Agency), who served as models for the fitness photos; Joseph T. Adams, for his assistance with the Index; Mrs. Beth Jarmen for her typing assistance; Dr. Patrick M. Yeh for his computer assistance; Dr. and Mrs. George and Linda Pearson, Mr. and Mrs. Don and Sue Parker, Dr. and Mrs. Albert and Arla Funk, Mr. and Mrs. Boyd and Kim Wagstaff, Dr. and Mrs. Craig and Joan Anderson, Dr. Judy Norman, Ms. Dixie Hall, Mr. and Mrs. Gary and Debbie Felt, Mr. and Mrs. Mike and Bonnie Mihlberger, Dr. Blair Bybee, Dr. Dan Bellingham, Mr. and Mrs. Chris and Carolyn Hopkins, Mr. and Mrs. Kevin and Marlene Yates, Dr. and Mrs. John and LeeAnn Christensen, Dr. and Mrs. Alan and Marsha Morgan, Dr. and Mrs. Jay "Chip" and Colleen Yates, Mr. Roy D. Call, Mr. and Mrs. Roger and Callie Wilhelmsen, Dr. and Mrs. Charles and Jolynn Bean; Mrs. Ethel W. Adams, Judge and Mrs. Thornley and Dorothy Swan, Mr. and Mrs. Paul and Elizabeth Major, Mr. and Mrs. Les and Madge Green, Mr. Delbert Adams, Mr. and Mrs. Rusty and Mary Alice Pettit, Mrs. Alice Johnson, Mr. Joe Whitesides, Mrs. Ella D. McGlinch, Mr. and Mrs. Ike and Janine Swan, Mr. and Mrs. Gary and Margaret Wilmarth, Mr. Mark Robbins, Mr. David Funk, Mr. Melvin Endito, Mr. John Boden, Mr. and Mrs. Martell and Venice Bird, Mr. and Mrs. Wayne and Virginia Winegar, Miss Lugardis Marxer, Ms. LouJean Brown, Mr. Jack Vizzard, Mr. and Mrs. David and Helen Beardshall, and Mr. and Mrs. Gus and Helen Glissmeyer for their support and/or review of the manuscript; members of The Fitness Institute staff of LDS Hospital, Dr. Tom Rosenberg, Dr. Greg Elliott, Diane Marshall, Christopher M. Southwick, Kent Ririe, Chad Edgington, Michele Eccles, Eva McLellan, Alice Carling, Lesley Mason, Carrie Ryan, Tracy Vayo, Brenda Hughston, Paul Cummings, Aaron Billin, Debbie "Yosh" Yoshimura, Julie Metos, Peg Michael, and Karin Anderson; Dr. Jeffrey Anderson, Chief, Division of Cardiology at LDS Hospital; Brad Zollinger, Administrative Director of Rehabilitation at LDS Hospital; Richard Nash and Karyn Haeckel, Public Relations Department at LDS Hospital; Gary Farnes (IHC's CEO of Salt Lake Valley hospitals), Richard Cagen (LDS Hospital Administrator), Richard Smith, Wes Thompson, Scott Lloyd, Greg Spencer, and Earl Christison (Assistant Administrators), Richard A. Christenson (President of the Deseret Foundation), Melissa Phillips, and Lori Piscopo (Directors of the Deseret Foundation) for their continued support of the mission of The Fitness Institute; Dr. Gail P. Dalsky, University of Connecticut Health Center, Osteoporosis Center, for her information on osteoporosis; Dr. Steven Blair, Aerobic Research Center, Dallas, Texas, for his assistance with exercise ECG testing guidelines; Dr. Robert J. Farney and Dr. James M. Walker for their information on sleep disorders; Dr. Irena Tocino for her review of the information on breast cancer screening; Dr. John J. Christensen and Dr. Wallace B. Brown for their review of dental care information; and Dr. David W. Richards, Dr. Garner B. Meads, Sr., and Dr. Robert F. Bitner for their dedication as primary-care physicians.

We also express our thanks to Mr. James S. Poulter and Mr. and Mrs. Val and Laurie Sorensen for helping to find the "lost manuscript;" Mr. and Mrs. Vern and Jeannie Jensen for helping our kids at the ranch while we worked on the book; and to the "Sugar Bear" on Lake Powell where new hope for the book always seemed to emerge.

Finally, we acknowledge the great effort of primary-care physicians everywhere.

CHAPTER

1

Making The Difference –
Before It's Too Late

Any machine, whether the human body or an automobile,
*will obviously wear out **sooner** if it is overworked,*
mistreated, improperly lubricated or fed chemicals
that leave a residue of carbon around the valves!
So, treat your marvelous human machine far more
carefully than you would a Rolls Royce!

—Dr. George W. Crane

———————

Does our highly respected friend, Dr. Crane, jest in suggesting that a Rolls might get better attention than its successful owner? Hardly! In fact, the medical world faces daily the shocking reality that many vehicles in the hospital parking lot are maintained much better than are their rod-thrown owners lying beyond repair on hospital beds.

Why? What would account for an owner's giving better attention to his auto than to his own well-being; and what explains the too frequent neglect of what Dr. Crane calls: "the marvelous human machine?"

At least in part the answer lies in this harsh reality: Neglected automobiles strand their owners and obligate them to huge towing and repair bills. Every hood raised at the side of the road is a jarring reminder that maintenance must not be neglected. Fortunately, these motivating roadside reminders are effectively supported by user-friendly maintenance manuals that permit even the least mechanically minded driver to track with ease the services needed as the miles roll by. Vehicles get attention because their maintenance needs demand it and because effective manuals provide check-list guidance. The combination works!

In contrast, we neglect maintaining the human machine because the reminders are seldom found lying in full view at the side of the road; instead, they are out of sight and often out of mind in the privacy of a hospital room. Further, the incredibly complex and miraculous human machine tends to "make do" despite our neglecting it. Rather than giving a flashing red light on the dash panel, it often compensates for neglect by drawing down resources from other body strengths, offering splendid service despite its being irreparably abused.

While the body miraculously compensates for its owner's neglect, the valuable warning pains or signs it frequently provides are often ignored or repressed with the notion: "This is not serious; I'll be better soon." Regrettably, in many instances, little if any warning is given to the owner until the body "blow-out" occurs.

Unlike the motorist who can reach for the manual, the owner of the human machine fears a huge chasm that seems to lie between what he knows about his condition and the medical community that seems too unapproachable, time-consuming and expensive. Until now, we have had no manual in the glove compartment to tell the owner what to do and when.

Without question, the service given to the human body will eventually determine the length and quality of its service to us. While modern medicine may help many of us celebrate more birthdays, the quality of those years will largely be determined by our punctual response to *every* maintenance need the body requires. The upshot of all of this concern: We need a manual that will get our attention and that will systematically guide us through the "checks and services" the human machine requires and deserves.

I Meant To *or* Penalty for Neglect

While owning a maintenance manual is a giant stride toward exceptional performance, actually tracking *every* service to its documented completion is essential. Unfortunately, most of us can identify with our energetic, do-it-yourselfer friend, Ed, who now has an increased respect for his maintenance manual.

Planning a trip to the East recently, Ed pulled every manual-listed maintenance check on his diesel Suburban and paid extra to have even not-quite-due services attended. Enroute, Ed made certain that even simple petrol stops included careful checking of all fluid levels and gauges; the successful trip concluded in October.

In January, hundreds of miles later, his $23,000 machine almost made it to the top of Quail Valley Drive before its grinding metallic sounds loudly announced that a $2,800 engine had just seized for lack of oil. Impossible! Immediately, frustrated Ed turned to the maintenance manual to discover what the family didn't want to learn.

The son who had been charged with taking the vehicle in for service at the end of the trip had taken the rig to the shop, but finding a waiting line, he had returned home with the work not done. After all, the long trip had not used all the miles allowed between services; Ed was actually a tad ahead of schedule, wanting to care well for a vehicle that had been under the strain of an extended journey. Intentions were firm to return the following day.

Aware? Yes! Conscientious? To the point of both planning and initiating action — but *not* to the required point of documenting the actual completion of the services.

The family's in-city jaunts in the weeks following the vacation were just a few miles at a time, logging a shocking number of miles in a manner very similar to the miles quietly logged on the human body. The damaging additional miles ruined an engine while Ed was enjoying the euphoria that accompanies knowing that you couldn't care more! Good intentions and over-confidence crowded out frequent, consistent checking of the maintenance record.

Was it painful to pay $3,000 (with no insurance assistance) when a $19 lube and oil job would have preserved that almost-new diesel engine for thousands of trouble-free miles? Ed thought so; in fact, he still does! Has he learned his lesson regarding using the car's maintenance manual every time he approaches the vehicle? Painfully he has! Have the rest of us?

We Are In Charge

This manual revolves around two premises: *First, we all want good health!* Absolutely *no* possession ever equals the gift of good health. From Ponce de Leon's pilgrimage to find the Fountain of Youth to every aspect of our modern-day medical pursuits, the quest is ever and urgently towards good health.

The second premise is that *as individuals we must be more responsible for our own health.* This statement has not always been true!

At the turn of this century the major cause of death in the U.S. was attributed to acute, largely infectious diseases such as smallpox, tuberculosis, diphtheria, rheumatic fever, tetanus and polio[1,2] — illnesses generally beyond the control of the victim. In a matter of days, perfectly healthy individuals contracting these diseases faced serious illness and the potential of lifetime disabilities or death.

No longer are we dying from these diseases. In fact, acute illnesses now account for less than two percent of the health concerns in 1900, and smallpox has been entirely eliminated from our planet.[1,3]

Today, the major cause of death and disability is the result of lifestyle-caused illnesses that are generally preventable through proper attention to diet, exercise, smoking elimination, seat belt usage and periodic medical screening. In fact, personal health practices are the vital and paramount component of preventive health. Unfortunately, we live in a society in which *NEGLECT OF SELF IS THE PRIMARY CAUSE OF SUCH ILLNESSES AS*:

Coronary Heart Disease

Cancer

Diabetes

Lung Disease

Liver Disease

High Blood Pressure

Stroke

Osteoporosis

The good news is that we can have a direct and positive effect on all of these; we *are* in charge of our own health. But just as proper maintenance of our car requires consistent effort, the same attention is necessary to maintain our bodies and promote optimal health.

Unfortunately, individual concern for our health does not always receive deserved priority, especially in a world of tight schedules and unrelenting demands. We all want good health; we all mean well, and we all suppose that our caring will see us through. But in all this we urgently need to use effectively a health manual that will visibly spell out for us what must be done and when — to plot for the user how to avoid the penalty of neglect.

An Urgent Need –
The Maintenance Manual

Working in preventive health care for the past two decades, we have been made keenly aware of the need for a maintenance manual. Individuals ask us daily what they should do to guarantee good health and prevent early death. Unfortunately, all too often the inquirer comes to us much too late, when "What can I do?" should have been asked years earlier at a time when the preventive steps could have made all the difference.

Daily we agonize as patients face the painful consequences of poor lifestyle habits and of wide-spread failure to conduct periodic medical screening.

This critically important need for a maintenance manual for the human body has motivated us to research exactly what is required to promote and maintain one's health. As we began a review of the current medical research relating to the length and quality of life, we concluded that individuals must follow a well-designed checklist of lifestyle habits of exercise, diet, and medical screenings, such as a periodic mammogram or blood cholesterol test.

How to organize a systematic, easy-to-follow schedule that incorporated these current health recommendations came easily when we recognized that for years the car owner's manual has offered to motorists the periodic maintenance schedule for successfully maintaining their automobiles. Has not the conscientious auto owner been promised that his well maintained machine would:

Run Smoother

Last Longer, and

Cost Less to Operate ?

Are these not the very qualities we're seeking for the human machine? Would we not be foolish to neglect a well established method that has been proven sound?

This book, then, develops a personal manual for both *promoting* and *maintaining* good health and provides an up-to-date, medically sound plan to further ensure that our bodies will:

Run Smoother

Last Longer, and

Over the Lifetime,
Cost Much Less to Operate

Further, a substantial bonus for following the manual is increased productivity and improved quality of life. As a result of following this maintenance manual we will:

1) Do all we can to eliminate early death and disability — detecting disease before it's too late;
2) Identify and modify individual risk factors for heart disease and cancer;
3) Determine our current fitness status and learn how to implement practical exercise, nutrition, weight control and stress management;
4) Learn how, why and when health tests are recommended and performed by us and our doctors;
5) Receive the peace of mind, confidence and even joy of knowing we are doing all we can to maintain our bodies and attain optimal health.

In essence, the manual puts us behind the wheel *and* gives clear direction for trouble-free travel. We look forward to a long and successful journey as we continue to maintain the miracle — a miracle that must last a lifetime.

CHAPTER

2

Using The
Maintenance Manual

*We can no longer afford **not** to invest in prevention.*
From the perspective of avoiding human suffering
as well as saving wasteful costs for treating diseases
and injuries that could have been prevented,
the 1990s should be the decade of prevention in the United States.

— James O. Mason, M.D., Dr. P.H.
U.S. Assistant Secretary for Health

It Works!

Two years prior to his lift off into space, Senator Jake Garn was tested in our hospital's Fitness Institute and informed that certain health improvements were needed. His demanding schedule had somewhat crowded out attention to a fitness lifestyle. However, with an activity log in hand, the senator left our facility determined to make methodic changes!

Returning months later for follow-up tests, Senator Garn proudly displayed his activity log. Without fail, he had faithfully recorded the details of his regular exercise. One entry was made from a hotel lobby in Sydney, Australia, where he had jogged in place because a typhoon was raging. Keeping the log had been the critical factor for the senator in establishing consistent and effective lifestyle changes.

The results were as impressive as the fitness log: a 30 percent improvement in the treadmill fitness test—greater than the 99th percentile for men his age. Upper-body strength had increased to the "excellent" category, and his weight was equal to his high school weight, with a recorded body fat of 15 percent — excellent.

The senator had lowered his cholesterol by 15 mg percent and had increased his "good" cholesterol, HDL, from 30 to 46. The day of his follow-up treadmill test the senator announced to our staff that because he was now in such excellent shape, he had decided to "go into space."

The rest is history! Senator Garn met the demanding physical tests required of an astronaut and on April 12, 1985, he flew aboard the space shuttle *Discovery*, Flight 51D. In fact, while orbiting the earth for seven days, the senator performed several physiological/medical experiments — tests done for the first time in space.

Faithfully using a maintenance log worked for the senator; let it work for you!

Following the Manual: Five Easy Steps

To begin using your maintenance manual, follow these five steps:

STEP 1: SELECT YOUR HEALTH CHECK TABLE

The centrum of this manual is your **HEALTH CHECK TABLE**. This easy-to-follow table clearly identifies when you need to perform each health check to promote and maintain your good health. Five health check tables have been carefully designed for each of the following age groups:

STEP 2: USE YOUR HEALTH CHECK TABLE'S SUB-SECTIONS

To make your Health Check Table user friendly, we've divided each table into five Health Check sections (A through E).

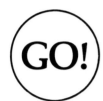 *SECTION A* includes **DAILY HEALTH CHECKS** (such as proper nutrition or physical activity) — symbolized with a "go" sign to suggest you *go forward without any delay.*

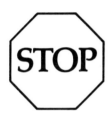 *SECTION B* includes **MONTHLY HEALTH CHECKS** (such as breast self-exam) — symbolized with a "stop" sign to recommend strongly that you *stop* and perform the self-exams.

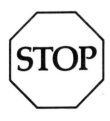 *SECTION C* includes **YEARLY OR PERIODIC HEALTH CHECKS** you and your doctor perform (such as a physical examination and blood cholesterol test) — also symbolized with a "stop" sign to recommend strongly that you and your doctor *stop when recommended* and perform the medical health checks.

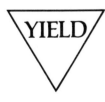 *SECTION D* includes **LIFESTYLE COUNSELING HEALTH CHECKS** that cover topics like substance abuse or injury prevention — symbolized with a "yield" sign to suggest you *yield when appropriate,* and participate by following the recommendations.

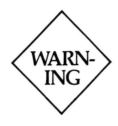 *SECTION E* includes **HEALTH CHECKS FOR HIGH-RISK PERSONS** — symbolized with a "warning" sign to give *warning* of high-risk groups who may require additional health checks or counseling because of personal or family risk (such as a strong family history of colon or breast cancer). **DON'T FAIL TO REVIEW HIGH-RISK ITEMS.**

STEP 3: EXPANDED HEALTH CHECK GUIDANCE

The Health Check Tables don't stand alone. Your table provides the page numbers for the expanded health check guidance placed in **Chapter Three: Expanded Health Check Information.**

For example, in your Health Check Table, listed under *Section C: Yearly or Periodic Health Checks* is *Health Check #1: Physical Exam and Health History (Initial/Interim)*. Note that page 76 is listed by this health check. To learn more about the physical exam, refer to Chapter Three, page 76.

STEP 4: MEDICAL HISTORY QUESTIONNAIRE

A detailed medical questionnaire is also included to assist you and your doctor with your medical history record. **The questionnaire will serve as a basis for your maintenance manual for the remainder of your life.** Keep it current.

STEP 5: MAKING IT WORK FOR YOU

Working through the four steps above may have left you feeling a little overwhelmed — there is, after all, an overwhelming amount of critically important information in this manual. We suggest a sensible and **gradual** approach to making your maintenance manual work.

First, set aside some time and complete the medical questionnaire found in Appendix A, page 170. The process of completing the questionnaire will give you a better idea of what health checks you need first. The questionnaire will also be *critical* in assisting you and your doctor in identifying whether you need to consider the *High-Risk Health Checks*, or the *Lifestyle Counseling Health Checks*.

Further instructions designed to help you complete the questionnaire are found on page 77. When you have completed the questionnaire, we suggest you make a copy to take to your primary-care physician.

Second, in approaching the **Daily Health Checks**, choose one or two items, read the expanded material written about those health checks in Chapter Three, and then gradually begin to practice those particular health checks. Keep in mind that you may already be practicing many of these health checks.

Third, based upon your medical questionnaire, determine when you last had a physical examination. Next, turn to the *Yearly or Periodic Health Check #1, Physical Examination and Health History* (page 76), and follow the instructions for scheduling a physical examination.

Recognize that although the **Yearly or Periodic Health Checks** appear to be quite numerous, the procedures are only performed on a periodic basis; your doctor will assist you in completing most of these health checks.

Important: We strongly urge you to record in the spaces provided on your *Health Check Table* the **Yearly or Periodic Health Checks** and, where appropriate, the value (such as height, weight, blood pressure or cholesterol). For example, if you are 44 years of age and you have just had a physical examination, you should open your *Health Check Table* (for ages 40–49) to pages 22–23, and under the column "**Age 44**" record the date of the physical exam. Under this same column you should record any other health checks that were performed in conjunction with your physical exam. Also, record any values that correspond to the health check, such as your blood pressure reading, your height and weight, or your cholesterol level.

Having recorded the date you participated in the health check, you can now refer to the **Frequency** column of your **Yearly or Periodic Health Checks** to determine when to schedule your next health check. In the above example, the next physical examination would normally be performed at age 47. The **Lifestyle Counseling Health Checks** and the **High-Risk Health Checks** should also be recorded if you participate in these items.

The **Monthly Health Checks** should be recorded in the *Health Check Table* when each self-exam is performed. Although we have included only enough lines to record six months of activity, after you have consistently performed monthly self-exams for six months, the activities should be a habit and further recording should not be necessary.

Many of the **Daily Health Checks** do not require daily records, but for those health checks that do (physical activity, nutrition, weight control and stress management), a daily log or record is located in the Appendix, page 195.

Staggering Costs?

You may be concerned about costs generated by following the maintenance manual. Be assured that every effort has been made to recommend *only* medical screening health checks that will insure early disease detection.

Further, most of the health checks in your maintenance manual are to be performed *on your own* at no expense: lifestyle practices that have tremendous impact on *lowering* personal health care costs. In addition, the cost of the recommended medical screening is very small compared to the expense of a major medical problem — a problem that is more likely to result when health checks are neglected.

A final word about costs. By establishing a partnership with your doctor while following your maintenance manual, you become an active participant in determining the appropriateness of recommended medical tests or procedures. This partnership can have a definite impact on medical expenses; your doctor will better understand what's normal for you, and you'll feel more comfortable taking part in the process of medical decision making.

Get Going!

You are already inescapably behind the wheel of a miraculous human machine. The real payoff for carefully following your manual is the difference you'll be making in the *quality and length* of your life. Turn to the Health Check Table appropriate for your age, and get going!

(*CAUTION:* The recommended health checks are generally intended for the apparently healthy individual who is without major medical problems and/or symptoms of disease. Those individuals who currently have symptoms or major medical problems may need, with the assistance of their physician, to alter the Health Check Table. Even apparently healthy individuals should alter the frequency of the recommended health check procedures or activities if genetic (family history) or environmental factors (including personal lifestyle) would suggest they are at an increased risk for a given disease or disability. For example, knowing your father and older brother had colon cancer should cause you to discuss with your personal physician the wisdom of adjusting your health check table to pursue additional types of medical procedures such as a colonoscopy exam. In addition, your primary-care physician may recommend screening tests that are in addition to those outlined in your Health Check Table.)

Ages 19 to 29

• Health Check Table •

LEADING CAUSES OF DEATH — AGES 19 TO 29 ARRANGED IN ORDER OF INCIDENCE

Men

Motor Vehicle Accidents
Homicide/Legal Intervention
Suicide
Non-Vehicle Accidents
AIDS
Heart Disease

Women

Motor Vehicle Accidents
Homicide/Legal Intervention
Suicide
Non-Vehicle Accidents
Heart Disease
AIDS

A. (GO!) Daily Health Checks

Daily logs or record sheets for Daily Health Checks are located with the expanded sections (see pages listed).

C. (STOP) Yearly or Periodic Health Checks

Record the month and year (e.g. 8/92) when the Health Check is performed and, where appropriate, the value (such as blood pressure,120/80). Record this information in the column that corresponds with your age at the time the Health Check is performed. (NOTE: M = male; F = female)

	Reference	Frequency	Age 19	Age 20
① Physical Examination & History (Initial/Interim) (M, F) ...page 76		Every 5 years		
② Cardiac Risk Factor Screening[†] (M, F)	page 79	Every 1 – 3 years		
③ Blood Pressure Screening[†] (M, F)	page 84	Every 2 years		
⑤ Clinical Skin Exam[†] (M, F)	page 92	Every 5 years		
⑥ Clinical Testicular Exam[†] (M)	page 98	Every 5 years		
⑦ Examine for Thyroid Nodules[†] (M, F)	page 101	Every 5 years		
⑧ Clinical Oral Cavity Exam[†] (M, F)	page 103	Every 5 years		
⑨ Total Blood Cholesterol (M, F)	page 105	Every 5 years		
⑫ Pap Test/Pelvic Exam[†] (F)	page 109	Every 1 – 3 years[*]		
⑬ Clinical Breast Exam[†] (F)	page 111	Every 5 years		
⑱ Blood Test (CBC, SMAC) and Urinalysis (M, F)	page 119	Optional[§]		
⑲ Dental Checkup (M, F)	page 132	Yearly		
⑳ Tetanus-Diphtheria Vaccination (M, F)	page 121	Every 10 years		
㉓ Height and Weight (M, F)	page 76	Every 2 years		

[†] These health checks are often performed in concert with a periodic physical examination.

[*] Pap test every 1 – 3 years, following two initial negative Pap tests.

[§] Routine blood tests (CBC, SMAC) and urinalysis are generally not recommended by most adult health maintenance organizations. The frequency of performing this health check is left to the discretion of you and your physician.

B. (STOP) Monthly Health Checks

Record the day and month (d/m) when these Health Checks are performed. (NOTE: M = male; F = female)

	d/m	d/m	d/m	d/m	d/m	d/m
① Breast Self-Exam (F) ....page 111						
② Skin Self-Exam (M, F) ....page 92	d/m	d/m	d/m	d/m	d/m	d/m
③ Testicular Self-Exam (M) ....page 98	d/m	d/m	d/m	d/m	d/m	d/m

Age 21	Age 22	Age 23	Age 24	Age 25	Age 26	Age 27	Age 28	Age 29

Continued next page

D. ▽YIELD Lifestyle Counseling

Review the Lifestyle Counseling information every one to three years and record the date.

E. ◇WARN-ING High-Risk Health Checks

The frequency of these tests should be based on your medical history and other individual circumstances (see specific pages listed below).

When additional High-Risk Health Checks are recommended, use this space to record pertinent information.

Recommended Health Check	Date	Date	Date	Comments
1.				
2.				
3.				
4.				
5.				
6.				
7.				
8.				
9.				
10.				
11.				
12.				
13.				
14.				
15.				
16.				
17.				
18.				

REMAIN ALERT FOR SIGNS IN SELF AND OTHERS:

Source material for this *Health Check Table* has included:
- The "Age-Specific Charts" of the U.S. Preventive Services Task Force (USPSTF);
- The cancer screening recommendations of the National Cancer Institute and the American Cancer Society;
- The screening test guidelines of the American College of Physicians;
- The periodic health evaluation guidelines by Dr. John H. Holbrook;
- The National Cholesterol Education Program Committee;
- Other medical organizations and medical scientists as set forth in the references of this book.

Ages 30 to 39

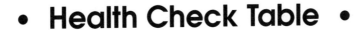

• Health Check Table •

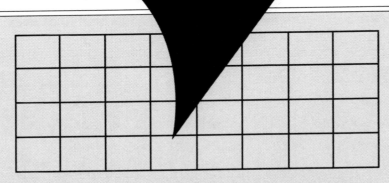

**LEADING CAUSES OF DEATH — AGES 30 TO 39
ARRANGED IN ORDER OF INCIDENCE**

Men	Women
Motor Vehicle Accidents	Motor Vehicle Accidents
AIDS	Breast Cancer
Heart Disease	Heart Disease
Non-Vehicle Accidents	Homicide/Legal Intervention
Suicide	Suicide
Homicide/Legal Intervention	Non-Vehicle Accidents

A. (GO!) Daily Health Checks

Daily logs or record sheets for Daily Health Checks are located with the expanded sections (see pages listed).

C. (STOP) Yearly or Periodic Health Checks

Record the month and year (e.g. 8/92) when the Health Check is performed and, where appropriate, the value (such as blood pressure, 120/80). Record this information in the column that corresponds with your age at the time the Health Check is performed. (NOTE: M = male; F = female)

	Reference	Frequency	Age 30	Age 31
(1) Physical Examination & History (Initial/Interim) (M, F)	page 76	Every 4 years		
(2) Cardiac Risk Factor Screening[†] (M, F)	page 79	Every 1 – 3 years		
(3) Blood Pressure Screening[†] (M, F)	page 84	Every 2 years		
(5) Clinical Skin Exam[†] (M, F)	page 92	Every 4 years		
(6) Clinical Testicular Exam[†] (M)	page 98	Every 4 years		
(7) Examine for Thyroid Nodules[†] (M, F)	page 101	Every 4 years		
(8) Clinical Oral Cavity Exam[†] (M, F)	page 103	Every 4 years		
(9) Total Blood Cholesterol (M, F)	page 105	Every 5 years		
(12) Pap Test/Pelvic Exam[†] (F)	page 109	Every 1 – 3 years[*]		
(13) Clinical Breast Exam[†] (F)	page 111	Every 4 years		
(18) Blood Test (CBC, SMAC) and Urinalysis (M, F)	page 119	Optional[§]		
(19) Dental Checkup (M, F)	page 132	Yearly		
(20) Tetanus-Diphtheria Vaccination (M, F)	page 121	Every 10 years		
(23) Height and Weight (M, F)	page 76	Every 2 years		

[†] These health checks are often performed in concert with a periodic physical examination.

[*] Pap test every 1 – 3 years, following two initial negative Pap tests.

[§] Routine blood tests (CBC, SMAC) and urinalysis are generally not recommended by most adult health maintenance organizations. The frequency of performing this health check is left to the discretion of you and your physician.

B.　STOP　Monthly Health Checks

Record the day and month (d/m) when these Health Checks are performed.　(NOTE: M = male; F = female)

① Breast Self-Exam (F) ....page 111	d/m	d/m	d/m	d/m	d/m	d/m
② Skin Self-Exam (M, F) ....page 92	d/m	d/m	d/m	d/m	d/m	d/m
③ Testicular Self-Exam (M) ....page 98	d/m	d/m	d/m	d/m	d/m	d/m

Age 32	Age 33	Age 34	Age 35	Age 36	Age 37	Age 38	Age 39

Continued next page

D. ▽YIELD Lifestyle Counseling

Review the Lifestyle Counseling information every one to three years and record the date.

mo / yr	mo / yr	mo / yr
mo / yr	mo / yr	mo / yr
mo / yr	mo / yr	mo / yr
mo / yr	mo / yr	mo / yr
mo / yr	mo / yr	mo / yr
mo / yr	mo / yr	mo / yr
mo / yr	mo / yr	mo / yr
mo / yr	mo / yr	mo / yr
mo / yr	mo / yr	mo / yr

E. ◇WARN-ING High-Risk Health Checks

The frequency of these tests should be based on your medical history and other individual circumstances (see specific pages listed below).

When additional High-Risk Health Checks are recommended, use this space to record pertinent information.

Recommended Health Check	Date	Date	Date	Comments
1.				
2.				
3.				
4.				
5.				
6.				
7.				
8.				
9.				
10.				
11.				
12.				
13.				
14.				
15.				
16.				
17.				
18.				

REMAIN ALERT FOR SIGNS IN SELF AND OTHERS:

Source material for this *Health Check Table* has included:

- The "Age-Specific Charts" of the U.S. Preventive Services Task Force (USPSTF);
- The cancer screening recommendations of the National Cancer Institute and the American Cancer Society;
- The screening test guidelines of the American College of Physicians;
- The periodic health evaluation guidelines by Dr. John H. Holbrook;
- The National Cholesterol Education Program Committee;
- Other medical organizations and medical scientists as set forth in the references of this book.

Ages 40 to 49

• Health Check Table •

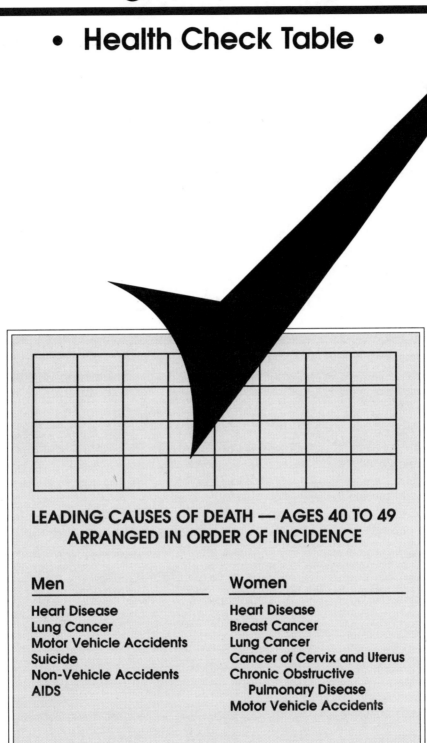

**LEADING CAUSES OF DEATH — AGES 40 TO 49
ARRANGED IN ORDER OF INCIDENCE**

Men	Women
Heart Disease	Heart Disease
Lung Cancer	Breast Cancer
Motor Vehicle Accidents	Lung Cancer
Suicide	Cancer of Cervix and Uterus
Non-Vehicle Accidents	Chronic Obstructive
AIDS	Pulmonary Disease
	Motor Vehicle Accidents

A. (GO!) Daily Health Checks

Daily logs or record sheets for Daily Health Checks are located with the expanded sections (see pages listed).

C. (STOP) Yearly or Periodic Health Checks

Record the month and year (e.g. 8/92) when the Health Check is performed and, where appropriate, the value (such as blood pressure,120/80). Record this information in the column that corresponds with your age at the time the Health Check is performed. (NOTE: M = male; F = female)

	Reference	Frequency	Age 40	Age 41
(1) Physical Examination & History (Initial/Interim) (M, F)	page 76	Every 3 years		
(2) Cardiac Risk Factor Screening[†] (M, F)	page 79	Every 1 – 3 years		
(3) Blood Pressure Screening[†] (M, F)	page 84	Yearly		
(4) Digital Rectal Exam[†] (M, F)	page 87	Yearly		
(5) Clinical Skin Exam[†] (M, F)	page 92	Every 3 years		
(6) Clinical Testicular Exam[†] (M)	page 98	Every 3 years		
(7) Examine for Thyroid Nodules[†] (M, F)	page 101	Every 3 years		
(8) Clinical Oral Cavity Exam[†] (M, F)	page 103	Every 3 years		
(9) Total Blood Cholesterol (M, F)	page 105	Every 5 years		
(12) Pap Test/Pelvic Exam[†] (F)	page 109	Every 1 – 3 years[*]		
(13) Clinical Breast Exam[†] (F)	page 111	Yearly		
(14) Mammogram (F)	page 111	Every 1 – 2 years[#]		
(16) Tonometry (M, F)	page 117	Every 2 – 4 years[∞]		
(18) Blood Test (CBC, SMAC) and Urinalysis (M, F)	page 119	Optional[§]		
(19) Dental Checkup (M, F)	page 132	Yearly		
(20) Tetanus-Diphtheria Vaccination (M, F)	page 121	Every 10 years		
(23) Height and Weight (M, F)	page 76	Yearly		

[†] These health checks are often performed in concert with a periodic physical examination.

[*] Pap test every 1 – 3 years, following two initial negative Pap tests.

[#] This frequency is recommended by the National Cancer Institute and the American Cancer Society. The American College of Physicians and the USPSTF recommend yearly mammograms for women in their 40s only if they have a family history of breast cancer or if they are otherwise at increased risk.

B. (STOP) Monthly Health Checks

Record the day and month (d/m) when these Health Checks are performed. (NOTE: M = male; F = female)

① Breast Self-Exam (F) ....page 111	d/m	d/m	d/m	d/m	d/m	d/m
② Skin Self-Exam (M, F) ....page 92	d/m	d/m	d/m	d/m	d/m	d/m
③ Testicular Self-Exam (M) ....page 98	d/m	d/m	d/m	d/m	d/m	d/m
④ Oral Cavity Self-Exam (M, F) ....page 103	d/m	d/m	d/m	d/m	d/m	d/m

Age 42	Age 43	Age 44	Age 45	Age 46	Age 47	Age 48	Age 49

∞ This recommendation is by the American Academy of Ophthalmology.

§ Routine blood tests (CBC, SMAC) and urinalysis are generally not recommended by most adult health maintenance organizations. The frequency of performing this health check is left to the discretion of you and your physician.

Continued next page

D. Lifestyle Counseling

Review the Lifestyle Counseling information every one to three years and record the date.

mo / yr	mo / yr	mo / yr
mo / yr	mo / yr	mo / yr
mo / yr	mo / yr	mo / yr
mo / yr	mo / yr	mo / yr
mo / yr	mo / yr	mo / yr
mo / yr	mo / yr	mo / yr
mo / yr	mo / yr	mo / yr
mo / yr	mo / yr	mo / yr
mo / yr	mo / yr	mo / yr

E. High-Risk Health Checks

The frequency of these tests should be based on your medical history and other individual circumstances (see specific pages listed below).

When additional High-Risk Health Checks are recommended, use this space to record pertinent information.

Recommended Health Check	Date	Date	Date	Comments
1.				
2.				
3.				
4.				
5.				
6.				
7.				
8.				
9.				
10.				
11.				
12.				
13.				
14.				
15.				
16.				
17.				
18.				

REMAIN ALERT FOR SIGNS IN SELF AND OTHERS:

Source material for this *Health Check Table* has included:
- The "Age-Specific Charts" of the U.S. Preventive Services Task Force (USPSTF);
- The cancer screening recommendations of the National Cancer Institute and the American Cancer Society;
- The screening test guidelines of the American College of Physicians;
- The periodic health evaluation guidelines by Dr. John H. Holbrook;
- The National Cholesterol Education Program Committee;
- Other medical organizations and medical scientists as set forth in the references of this book.

Ages 50 to 59

• Health Check Table •

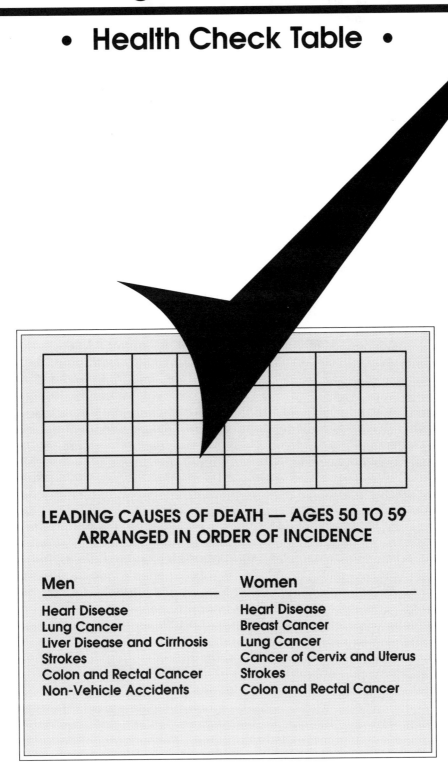

**LEADING CAUSES OF DEATH — AGES 50 TO 59
ARRANGED IN ORDER OF INCIDENCE**

Men	Women
Heart Disease	Heart Disease
Lung Cancer	Breast Cancer
Liver Disease and Cirrhosis	Lung Cancer
Strokes	Cancer of Cervix and Uterus
Colon and Rectal Cancer	Strokes
Non-Vehicle Accidents	Colon and Rectal Cancer

A. (GO!) Daily Health Checks

Daily logs or record sheets for Daily Health Checks are located with the expanded sections (see pages listed).

C. (STOP) Yearly or Periodic Health Checks

Record the month and year (e.g. 8/92) when the Health Check is performed and, where appropriate, the value (such as blood pressure,120/80). Record this information in the column that corresponds with your age at the time the Health Check is performed. (NOTE: M = male; F = female)

	Reference	Frequency	Age 50	Age 51
① Physical Examination & History (Initial/Interim) (M, F)	page 76	Every 2 years		
② Cardiac Risk Factor Screening† (M, F)	page 79	Every 1 – 2 years		
③ Blood Pressure Screening† (M, F)	page 84	Yearly		
④ Digital Rectal Exam† (M, F)	page 87	Yearly		
⑤ Clinical Skin Exam† (M, F)	page 92	Every 2 years		
⑥ Clinical Testicular Exam† (M)	page 98	Every 2 years		
⑦ Examine for Thyroid Nodules† (M, F)	page 101	Every 2 years		
⑧ Clinical Oral Cavity Exam† (M, F)	page 103	Every 2 years		
⑨ Total Blood Cholesterol (M, F)	page 105	Every 5 years		
⑩ Sigmoidoscopy (M, F)	page 87	Every 3 – 5 years (if first exam is normal)		
⑪ Blood Stool Test† (M, F)	page 87	Yearly		
⑫ Pap Test/Pelvic Exam† (F)	page 109	Every 1 – 3 years*		
⑬ Clinical Breast Exam† (F)	page 111	Yearly		
⑭ Mammogram (F)	page 111	Yearly		
⑯ Tonometry (M, F)	page 117	Every 2 – 4 years∞		
⑱ Blood Test (CBC, SMAC) and Urinalysis (M, F)	page 119	Optional§		
⑲ Dental Checkup (M, F)	page 132	Yearly		
⑳ Tetanus-Diphtheria Vaccination (M, F)	page 121	Every 10 years		
㉓ Height and Weight (M, F)	page 76	Yearly		

† These health checks are often performed in concert with a periodic physical examination.
* Pap test every 1 – 3 years, following two initial negative Pap tests.
∞ This recommendation is by the American Academy of Ophthalmology.

B. [STOP] Monthly Health Checks

Record the day and month (d/m) when these Health Checks are performed. (NOTE: M = male; F = female)

(1) Breast Self-Exam (F) ....page 111 ....

d/m	d/m	d/m	d/m	d/m	d/m

(2) Skin Self-Exam (M, F) ....page 92 ....

d/m	d/m	d/m	d/m	d/m	d/m

(4) Oral Cavity Self-Exam (M, F) ....page 103 ....

d/m	d/m	d/m	d/m	d/m	d/m

Age 52	Age 53	Age 54	Age 55	Age 56	Age 57	Age 58	Age 59

§ Routine blood tests (CBC, SMAC) and urinalysis are generally not recommended by most adult health maintenance organizations. The frequency of performing this health check is left to the discretion of you and your physician.

Continued next page

D. ▽YIELD Lifestyle Counseling

Review the Lifestyle Counseling information every one to three years and record the date.

1 Substance Use .... page 123 ..
2 Injury Prevention .... page 127 ..
3 Dental Health .... page 132 ..
4 Preventing Sexually Transmitted Diseases ..... page 135 ..
5 Preventing Low-Back Injury .... page 138 ..
6 Choosing a Doctor .... page 142 ..
7 Choosing a Health Care Plan .... page 144 ..
8 Assessing Genetic and Environmental Risk ... page 147 ..
9 Proper Sleep Hygiene .... page 149 ..

(mo / yr columns x3)

E. ◇WARN-ING High-Risk Health Checks

The frequency of these tests should be based on your medical history and other individual circumstances (see specific pages listed below).

1 Fasting Plasma Glucose .... page 152
2 Urinalysis for Bateriuria .... page 153
3 Hearing Screening .... pages 115, 154
4 Colonoscopy .... pages 87, 154
5 Resting Electrocardiogram .... page 79
6 Exercise Electrocardiogram .... page 79
8 Tuberculin Skin Test .... page 156
9 Bone Mineral Content .... page 157
10 Estrogen Replacement .... page 157
11 Osteoporosis Risk .... page 157
12 Aspirin Therapy .... page 159

14 Injuries in the Elderly .... page 127
15 Prevention of Childhood Injuries .... page 127
16 Hepatitis B Vaccine .... page 162
19 Pneumococcal Vaccine .... page 121
20 Influenza Vaccine .... page 121
21 Auscultation for Carotid Bruits .... page 164
22 Chlamydial Test .... page 165
23 Gonorrhea Culture .... page 166
24 VDRL (Syphilis Screen) .... page 166
25 Testing for AIDS Virus (HIV) .... page 167
27 Prostate Specific Antigen Test .... pages 87, 168

When additional High-Risk Health Checks are recommended, use this space to record pertinent information.

Recommended Health Check	Date	Date	Date	Comments
1.				
2.				
3.				
4.				
5.				
6.				
7.				
8.				
9.				
10.				
11.				
12.				
13.				
14.				
15.				
16.				
17.				
18.				

REMAIN ALERT FOR SIGNS IN SELF AND OTHERS:

Source material for this *Health Check Table* has included:
- The "Age-Specific Charts" of the U.S. Preventive Services Task Force (USPSTF);
- The cancer screening recommendations of the National Cancer Institute and the American Cancer Society;
- The screening test guidelines of the American College of Physicians;
- The periodic health evaluation guidelines by Dr. John H. Holbrook;
- The National Cholesterol Education Program Committee;
- Other medical organizations and medical scientists as set forth in the references of this book.

Ages 60 and Older

• Health Check Table •

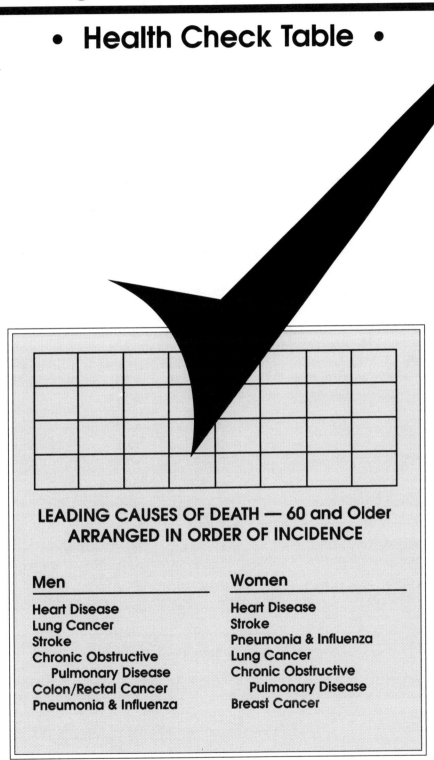

**LEADING CAUSES OF DEATH — 60 and Older
ARRANGED IN ORDER OF INCIDENCE**

Men	Women
Heart Disease	Heart Disease
Lung Cancer	Stroke
Stroke	Pneumonia & Influenza
Chronic Obstructive Pulmonary Disease	Lung Cancer
Colon/Rectal Cancer	Chronic Obstructive Pulmonary Disease
Pneumonia & Influenza	Breast Cancer

A. (GO!) Daily Health Checks

Daily logs or record sheets for Daily Health Checks are located with the expanded sections (see pages listed).

C. (STOP) Yearly or Periodic Health Checks

Record the month and year (e.g. 4/92) when the Health Check is performed and, where appropriate, the value (such as blood pressure,120/80). Record this information in the column that corresponds with your age at the time the Health Check is performed. (NOTE: M = male; F = female)

	Reference	Frequency	60 / 70 / 80	61 / 71 / 81
① Physical Examination & History (Initial/Interim) (M, F)	page 76	Yearly		
② Cardiac Risk Factor Screening[†] (M, F)	page 79	Yearly		
③ Blood Pressure Screening[†] (M, F)	page 84	Yearly		
④ Digital Rectal Exam[†] (M, F)	page 87	Yearly		
⑤ Clinical Skin Exam[†] (M, F)	page 92	Yearly		
⑥ Clinical Testicular Exam[†] (M)	page 98	Yearly		
⑦ Examine for Thyroid Nodules[†] (M, F)	page 101	Yearly		
⑧ Clinical Oral Cavity Exam[†] (M, F)	page 103	Yearly		
⑨ Total Blood Cholesterol (M, F)	page 105	Every 5 years		
⑩ Sigmoidoscopy (M, F)	page 87	Every 3 – 5 years (if initial exam is normal)		
⑪ Blood Stool Test[†] (M, F)	page 87	Yearly		
⑫ Pap Test/Pelvic Exam[†] (F)	page 109	Every 1 – 3 years[*]		
⑬ Clinical Breast Exam[†] (F)	page 111	Yearly		
⑭ Mammogram (F)	page 111	Yearly		
⑮ Hearing and Hearing Aids (M, F)	page 115	Yearly		
⑯ Tonometry and Visual Acuity (M, F)	page 117	Every 1 – 2 years[∞]		
⑰ Dipstick Urinalysis (M, F)	page 119	Yearly		
⑱ Blood Test (CBC, SMAC) (M, F)	page 119	Optional[§]		
⑲ Dental Checkup (M, F)	page 132	Yearly		
⑳ Tetanus-Diphtheria Vaccination (M, F)	page 121	Every 10 years		
㉑ Pneumococcal Vaccination (M, F)	page 121	At 65		
㉒ Influenza Vaccination (M, F)	page 121	At 65 (yearly thereafter)		
㉓ Height and Weight (M, F)	page 76	Yearly		

[†] These health checks are often performed in concert with a periodic physical examination.
[*] Pap test every 1 – 3 years, following two initial negative Pap tests.   [∞] American Academy of Ophthalmology recommendation.

B. [STOP] Monthly Health Checks

Record the day and month (d/m) when these Health Checks are performed. (NOTE: M = male; F = female)

(1) Breast Self-Exam (F) ....page 111 ....

d/m	d/m	d/m	d/m	d/m	d/m

(2) Skin Self-Exam (M, F) ....page 92 ....

d/m	d/m	d/m	d/m	d/m	d/m

(4) Oral Cavity Self-Exam (M, F) ....page 103 ....

d/m	d/m	d/m	d/m	d/m	d/m

62 / 72 / 82	63 / 73 / 83	64 / 74 / 84	65 / 75 / 85	66 / 76 / 86	67 / 77 / 87	68 / 78 / 88	69 / 79 / 89

§ Routine blood tests (CBC, SMAC) are generally not recommended by most adult health maintenance organizations.
The frequency of performing this health check is left to the discretion of you and your physician.   Continued next page

D. Lifestyle Counseling

Review the Lifestyle Counseling information every one to three years and record the date.

mo / yr	mo / yr	mo / yr
mo / yr	mo / yr	mo / yr
mo / yr	mo / yr	mo / yr
mo / yr	mo / yr	mo / yr
mo / yr	mo / yr	mo / yr
mo / yr	mo / yr	mo / yr
mo / yr	mo / yr	mo / yr
mo / yr	mo / yr	mo / yr
mo / yr	mo / yr	mo / yr

E. WARN-ING High-Risk Health Checks

The frequency of these tests should be based on your medical history and other individual circumstances (see specific pages listed below).

When additional High-Risk Health Checks are recommended, use this space to record pertinent information.

Recommended Health Check	Date	Date	Date	Comments
1.				
2.				
3.				
4.				
5.				
6.				
7.				
8.				
9.				
10.				
11.				
12.				
13.				
14.				
15.				
16.				
17.				
18.				

REMAIN ALERT FOR SIGNS IN SELF AND OTHERS:

Depression ....page 67
Suicide Risk Factors ....page 67
Abnormal Bereavement ....page 67
Signs of Physical Abuse or Neglect ....page 127
Peripheral Arterial Disease ....page 83
Possible Skin Cancer ....page 92
Tooth Decay, Gingivitis, Loose Teeth ....page 132

Source material for this *Health Check Table* has included:

- The "Age-Specific Charts" of the U.S. Preventive Services Task Force (USPSTF);
- The cancer screening recommendations of the National Cancer Institute and the American Cancer Society;
- The screening test guidelines of the American College of Physicians;
- The periodic health evaluation guidelines by Dr. John H. Holbrook;
- The National Cholesterol Education Program Committee;
- Other medical organizations and medical scientists as set forth in the references of this book.

CHAPTER

3

Expanded
Health Check
Material

Daily Health Check #1
PHYSICAL ACTIVITY PROGRAMS

There is no drug in current or prospective
use that holds as much promise for sustained health
as a lifetime program of physical exercise.

— Journal of the American Medical Association, 1982

RECOMMENDATIONS

1. Participate in structured exercise three to five days per week for 20 to 60 minutes at 60 to 90 percent of maximal heart rate (pages 42 to 44).
   ### and/or
2. Pursue active leisure-time activities at least three times per week for at least 60 minutes (page 44).

3. Participate in one set of 8 to 12 repetitions of 8 to 10 muscle resistance exercises at least twice a week[16] (include the major muscle groups). See *Health Check #2, Body Strength Program*, page 47.

4. Participate in four to five stretching exercises at least three to five times per week (daily stretching is acceptable). See *Health Check #3, Body Flexibility Program*, page 53.

5. Maintain at least an **average** fitness score (as measured from the Rockport Fitness Walking Test located in Appendix B, page 184), and an **average** body strength and flexibility score (see strength and flexibility tests located in Appendix D, page 201, and Appendix E, page 204).

6. Keep a log of your physical activity. How to use your log is discussed on page 46, and six months of activity logs are found in Appendix C, page 195.

7. For additional safety tips for participation in physical activity, refer to Appendix I, page 225.

Why Perform

Physical activity has been shown to:
- Decrease risk of death from coronary heart disease; physically inactive people are twice as likely to develop heart disease;[4-7]
- Lower death rate;[7, 8]
- Prevent or control: high blood pressure, osteoporosis, obesity, mental health problems, and diabetes;[9, 10]
- Improve the structure and function of ligaments, tendons, and joints;[11, 12]
- Increase muscular strength;[11, 13, 14]
- Maintain functional capacity and contributes to continued independent living with increasing age.

How Performed

Physical activity can be viewed as activities that result in calories being burned.[15] As illustrated on the next page in Figure 1, there are two physical activity approaches.

(*Note:* Ask yourself whether or not it is safe at this time to begin pursuing a structured exercise program and/or engage in vigorous leisure time activities. We encourage you to first check with your primary-care physician before undertaking a vigorous exercise program. Walking is generally not considered to be a vigorous activity and if started gradually and performed with common sense, it can usually be enjoyed by all. Refer also to *Yearly or Periodic Health Check #2, Cardiac Risk Factor Screening*, page 79, before beginning your physical activity program. The guidelines in this health check will help you and your physician determine if you need an exercise stress test.

Figure 1. Physical Activity Programs

Exercise Program
- Structured, planned, repetitive

Leisure/Occupational Time (LOT) Activity Program
- Less structured (may include leisure, occupational, household activities)

Examples:
- Walking
- Jogging
- Aerobic dance
- Stationary cycling

Plus
- Muscle-resistance exercises
- Flexibility exercises

Examples
- Walking
- Yard work
- Stair climbing
- Hiking
- Housework

Guidelines
- 3–5 days/week for 20–60 minutes (cardiovascular activity)
- 8–10 muscle resistance exercises (at least 2 days/week)
- 4–5 stretching exercises (at least 3–5 days/week)

Guidelines
- At least 3 days/week (preferably 3–5 days/week) for at least 60 minutes per day

Benefits
1. Decreased risk of death from coronary heart disease (physically inactive people are twice as likely to develop heart disease). [4–7]
2. Lower death rate. [7,8]
3. Prevention or control of high blood pressure, osteoporosis, obesity, mental health problems, and diabetes. [9,10]
4. Improvement in structure and function of ligaments, tendons, and joints. [11,12]
5. Increased muscular strength. [11,13,14]
6. Continued independent living with increasing age.

Starting a Structured Exercise Program

The *structured exercise program* is planned and repetitive and includes activities such as brisk walking, swimming, jogging, rowing, aerobic dancing, and stationary cycling performed *three to five days per week* for a period of *30 to 60 minutes* per session.[16] In addition, muscle strengthening activities such as resistive weight training and flexibility exercises should be performed at least *two to three days per week*. The structured exercise program has been shown to result in improved health status as well as improved physical fitness levels such as aerobic power, body fat percentage and muscle endurance.

The structured exercise program consists of three components:

- **CARDIOVASCULAR**
- **MUSCLE RESISTANCE**
- **STRETCHING**

CARDIOVASCULAR COMPONENT

This component includes **five steps**:
- Choosing the **type** of exercise activity;
- Determining how **hard**, how **long**, and how **often** you should exercise;
- **Warming-up/cooling-down.**

Step One – Type of Exercise Activity. The activity should include the use of *large muscle groups* (primarily the large leg muscles) moving in a *rhythmic fashion* (the activity is repeated over and over again) and performing in a *continuous nature*. If these **three criteria are met**, the activity is considered "aerobic" and will promote cardiovascular fitness. Examples of appropriate aerobic activities include: brisk walking, jogging/running, swimming, and aerobic dancing.

Step Two – Intensity or *How Hard You Should Exercise.* Three methods — the talk test, relative perceived exertion, and the heart rate — can be used to determine if you are exercising with sufficient intensity or with too much vigor.

"Talk Test." If, while exercising, you can carry on a conversation with your friend, your partner, or the dog, you are probably exercising at a safe intensity. If, on the other hand, you are unable to communicate because you are so out of breath, then you are working too hard; reduce the intensity. The old adage that "to get the benefit you must hurt" is simply not true.

Relative Perceived Exertion. While performing physical activity, ask yourself if the activity is light, somewhat hard, hard, or very hard. Listen to your whole body, such as your breathing and how your muscles are feeling. Try to maintain your activity level at the "somewhat hard" level (you shold be breathing harder but still able to talk). Learn to distinguish the somewhat hard exertion level from the hard or very hard level.

Taking Your Heart Rate. The structured exercise program suggests you exercise at 60-90 percent of *maximum heart rate*. This range is often referred to as the "**target zone.**" To find your zone, refer to Table 1 on the next page and locate in the left-hand column your age to the nearest five years. Scan this row to find your target heart range for moderate activity (60–75 percent of maximum) and for intense exercise (75–90 percent of maximum) in beats/10 seconds.

As an example, let's assume you are 43 years old and just beginning an exercise program. The closest age on Table 1 is 45. The target zone is 18–22 beats per 10 seconds for the 60–75 percent heart rate target zone (for lower intensity activities, i.e., walking) and 22–26 beats for 10 seconds [75–90 percent] for more intense exercise (i.e., jogging or stationary cycling with applied tension).

If you have been sedentary for some time, you should consider exercising in the lower heart rate range (60– 75 percent) for the first two to four weeks of your exercise program. Thereafter, depending on the type of activity you choose, you can continue in this range (60–75 percent) or you can increase to the 75–90 percent range.

During the early weeks of your exercise program, we encourage you to take your heart rate halfway through your exercise session. If you need to stop exercise momentarily to take your pulse, quickly find your pulse and take it for only 10 seconds. Most individuals soon learn to "listen to their body" and avoid the taking of the pulse during every exercise session. In fact, the talk test and relative perceived exertion are good ways to monitor exercise intensity because the predicted maximal heart rate has a high degree of variability.

Taking the pulse. Two common places to take your pulse are at the neck and the wrist. To take your pulse at the neck, place your finger (not the thumb) **gently** to the right or left of the Adam's apple, generally located in the "natural" groove in your neck. Count the number of beats you feel in 10 seconds.

To take your pulse at the wrist, place the middle and index fingers in the soft area of the wrist, just under the thumb. There is a natural groove in which to place your fingers. Elderly people should **avoid** taking their pulse at the neck because there may be plaque build-up in the large arteries of the neck (the carotid arteries).

Table 1. *Taking Your Heart Rate*

Age	Ave. Max. Heart Rate (Beats/Min.)	60-75% Target Zone (Beats/10 sec.)	(Beats/min.)	75-90% (Beats/10 sec.)	(Beats/min.)
20 years	200	20-25	(120-150)	25-30	(150-180)
25 years	195	20-24	(117-146)	24-29	(146-176)
30 years	190	19-24	(114-143)	24-29	(143-171)
35 years	185	19-23	(111-139)	23-28	(139-167)
40 years	180	18-23	(108-135)	23-27	(135-162)
45 years	175	18-22	(105-131)	22-26	(131-158)
50 years	170	17-21	(102-128)	21-26	(128-153)
55 years	165	17-21	(99-124)	21-25	(124-149)
60 years	160	16-20	(96-120)	20-24	(120-144)
65 years	155	16-19	(93-116)	19-23	(116-140)
70 years	150	15-19	(90-113)	19-23	(112-135)
75 years	145	15-18	(87-109)	18-22	(109-131)
80 years	140	14-18	(84-105)	18-21	(105-126)

NOTE: The heart rate figures are averages and should only be used as a guideline. Some individuals are taking medications which lower their heart rates (i.e., beta blocking medications, like Inderal), and so the target zone heart rate ranges in Table 1 would not be appropriate. Ask your physician or a qualified consultant if this applies to your situation.

***Step Three – Duration** or **How Long You Should Exercise**.* The duration of each exercise session will depend upon the intensity of the activity (or how high the heart rate is). For example, the recommended duration of walking will be longer than the time suggested for jogging or riding your stationary bike (with moderate tension applied). Although your target heart rate zone will be lower with the walking as compared to jogging, you can get the same cardiovascular benefits by increasing the duration of your walk.

The exercise duration is low when starting an exercise program, and is *gradually* increased every week or two. The exact recommendations for duration will be discussed later in the detailed sample exercise schedules.

A rule of thumb. If you haven't fully recovered one hour after an exercise session, you've probably pushed too hard. Decrease the pace or the mileage (or both) during your next exercise session. *The key is that you **do not** push too hard or exercise too long, too soon.*

Step Four - Frequency Or How Often You Should Exercise. The *minimal* number of exercise sessions per week necessary to attain and maintain cardiovascular fitness is *three*, preferably every other day. We recommend *four to five days per week* as an optimal number of exercise sessions per week.

Step Five - Warm-Up and Cool-Down. The warm-up activity should include some light stretching, followed by the same activity you will be doing for your regular fitness program, but at a reduced intensity.

For example, if your activity is stationary cycling, you should mount the bike (following a couple of minutes of light stretching), and begin pedaling **without** any tension. Over the next four to five minutes, gradually increase the tension until you are at or near your target heart rate.

A proper warm-up will help to reduce the strain on the cardiovascular and musculature systems of the body. (An additional tip: Never start your walking or jogging by ascending a hill.)

If you have been riding a stationary bicycle, release the tension for your cool-down, and pedal freely for several minutes until you are back to normal breathing. If your activity has included brisk walking, cool down with a slower walk. A gradual five-minute cool-down keeps the large leg muscles pumping much needed blood back to the heart and prevents the blood from pooling in the lower extremities. Failing to cool down may cause you to become light-headed, dizzy or even to faint.

(NOTE: Many individuals perform heavy stretching activities following the exercise session. We encourage this procedure because the muscles are warm and less likely to experience muscle pulls.)

TWO SAMPLE 16-WEEK CARDIOVASCULAR EXERCISE SCHEDULES

Two sample 16-week cardiovascular exercise schedules (for all ages) are given in Tables 2 and 3 (see next page). (In addition, a sample **walking** schedule, designed to accompany the **Rockport Fitness Walking Test**, is outlined in Appendix B, page 184.) If you are already involved in a structured exercise program, you can begin at your current duration as listed on the charts.

Table 2 — Description of Lower Intensity 16-Week Schedule. The schedule outlined in Table 2 is for lower intensity activities. Notice that a blank column is included in the table for entering your 10-second target heart rate (60 to 75 percent taken from Table 1 on page 43). Rather than using heart rate, you may choose to use the **Talk Test** or to monitor your perceived exertion (see page 42).

Every two weeks, adjustments in the exercise program should be made.

- **First two weeks**: warm-up (five minutes); exercise (15-20 minutes); and cool-down (five minutes).
- **Every two weeks**: Increase the exercise time (duration) by about five minutes.
- **Duration Goal**: 50 to 60 minutes (you may choose to break the exercise time into two 30-minute sessions).
- **Frequency**: Initially, three to four days per week, eventually increase to **four to five days** per week. (Lower intensity exercise activities such as brisk walking can be performed **daily**.)

Having reached a goal of 50 to 60 minutes of lower intensity exercise, you may continue with this duration of exercise for the remainder of your life or you may want to consider the more intense exercise recommendations outlined in Table 3 and discussed in the next paragraph.

Table 3 — Description of More Intense Activities. Table 3 is for the more intense activities in which the heart rate will naturally be higher during exercise (75 to 90 percent of maximum). Please note the blank column for you to record your 10-second heart rate range (75 to 90 percent of maximum), taken from *Table 1, Taking Your Heart Rate*, page 43.

Every two weeks, adjustments in the exercise program should be made.

- **First two weeks**: warm-up (five minutes); exercise (10-15 minutes); cool-down (five minutes).
- **Every two weeks**: Increase the exercise time (duration) by about five minutes.

- **Duration Goal**: 30 to 35 minutes.
- **Frequency**: Initially, three to four days per week, eventually increase to **four to five days** per week.

Having completed the 16-week exercise program, you can follow the recommendations that are listed in the "15-16 week" column for the remainder of your life.

MUSCLE RESISTANCE COMPONENT

To begin a muscle-resistance program, refer to *Daily Health Check #2*, **page 47**.

STRETCHING (FLEXIBILITY) COMPONENT

To begin a flexibility program, refer to *Daily Health Check #3*, **page 53.**

Starting a Leisure/ Occupational Time (LOT) Program

The *leisure/occupational time (LOT) program* is less structured and generally less continuous in nature, and suggests you participate in activities such as stair climbing, yard work, housework, hiking, and sporting activities *at least three days per week* or have a physically demanding occupation. The amount of cumulative time spent in these activities should be approximately *60 minutes.*[11]

Studies involving large population groups have shown that individuals participating in leisure activities or occupations that burn extra calories have a reduced risk for heart attack and other chronic diseases.

Hopefully, this amount of LOT activity will be adequate for achieving and maintaining at least an **average** fitness level. The Rockport Fitness Walking Test (located in Appendix B, page 184) can be used to monitor your fitness level. If you fall below the **average fitness level** when you take this fitness test, you may need to increase the leisure time activity and/or consider the structured exercise program discussed earlier.

We should mention that leisure time activity research data is still somewhat unclear regarding the degree of benefit this program has for weight loss. If your main objective in becoming more active is for weight loss, and you find that over time the leisure time activity prescription isn't producing the desired results — you may want to participate in the more structured exercise program that has been previously detailed.

GO!
Daily #1

Table 2. *For Lower Intensity Activities*

Brisk Walking, Mini-Tramping, Country Bicycling, Roller Skating, Stationary Cycling (with very little or zero tension).

Week	% of Maximal Heart Rate Target Zone	Heart Rate (Beats/10 sec.) Target Zone	Warm-Up	Duration (Exercise Time)	Cool-Down	Frequency (Days/Week)
1–2	60–75%		5 min.	15–20	5 min.	3–4
3–4	60–75%		5 min.	20–25	5 min.	3–4
5–6	60–75%		5 min.	25–30	5 min.	4–5
7–8	60–75%		5 min.	30–35	5 min.	4–5
9–10	60–75%		5 min.	35–40	5 min.	4–5
11–12	60–75%		5 min.	40–45	5 min.	4–5
13–14	60–75%		5 min.	45–50	5 min.	4–5
15–16	60–75%		5 min.	50–55	5 min.	4–5

(*Note:* You may want to consider using the Talk Test or Relative Perceived Exertion [see page 42] in place of the heart rate target zone.)

Table 3. *For Higher Intensity Activities*

Jogging, Swimming, Aerobic Dancing, Cross-Country Skiing, Stationary Cycling (with tension).

Week	% of Maximal Heart Rate Target Zone	Heart Rate (Beats/10 sec.) Target Zone	Warm-Up	Duration (Exercise Time)	Cool-Down	Frequency (Days/Week)
1–2	75–90%		5 min.	10–15	5 min.	3–4
3–4	75–90%		5 min.	15–20	5 min.	3–4
5–6	75–90%		5 min.	20–25	5 min.	4–5
7–8	75–90%		5 min.	25–30	5 min.	4–5
9–10	75–90%		5 min.	30–35	5 min.	4–5
11–12	75–90%		5 min.	30–35	5 min.	4–5
13–14	75–90%		5 min.	30–35	5 min.	4–5
15–16	75–90%		5 min.	30–35	5 min.	4–5

(*Note:* You may want to consider using the Talk Test or Relative Perceived Exertion [see page 42] in place of the heart rate target zone.)

Combining the Two Activity Programs

Dr. Per Olf Astrand (a father of sports medicine), recommends that people follow a **combination** of the structured and LOT activity programs. He encourages people to be up and about, on their feet, walking, climbing stairs, moving — for 60 minutes a day. This includes "one minute 60 times a day, 12 minutes five times a day, or any combination totaling 60 minutes."[11] In addition, Dr. Astrand recommends 30 to 45 minutes, three days per week, of exercise such as brisk walking, jogging, swimming, or aerobic dance.

Setting a Date and Keeping An Activity Log

The most difficult component of a physical activity program is "getting started." The next most difficult step is remaining consistent in your physical activity. To help overcome these two barriers, we suggest you set a date for beginning your physical activity program and then consistently keep a physical activity log. Outlined below in Table 4 is information on how to keep a physical activity log. Keep your log for *at least* 16 weeks. Appendix C includes a six month supply of physical activity logs (see Appendix C, page 195).

Conclusion: Does Physical Activity Work?

I first met Senator Wallace F. Bennett in his Washington, D.C., office. I was a 17-year-old high school student and the senator was 69.

I next met the Senator 14 years later at The Fitness Institute at LDS Hospital. Senator Bennett (then 82) was undergoing a complete fitness evaluation. The senator's results were impressive: percent body fat, 20.8 percent – excellent; blood pressure, 125/78 – excellent; and total blood cholesterol, 201 mg percent and an HDL-cholesterol (the "good" cholesterol), 50 mg percent – both excellent. His exercise treadmill test revealed a fitness level well above average. We asked the senator about his secret for good health.

He told us he was first elected to Congress in 1950. During his first medical evaluation his physician said, "You need exercise, but believe me, your senate schedule will always interfere with a consistent exercise routine. Whenever possible, I suggest you *walk*."

The senator took his doctor's advice, and for the next 24 years of congressional service, Senator Bennett became the "walking senator." He walked to the Senate Chamber and to committee meetings; when the weather allowed, he walked throughout his Washington neighborhood.

When the senator retired from public office, the walking continued. At age 82 when we tested the senator, he was walking six days per week, 60-90 minutes per day, and at an 18-minute-per-mile pace. Now, at age 92, he's still walking.

Table 4: Sample Physical Activity Log

Days	Date	Exercise Type	Minutes			Distance (optional)	Target Heart Rate (10 sec.)	Weight (pounds)	Meditation/ Relaxation (Yes or No)	Did Something For Self (Yes or No)
			Warm-up	Exercise	Cool-Down					
1	6/3	Walking	5	45	4	—	19	165	yes	no
2	6/4	Strength Exer	3	40	3					
3	6/5	Walk/Stretch	4	47	5 & 15	2-1/2 mi.	18	164	yes	yes
4	6/6	Walking	5	45	5	—	—	164	no	yes
5	6/7	Strength Exer	3	40	3					
6	6/8	Walk/Stretch	5	48	4 & 15	2-1/2 mi.	18	164	yes	yes
7										
8										
9										

Daily Health Check #2
BODY STRENGTH PROGRAM

RECOMMENDATIONS

1. Participate in one set of 8 to 12 repetitions of 8 to 10 muscle resistance exercises at least two times per week[16] (include the major muscle groups).

2. In addition to the recommendation above, we encourage individuals to participate in a structured and/or leisure-time activity program as outlined in *Daily Health Check #1*, page 40, and a flexibility program as outlined in *Daily Health Check #3*, page 53.

3. Maintain at least an **average** body strength score (see strength tests in Appendix D, page 201).

4. Record your participation in muscle strengthening activities in your activity log. How to use the activity log is found on page 46 and six months of logs are located in Appendix C, page 195.

CAUTION: **If you have a history of heart trouble, are over age 35 or have questions about your current health, check with your physician prior to starting a weight resistance program. Also, start and progress slowly. Never hold your breath while you are performing weight resistance exercises (whether using your own weight or gym-type weights). Instead, breathe freely during each repetition of the resistance exercise. And finally, when lifting weights, always have someone present.**

Why Perform

- The American College of Sports Medicine has recently recommended that all individuals include weight resistance training as part of their regular exercise program.[16]
- Daily weight resistance actvities have been shown to improve the structure and function of ligaments, tendons, and joints;[11, 12] decrease low-back pain; and increase muscular strength.[11, 13, 14]
- Inadequate muscular strength can result in serious musculoskeletal problems which can lead to poor posture, excessive pain, disability, and early retirement.[17]
- Lack of weight resistance activities can lead to bone loss that can eventually lead to osteoporosis.[17]

The popularity of strength training is increasing among both men and women. Women are realizing weight resistance training will **not** produce large bulky muscles. Instead, the exercises improve physical attractiveness by decreasing body fat, increasing lean body mass and improving muscle tone.

This section discusses how to strengthen skeletal muscles. In addition, self-administered body-strength tests are included in Appendix D, page 201. We recommend individuals attain at least an **average** score when taking these strength tests.

How Performed

STRENGTHENING SKELETAL MUSCLES USING YOUR OWN WEIGHT

Located on the following pages are photographs of the basic muscle resistance exercises. Eight to 10 of these exercises should be done at least two days per week. For each exercise you choose, begin by doing one set of three to five repetitions for the first week. Increase the number by two or three each week until you reach eight to 12 repetitions. Eventually you may want to increase the number of sets.

Listed below are one or more muscle-resistant exercises that can be used to strengthen the appropriate body parts. The numbers correspond to the **numbered** photographs on the following pages.

Shoulder	1a, 1b, 1c, 3, 4
Abdomen	5,6
Chest	1a, 1b, 1c
Legs	9, 10a, 10b, 11, 12
Back	3, 4, 7, 8
Biceps	1a, 1b, 1c, 2
Triceps	1a, 1b, 1c, 3

You may want to ask your physician or a physical therapist about other muscle resistance exercises that might be appropriate for your specific needs.

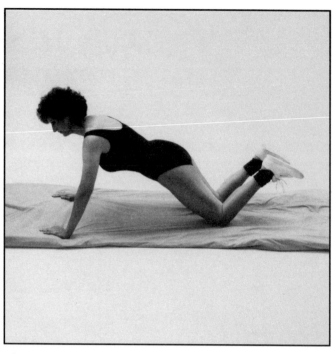

1b. Push-Up (Knee Pivot Position): Keeping hips and back straight, bend elbows to bring the chest to the floor and then return to starting position.

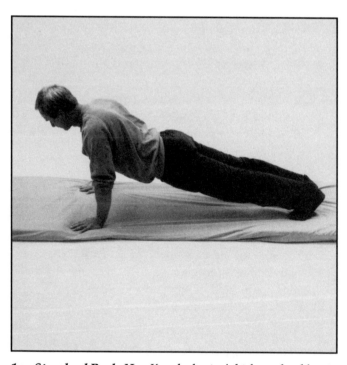

1c. Standard Push-Up: Keep body straight from shoulders to ankles, bend elbows to bring the chest to the floor and then return to starting position.

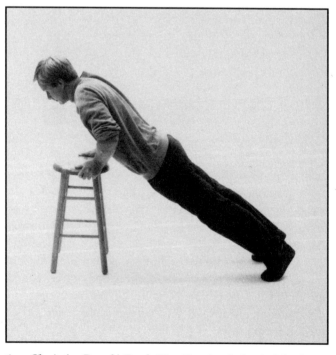

1a. Chair (or Bench) Push-Up: Keeping body straight, lower chest to level of hands and push back up.

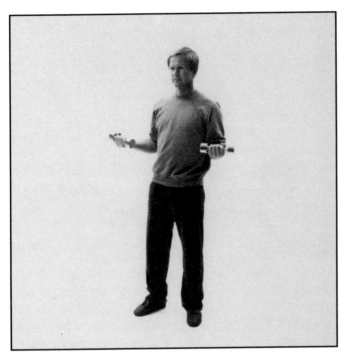

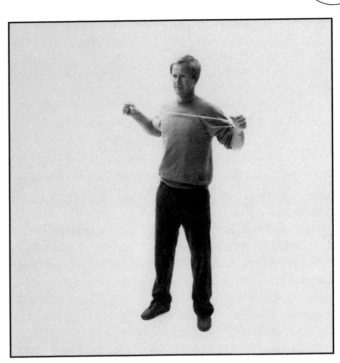

2. Biceps Curl: *Select a weight (such as light-weight barbell or soup cans) that can be easily lifted for three to five repetitions. Start with the arms to the side, elbows straight. Bend the elbow, pulling the hand up to the shoulder.*

4. Shoulder Pull: *Using a stretchy cord (such as Theraband, surgical tubing or elastic cord) held between the hands, pull the hands apart, bringing the elbows back and down and the shoulder blades together.*

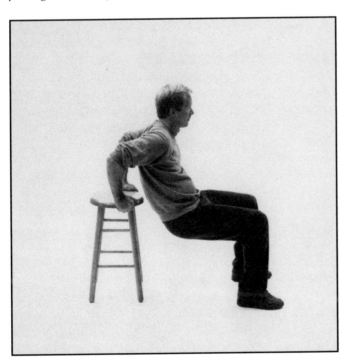

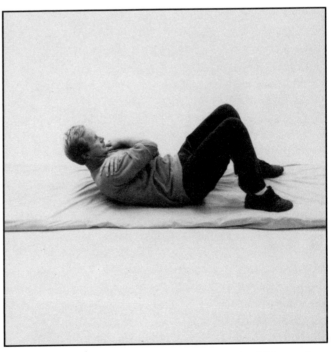

3. Chair Dip: *Placing the hands on the edge of a sturdy chair or the edge of a counter, lower your hips toward the floor as far as you feel comfortable. (Note: To adjust the degree of difficulty of this exercise, use chairs or counter of varying heights. The higher the chair surface is from the ground, the less difficult the exercise.)*

5. Partial Trunk Curl: *Lying on your back with knees bent (and not anchored), flatten the low-back onto the floor, using abdominal muscles. Holding this position throughout the exercise, curl the head and shoulders up until the shoulder blades clear the ground. Continue holding the low-back flat as you return to the starting position.*

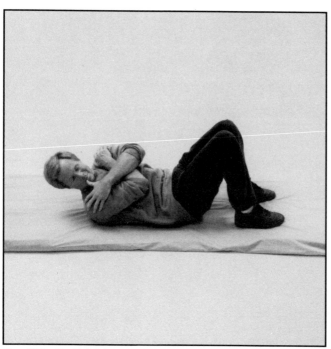

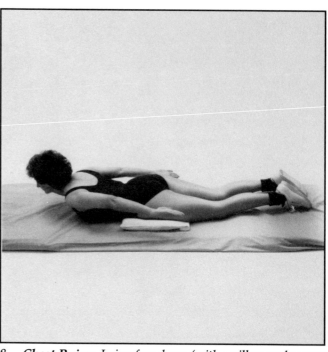

6. Side Curl: *Using the instructions given in the exercise #5, add a rotation as you curl up, bringing left shoulder towards right knee and vice versa.*

8. Chest Raise: *Lying face down (with a pillow under your hips, if desired), raise the head, chest, and arms up, squeezing the shoulder blades down and together.*

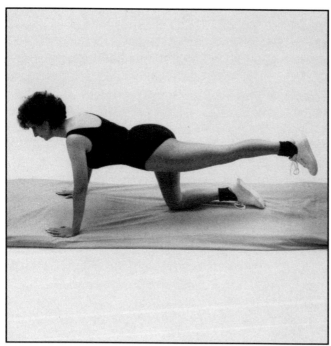

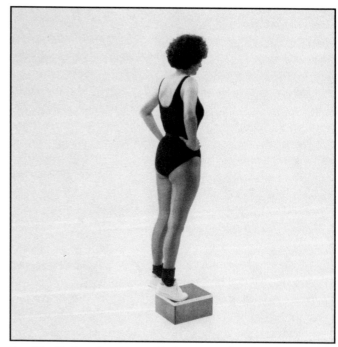

7. Kneeling Leg Raise: *From an all-fours position, raise one leg straight behind you from the floor to a horizontal position, and back down to the ground.*

9. Toe Raise: *Standing with the toes on the edge of a step, push yourself upwards onto your toes.*

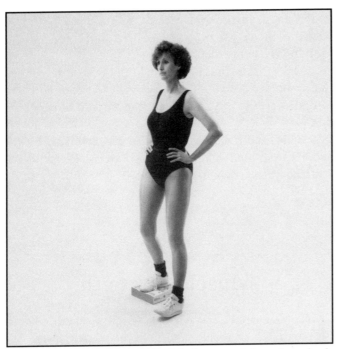

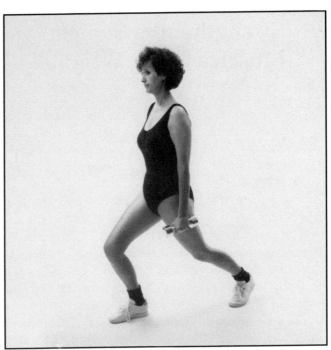

10a. **_Step Up:_** _Stand with the right foot on a stair or phone book. Keeping the left leg straight, push up with the right leg as in Figure 10b. Repeat the exercise with the left leg on the step._

11. **_Lunge:_** _Stand with the right foot a large stride ahead of the left. Keeping the right knee over the right toe, bend the right leg forward, lowering the body towards the ground._ **_Do not_** _go past a 90-degree angle at the knee. To increase the difficulty of the exercise, you may hold weights in your hands. Alternate legs._

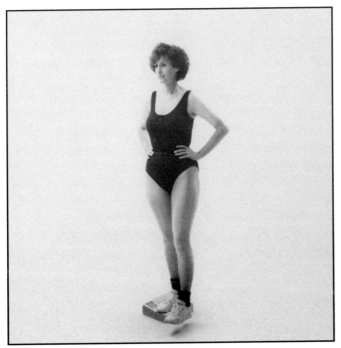

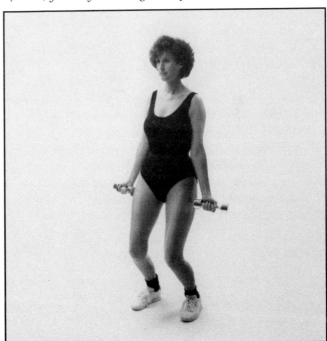

10b. **_Step Up._**

12. **_Partial Squats:_** _Stand with the feet shoulder-width apart; bend the knees forward over the toes (about a 40-degree angle), and straighten up again._

Strengthening Skeletal Muscles Using Weights

Just like aerobic exercise, weight resistance training has specific requirements. To develop greater strength, the muscles must be overloaded — you must work your muscle groups harder than they are accustomed to working. This principle of increased resistance is called the "overload principle."

There are two basic ways to use the overload principle: You can lift heavy weights a few repetitions and concentrate on muscular strength, or you can lift lighter weights for several repetitions and gain less strength while emphasizing muscle endurance and tone. The later approach is generally recommended as part of the structured exercise program.

To use weights for strengthening the skeletal muscles effectively, we suggest you purchase weight-lifting equipment for the home (this can be as simple as a few dumbbells and a chin-up bar) or visit a local health club. You may want to visit with an exercise specialist such as an exercise physiologist or a physical therapist for weight-training recommendations.

Make certain that you begin lifting with a weight that is appropriate for your initial strength. Also, be sure and progress slowly as you increase the amount of weight to lift.

Using hand-held weights is an excellent way for the elderly to strengthen their skeletal muscles. Remember to breathe freely as you use the weights.

Assessing Your Muscle Strength

To determine your current muscle strength, refer to Appendix D, page 201, and take the muscle tests. We suggest you maintain at least an **average** score on these tests.

Daily Health Check #3

BODY FLEXIBILITY PROGRAM

RECOMMENDATIONS

1. Participate in four to five stretching exercises at least three to five times per week (daily stretching is acceptable).

2. In addition to the recommendation above, we encourage individuals to participate in a structured and/or leisure-time activity program as outlined in *Daily Health Check #1*, page 40, and a body strength program as outlined in *Daily Health Check #2*, page 47.

3. Maintain at least an **average** body flexibility score (see flexibility tests in Appendix E, page 204).

4. Record your participation in flexibility activities in your activity log. How to use the activity log is found on page 46 and six months of logs are located in Appendix C, page 195.

Why Perform

- Individuals involved in flexibility activites have been shown to have a lower risk for orthopedic injuries and fewer low-back problems.
- Inadequate flexibility may result in serious musculoskeletal problems that can lead to poor posture and excessive pain.[17]

How Performed

Flexibility is measured by your ability to move a joint through its full range of motion. As you properly and regularly stretch major muscle groups, your body movements will seem easier. The process takes time, however, so be consistent and patient.

All stretching should be slow and deliberate. **Never** bounce or force joint movement. Bouncing makes the muscles respond with a reflex contraction (such as when the doctor taps the tendon directly under your knee) and may injure the muscle being stretched.

When stretching, move slowly to the suggested position until you begin to feel mild tension. At this point, hold your position for 10–15 seconds. Then attempt to gradually move forward (about one-fourth of an inch).

Hold the new position for 10–15 seconds and return to your original position and repeat the procedure. You should work on each stretching exercise for two or three minutes.

The entire time spent on stretching will vary from person to person. Try to spend at least 10–15 minutes stretching (preferably after physical activity when the muscles are warm).

SUGGESTED FLEXIBILITY (STRETCHING) EXERCISES

Listed in this section are recommended stretches. In addition, self-administered body flexibility tests can be found by referring to Appendix E, page 204.

For each body part listed, there are one or more exercises that can be used to stretch the appropriate muscles. The numbers correspond to the **numbered** photographs on the following pages.

Low back 1, 2, 3
Quadriceps.....................................11
Hamstrings 5
Upper back.....................................4, 6
Trunk rotators 4
Shoulders 6, 7
Achilles Tendon 3, 10
Chest 7, 8, 9
Hip flexor 2, 3
Groin 3, 12

You may want to ask your physician or a physical therapist about other body stretches that might be appropriate for your specific needs.

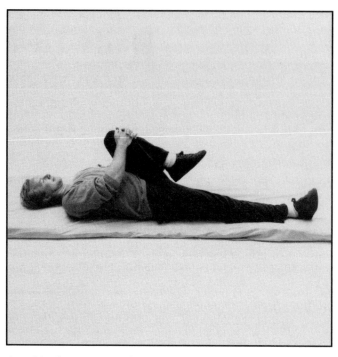

2. *Single Knee-to-Chest: Repeat exercise #1, using only one leg. Keep the leg that is not brought to the chest flat to the floor. A modification of this exercise can be performed by bringing the knee across diagonally towards the opposite shoulder.*

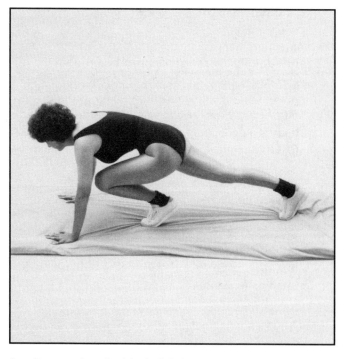

3. *Lunge: Stand with the left foot a large stride ahead of the right. Keeping the left knee over the left toe, bend the left leg forward, lowering the body towards the ground. Place the hands on the floor and lower the hips towards the ground. Alternate feet.*

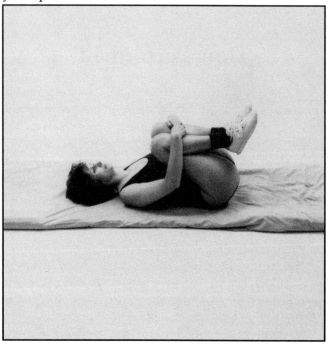

1. *Double Knee-to-Chest: Lying on your back, bring your knees upward, grasp them with your hands, and pull them towards your chest.*

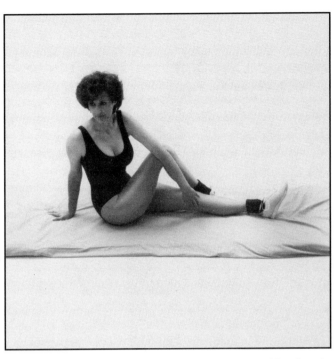

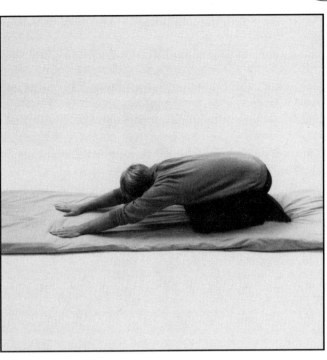

4. Twist: *Sitting as shown, rotate the torso and head to the right and then to the left.*

6. Prayer Stretch: *Sit on the heels of your feet and stretch the hands out in front of you, placing your chest on your knees.*

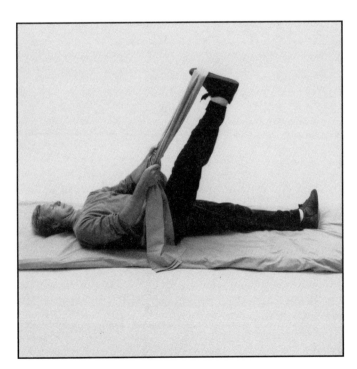

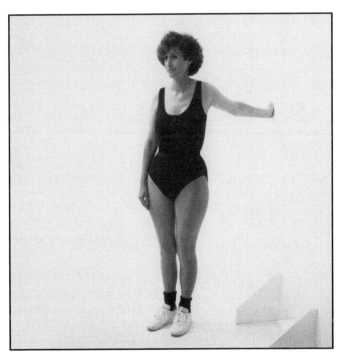

5. Hamstrings: *Placing a rolled sheet or rope across the ball of the right foot, raise the right leg with the knee straight. Alternate legs.*

7. Corner Stretch: *Place the left hand on a door jamb or a wall corner below shoulder height, and turn the body to the right. Alternate positions.*

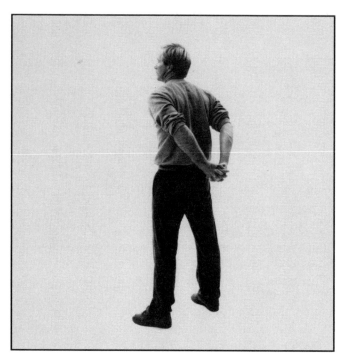

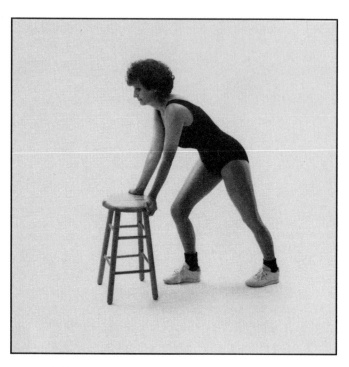

8. **Chest Opener:** *With the fingers laced together behind you, straighten the elbows and raise the arms up.*

10. **Achilles Tendon:** *Place the right foot ahead of the left foot, toes pointing straight ahead, and bend forward at the ankle. Lean against a wall with your arms outstretched. Alternate legs.*

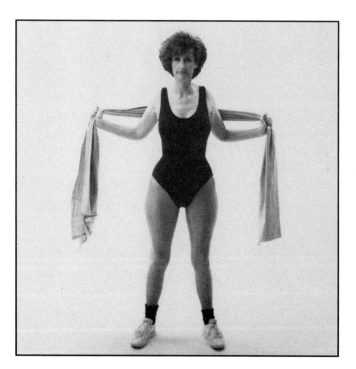

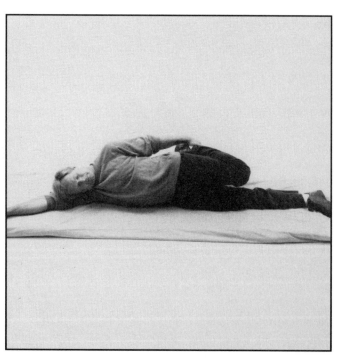

9. **Pull Down:** *Using a rolled sheet or rope between your hands, pull the arms and sheet down behind your back.*

11. **Quadriceps:** *Lie on the right side, grasp the left ankle, and pull the heel towards the buttock. Keep the left knee down and avoid arching the back. Alternate legs.*

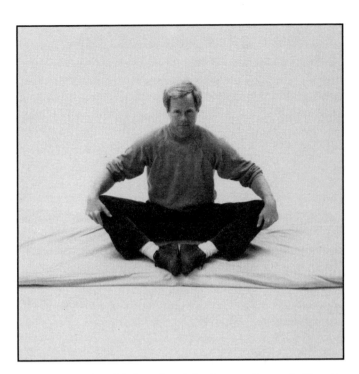

12. *Groin: Sit with the soles of the feet together and allow the knees to drop outward. Bring the feet as close to the groin as feels comfortable. Be certain to keep the back erect.*

Daily Health Check #4

PROPER NUTRITION PROGRAM

RECOMMENDATIONS [18-21]

1. Reduce consumption of fat to 30 percent or less of total daily calorie intake (saturated fat less than 10 percent of total calories) and reduce cholesterol intake to less than 300 mg/day. Use food preparations that contain little or no fat.

2. Increase consumption of fruits and vegetables (every day eat **five or more** servings) and increase the intake of whole grain foods, cereal products, dried beans and peas (**six or more** daily servings).

3. Reduce intake of sodium (six grams or less) by choosing foods relatively low in sodium and limiting the amount of salt added in food preparation and used at the table.

4. Alcohol consumption is not recommended. For those who drink alcoholic beverages, limit consumption to no more than two drinks per day.

5. Maintain adequate calcium intake. Refer to page 62 for specific calcium requirements.

6. Gradually work through the 11 dietary goal sheets located in Appendix F, page 206.

Why Perform

- The total amount and type of fat in our daily diet impact our risk for cardiovascular disease and for certain kinds of cancer (such as colon, breast and prostate).[18,19]
- Diets high in plant foods have been identified with a lower incidence of coronary heart disease and reduced rates of various forms of cancer (especially colon, esophagus, lung and stomach).[18]
- Good dietary habits can have a significant influence upon the prevention of obesity, high blood pressure, osteoporosis, adult-onset diabetes, dental diseases, and diverticular disease.[20,21]

How Performed

THE THREE FUELS: CARBOHYDRATES, FATS AND PROTEINS

Carbohydrates: Carbohydrates are an essential fuel of our daily diet, supplying **four calories** of food energy per gram.

Carbohydrates exist in two forms — simple carbohydrates (or sugars) and complex carbohydrates (starches and fiber). In nature, both simple sugars and complex starches come packaged in foods such as oranges, apples, corn, and wheat. Refined or processed carbohydrates are found in soft drinks, cookies, cakes, candy, and pies.

Fats (Saturated, Mono-unsaturated, and Polyun-saturated): Fats have more than twice the number of calories per gram as carbohydrates and proteins (one gram of fat = **nine calories**). In addition to providing calories, fat helps in the absorption of certain vitamins. Small amounts of fat are necessary for normal body function. Fats can be viewed in the following way:[22]

Total Fat — Is the sum of the three types of fat: saturated, mono-unsaturated, and polyunsaturated. A mixture of all three in varying amounts is found in most fat-containing foods.

Saturated Fat — This fat is found mostly in foods from animals such as meat, poultry, and whole-dairy products such as cream, milk, ice-cream, and cheese. Saturated fat easily raises blood cholesterol. Saturated fats are generally solid at room temperature.

Mono-unsaturated Fat — This fat is an unsaturated fat and is usually liquid at room temperature. This fat is found in plant foods such as peanut, olive, and canola (rapeseed) oils. When substituted for saturated fat, mono-unsaturated fat helps reduce blood cholesterol.

Polyunsaturated Fat — This fat is also liquid at room temperature and is a very unsaturated fat. The greatest amount of this fat is found in foods from plants such as safflower, sunflower, corn, and soybean oils. Plant fat contains **no** cholesterol. When substituted for saturated fat, polyunsaturated fat helps reduce blood cholesterol.

Protein: Protein supplies calories to the body (**four calories** per gram), and provides the structural components for our bones, muscles, enzymes, and hormones. Protein also carries the body's genetic information.

Unlike carbohydrate and fats, dietary protein requirements vary according to body size and age, and not activity. The recommended daily intake of protein is:
- **56 grams** for an adult male;
- **44 grams** for an adult female.

THE THREE-PHASE APPROACH TOWARD PROPER NUTRITION

The **best** fuel mixture is composed of:
- **Mostly** complex carbohydrates;
- **Adequate** amounts of protein;
- **Limited** amounts of fat;
- **Low** amounts of salt and refined sugars.

The vitamins and minerals which run our metabolism are present in the foods that comprise this fuel mixture.

This eating style (guaranteed to improve your health) is composed of a wide variety of foods from **six food groups**.
1. Vegetables
2. Fruits
3. Grains and cereals, emphasizing whole grain products.
4. Legumes (dried beans, peas and lentils)
5. Low fat dairy products, including skim milk, low fat yogurt, skim milk cheeses, and other milk products with the butterfat removed or reduced.
6. Fish, shellfish, poultry without skin, and lean meats.

This diet also includes vegetable oils, margarines and shortenings, sugar and other sweeteners in *small quantities*, and herbs and spices. These foods are used to enhance the flavors of the six groups listed above.

Most people will not be able to change abruptly their lifelong eating habits. We suggest **gradually** moving toward a more nutritious diet. Go at your own pace and progress with this diet in several small "steps." These steps can be summarized in **three phases**.

Phase I: Substitutions. The changes suggested in this phase are usually the easiest and the most painless. In fact, people in general are beginning to move through these dietary changes. In this phase, foods which are very high in saturated fats and cholesterol are replaced by substitute products which are very similar in appearance and taste, but which are lower in cholesterol and saturated fat. Examples of these changes include:
- Using margarine in place of butter;
- Using vegetable oils and shortenings in place of lard;
- Using skim milk instead of whole or 2% milk;
- Changing to "light" mayonnaise and spreads;
- Not using the egg yolks but using egg whites or egg substitutes;
- Using fish, poultry (without skin), and very lean cuts of meat to replace higher fat meats, and not using organ meats (liver, sweetbreads, etc.);
- Using salt substitutes and taking the salt shaker off the table.

Lowering the fat and cholesterol content of your favorite recipes can be a challenge. Remember that some recipes are easier to change than others, but all recipes can become "heart healthy," often with little change in taste, looks and quality.

In addition to the suggestions mentioned above, start reading the ingredients. Ask yourself if each ingredient serves a purpose. Identify any item you are trying to avoid or reduce and use one of the following methods:

1. **Elimination:** If the ingredient isn't essential, don't use it. For example, most package directions call for oil and salt added to water when cooking pasta or rice - they're not essential. Leave them out!

2. **Reduction:** If less will do - great! Try reducing sugar and fat by 1/3 to 1/2 in your recipe. Use nonstick pans and reduce the oil in casserole and skillet dishes.

3. **Substitution:** If you can find a healthier ingredient, use it! Try these easy substitutions:

1 EGG — 2 egg whites; *OR* 1/4 cup egg substitute (Eggbeaters*, Scramblers*, or Second Nature* can be found in the frozen food section of your grocery store); *OR* 1/4 cup homemade egg substitute (combine 6 egg whites, 1/4 cup nonfat powdered milk, 1 tablespoon oil and 6 drops of yellow food coloring. Stores in refrigerator up to one week.)

1 CUP BUTTER — 1/2 to 1 cup margarine (liquid, soft, or soft stick types); or Butter Buds*; or butter flavoring.

1 CUP LARD — 1/2 to 1 cup vegetable oil or vegetable shortening.

1 CUP WHOLE MILK — 1 cup skim milk.

1 CUP SHREDDED CHEESE — 1/2 to 1 cup lower-fat cheese like part-skim mozzarella, Countdown*, St. Otho* or Danbo*; *OR* 1/4 cup very sharp cheese; *OR* mix 1/2 cup low-fat cottage cheese with 1/2 cup lower fat or regular cheese for casseroles.

1 CUP WHIPPED CREAM — 1 cup homemade whipped topping. (Made by sprinkling 1/4 cup ice water with 1/4 cup non-fat milk powder. Beat until thick and add 1/4 teaspoon vanilla, 1/2 teaspoon lemon juice and 1/4 to 3/8 cup sugar.) *Note:* Most frozen non-dairy whipped toppings are not a good substitute because they are very high in saturated fats. Try using a low-fat vanilla yogurt as a topping for a change.

1 CUP SALAD DRESSING — 1 cup low calorie salad dressing.

1 CUP MAYONNAISE — 1 cup plain low-fat yogurt; *OR* 3/4 cup plain low-fat yogurt mixed with 1/4 cup or less low calorie mayonnaise; *OR* 1 cup low calorie imitation or "light" mayonnaise.

1 CUP SOUR CREAM — 1 cup plain low fat yogurt (take care not to boil this, or it will curdle); *OR* mix 1 cup "Mock Sour Cream" (Blend 1 cup low fat cottage cheese, 2 tablespoons buttermilk and 1/2 to 1 teaspoon fresh lemon juice in a blender or food processor until smooth. It's a great baked potato topper); *OR* 1 cup yogurt cheese made by straining 2 cups of low fat yogurt overnight in the refrigerator. (Line the strainer with several layers of cheesecloth and set over a bowl to catch the fluid).

1 OUNCE (SQUARE) BAKING CHOCOLATE — 3 tablespoons cocoa powder plus 1 tablespoon oil.

1 OUNCE CREAM CHEESE — 1 ounce Neufchatel cheese; *OR* 1 ounce Philadelphia Light*; *OR* 1 ounce low-fat ricotta cheese.

1 SLICE OF BACON — 2 teaspoons Bacon Bits*; *OR* a small amount of Lean Canadian bacon; *OR* Morningstar Farm Sizzlers*; *OR* Lean ham.

1 POUND GROUND BEEF — 1 pound or less **extra lean ground beef**; *OR* select a lean cut and have it ground for your use. Try lean ground turkey for a change. Use 1/4 pound or less per person and drain the fat after cooking.

1 CUP CRUSHED POTATO CHIPS OR CORN CHIPS — 1 cup rice crispies, cornflakes, or other cereal, crushed if desired.

1 TEASPOON SALT — 1/4 to 1/2 teaspoon regular salt; *OR* leave it out entirely. *Note:* Salt is not high in fat, but the American Heart Association recommends cutting it down to reduce another heart attack risk factor — high blood pressure.

Phase II: New Recipes. Ever decide to take a new route to work or perhaps travel to a new vacation spot? In this phase, people make changes by using some new food and cooking ideas. These changes can sometimes be difficult. Meals begin to look different. These changes include:

- Eat more whole grains, legumes, fruits and vegetables.
- Use less margarine, oil, salad dressing and other high fat condiments.
- Eat fish, shellfish, poultry and lean meats only

once per day, and cut the amount down to about six to eight ounce servings.

- Choose recipes that allow you to use low-fat cheeses, less fat, sugar and salt, and cocoa in place of chocolate.
- Avoid frying foods.

BREAKFAST. Most individuals find that they begin to like breakfasts which include cereal, fruit, toast or muffins, pancakes, French toast or waffles (made without egg yolks). Breakfasts no longer include the traditional bacon or sausage and eggs. Dinners are usually (but not necessarily) the meal when most people choose the one serving of fish, poultry or meat.

LUNCH. Lunch, on the other hand, becomes the challenge. A meatless lunch can include a peanut butter sandwich, a bowl of thick vegetable or other low-fat soup, salads topped with kidney beans or garbanzo beans, lots of fruits, vegetables, cereals and breads, and low-fat cottage cheese and yogurt.

DINNER. New recipe ideas are helpful. Ethnic foods are often centered around foods which have little or no meat. Mexican foods like bean burritos and tostados; Asian foods such as stir-fry dishes; Greek and Mediterranean dishes like tabouli, pita and others will fit in nicely when making recipe changes. New ideas for dishes based on legumes or whole grains are also helpful. Rather than always centering meals around the meat item, people begin to think of a grain or legume dish as the basis for their meals.

SNACKS AND DESSERTS. In this phase, new recipes are also needed for snacks and desserts that are lower in fat, sugar and salt. Snacks can include fruits and vegetables, low fat dips, low fat crackers, cookies and breadsticks, and low-fat chips (usually made at home). Low-fat desserts use the substitute products, with the fat, sugar and salt ingredients cut down. Desserts include sorbet and ice milks, quick breads, and fruit dishes like cobblers and crisps.

Phase III: Meat as a Condiment. This phase approaches the ideal diet. Meat (and poultry, fish and cheese) is de-emphasized and becomes a "condiment," a food used in small quantities to flavor the staples. The staples, or the main food sources, are the complex carbohydrate foods: legumes, grains, and cereals. The goals are as follows:

1. Meals are made up of large portions of legumes, grains, vegetables, fruits and low-fat dairy products.
2. Include only one serving per day of either six ounces of fish, three ounces of shellfish, poultry, or lean meat, or two ounces of regular cheese.

3. Only very small amounts of fats (margarines, oils or regular salad dressings) or sugars are added to foods.
4. For special occasions, the following foods are eaten only **rarely**: large servings of meats, rich desserts, chocolate, salty snacks, and other high-fat, salty foods.

Proportion Change. This phase is simply a change in proportions. Meat, fish, and poultry are still used, but in smaller amounts. The proportion of grains and legumes is increased. Pasta dishes, rice pilafs, bean soups, Chinese stir-fry dishes, Mexican recipes using tortillas, rice and beans, and many other dishes can be used in abundance.

The standard American format of meat, potato and salad can still be eaten, but with some changes in amounts. Lean cuts of beef could be used, but more often fish and poultry would be served. The serving of the meat would be small compared to the large serving of potato, rice, macaroni or other starches.

High fat condiments like sour cream, gravy, margarine or butter would not be spooned onto the potato or rice, but low fat sour cream substitute (made with cottage cheese or yogurt), low fat gravy, low fat sauces or other seasonings could be used for flavorings.

Large servings of vegetables would be served. Bread or muffins would be automatically put on the table, either eaten dry or with only a thin layer of margarine spread on them. The dinner could be rounded off with a low-fat dessert.

ASSESSING YOUR DIETARY HABITS

To help you assess your current dietary habits, refer to the Health Questionnaire in Appendix A (Section 4C, pages 178–179). This questionnaire information will also be helpful to your physician or nutritionist.

MAKING GRADUAL CHANGES USING GOAL SHEETS

To help individuals gradually implement the **Three Phase** diet, 11 easy-to-follow goal sheets have been prepared for your use. These goal sheets have been developed by Martha McMurry, R.D. Refer to **Appendix F**, page 206, and review the 11 goal sheets. After a brief review, consider choosing one or two of the goal sheets and begin experimenting with the gradual dietary changes that are recommended.

SODIUM, CALCIUM, VITAMINS AND MINERALS

Sodium. Although the body's daily **requirement** of sodium is 0.2 to 0.5 grams per day, the average person consumes six to 18 grams (approximately one to two teaspoonfuls) each day. Research has demonstrated that by reducing the amount of sodium in your diet, you may avoid high blood pressure or reduce an already existing condition of high blood pressure.

In the typical diet, approximately **half** of the intake of sodium comes from added salt. Other sodium sources come from the foods we eat, most of which is added to food during home and commercial processing. Some of the foods high in sodium include:

- Canned soups and vegetables;
- Pickles, hot dogs, sausages, bacon, cheese, ham, chips, crackers, and salted nuts;
- "Fast foods" and frozen foods.

Raw vegetables are generally low in natural sodium. Therefore, to be aware of both the "natural sodium" in foods as well as the sodium that is "added" in the food preparation is an important practice. Many different kinds of **sodium compounds** are added to foods. When these compounds are listed on food labels, the presence of added sodium is indicated. Be careful to watch for the words **soda** and **sodium** and the symbol **Na** on labels — these identify products that contain sodium compounds.

Calcium. Calcium is the most plentiful mineral in our bodies. Although 99 percent of calcium is found in our bones and teeth, the remaining one percent circulates in the bloodstream and is vital in the conduction of the nerve impulses, heart function, muscle contraction, blood clotting, and the activation of certain enzymes. Calcium also controls the response of cells to certain neurotransmitters and hormones.

With age, the body's natural system of regulation breaks down — especially in postmenopausal women. The overall absorption of calcium becomes less efficient, and the conversion of bone calcium to circulation calcium accelerates. The result is a condition known as osteoporosis, which is literally a thinning of the bones. (See *High Risk Health Checks #9-11*, page 157.)

There is some debate over the recommended daily allowances (RDA) for calcium. The government's official RDA is:

Adult Men	800 – 1,000 mg/day
Adult Women	800 – 1,000 mg/day

Pregnant or Breast Feeding

• Over age 19	1,200 mg/day
• Under age 19	1,600 mg/day

After Menopause

• Not on estrogen	1,500 mg/day
• On estrogen	1,000 mg/day

Low-fat dairy products are the best source of calcium. Vitamin D is required also to absorb calcium. Fortified dairy products, sunlight, and multi-vitamin supplements are good sources of vitamin D. Exercise, even in moderate amounts, has also proven to be an effective way to maintain bone mass.

Nicotine, caffeine, and an excessive intake of alcohol have a negative effect on bone formation. Prescription drugs such as corticosteriods, tetracycline, heparin, and dilantin can delete bone mass, as can non-prescription drugs such as some laxatives and antacids containing aluminum.

Vitamins and Minerals. Vitamins and minerals are essential for maintaining normal body functions. There are both fat-soluble and water-soluble vitamins.

- The fat-soluble vitamins include vitamins **A, D, E and K**.
- The water-soluble vitamins include vitamins **C** and those of the **B complex**.

To replace a well-balanced diet with vitamin supplements is impossible because all of the nutrients provided naturally have not been discovered. Vitamin and mineral supplements do not supply protein, and certain nutrients (vitamins and minerals) are absorbed by the body better if eaten in their natural foods.

The best way to get your daily requirements of vitamins and minerals is to eat a wide variety of foods. There is no "perfect" food which supplies all the necessary vitamins and minerals.

If you feel you are not eating a balanced diet, then you may consider a once-a-day vitamin. Your local pharmacist or primary-care physician can recommend a good vitamin tablet.

Daily Health Check #5

STRESS MANAGEMENT PROGRAM

THE FAR SIDE   By GARY LARSON

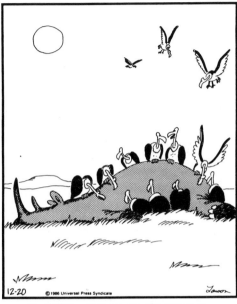

12-20   © 1986 Universal Press Syndicate   Larson

"Just think ... Here we are, the afternoon
sun beating down on us, a dead, bloated
rhino underfoot, and good friends flying
in from all over. ... I tell you, Frank,
this is the best of times."

RECOMMENDATIONS

1. Learn to distinguish appropriately between good and bad stress.

2. Spend **at least** 10 to 20 minutes each day of deep relaxing, deep breathing, or meditating. Consider recording your participation in this activity in your daily log (see Appendix C, page 195).

3. Make time to schedule and plan your day effectively.

4. Do **something for yourself** each day. Consider recording your participation in this activity in your daily log, see Appendix C, page 195.

5. Reduce or eliminate the impact of life's hassles and other self-defeating behavior, and develop personal hardiness.

6. Complete the "**psychological symptoms checklist**," located within your medical questionnaire found in Appendix A, page 181.

Why Perform

In the above cartoon, Gary Larsen captures "stress management" at its finest — a peaceful environment, caring friends, and a little time devoted to "self."

Unfortunately, the "best of times" is often viewed as being too few and too far between, and health-threatening stress results. In fact, the stresses of daily living, if not properly perceived and handled, can injure health and shorten life.

The good news is that individuals **can** learn to blend together the inherent powers of the body and the mind to achieve a peaceful balance in life. **To help you attain this balance, the boxed recommendations must be incorporated into a daily lifestyle.**

How Performed

EUSTRESS VS. DISTRESS

Stress alone doesn't endanger our health. Without stress, we would never feel challenged to tap our best resources. The stress which stimulates our most effective creative action is referred to as "eustress." This stress is mostly health enhancing and can be seen as the source of much personal achievement and satisfaction.

The stress most damaging to our well-being is called "distress." Daily situations can be potentially distressful if we **believe**:

- There are more **problems** than we can handle;
- We are **insufficient** to the task;
- We are the **victims** of extenuating circumstances.

The secret to living with stress seems to be largely dependent on *attitude*. The Greek stoic philosopher, Epictetus, pointed out in the first century A.D.: "**Man is not disturbed by the events of the world, but by the view he takes of them.**" You can manage stress effectively if:

- You are pursuing your own freely chosen goals;
- You have work that is satisfying;
- Your contributions in life result in receiving love and respect from persons around you.

TECHNIQUES FOR MANAGING STRESS

Recognizing that stress cannot and should not be totally avoided, there is virtue in having a variety of stress-management strategies available for different conditions. One of the major keys to becoming an effective stress manager is learning there are substitute ways of managing stressful situations.

Review the possibilities on the following page (Table 1) and check the column that best describes how you respond to a distressing situation. For the items that are checked **seldom or sometimes**, begin to experiment with these suggestions when faced with a stressful situation.

If despite your best coping efforts, you find yourself in a chronic, painful state of distress, consider the use of professional counseling. The need of such help does not mean you are weak, crazy or sick. It means you are only human. There are numerous types of counselors available including psychiatrists, psychologists, social workers and clergy. Often taking the initiative to seek appropriate help is the first courageous step required in pursuit of a more satisfying life. Refer below to *How Am I Doing?* to help you determine whether or not you should seek additional help.

HOW AM I DOING?
"PSYCHOLOGICAL SYMPTOMS CHECKLIST"

Part of the difficulty of managing stress is that people become insensitive to certain physical and emotional states to which they have become accustomed. Without question, various psychological and physical symptoms may signal serious distress.

To help you assess to what degree certain thoughts, emotions and behaviors have troubled you during the past month, Dr. Joan Borysenko has developed a simple **psychological symptoms checklist**. This checklist is contained within your medical questionnaire, found in Appendix A, page 170.

Turn to *Section 4E* of the questionnaire (Appendix A, page 181) and if you have not completed the psychological symptoms checklist, please do so at this time.

Dr. Borysenko has suggested that all of us encounter the symptoms listed in the psychological checklist **part of the time**. But, if you have checked **many** of the *often* or *frequent* columns (three or four), Dr. Borysenko suggests you consider "discussing your feelings with a psychotherapist (psychologist, psychiatrist, or social worker specifically trained in psychological counseling)." We also suggest you visit with your primary-care physician if you find many of your responses are found within the *often* or *frequent* columns (three or four).

As you develop new stress management skills, review the checklist again, looking for positive changes.

PSYCHOLOGICAL HARDINESS

Many people have the capacity to endure potentially stressful changes and yet remain healthy. The ability to cope with stressful events effectively and maintain health has been termed "psychological hardiness" and has been the major focus of exciting new research in behavioral medicine.

Since 1975 Drs. Salvatore R. Maddi and Suzanne C. Kobassa, both psychologists, have been conducting studies designed to isolate the components of psychological hardiness. The researchers point out that while many stressful life events are associated with illness and even death, the events themselves do not cause illness or death. Their view is that people are **not** the passive victims of life events. Instead, people are creative and use life events to generate stress and emotional strain **or** to generate personal growth and add meaning to life.

Their research supports the theory that the people who endure stress without damage to their health tend to score highly on the following personality traits they call the "three C's:" **Control, Commitment, and Challenge**.

Review the list in Table 2 and check whether or not you are practicing the specified hardiness techniques.

Table 1: Techniques for Managing Stress	Seldom	Sometimes	Often
1. **Change** the situation when possible. Prompt, effective action is a great stress reducer.			
2. **Examine** your assumptions about the situation. Is the circumstance really worth being upset about?			
3. **Accept** what you cannot change. All of our lives are influenced by events over which we have no control.			
4. **Remove** yourself from the stressful situation by: a) Choosing to involve yourself in a relaxing or pleasantly distracting pastime—daily doing **"something for yourself."** Record your participation in this activity in your daily log (see **Appendix C**, page 195).			
b) Try a change of scene. A vacation or even a one-day outing to someplace pleasant can be rejuvenating.			
c) Use some form of meditation technique to induce relaxation (**10 to 20 minutes each day**). To learn more about the "Relaxation Response," see page 67.			
5. **Dig-in** with full vigor and attack a job that needs to be done. Much distress is self-generated through procrastination.			
6. **Create** a peaceful environment for yourself. Have a quiet, private place for a retreat from the distractions and annoyances of daily living.			
7. **Anticipate** and prepare for new changes. Begin to regulate and execute personal influence on the rate of change in your life. Consider postponing new major decisions or changes if possible until you can regain your balance.			
8. **Simplify** your life if necessary. Consider making a decision to let go of some demands that may be complicating your life. The surest path to burn-out is to continue to insist on being **all things** to **all people** all of the time. Continue to invest in those activities that are most closely aligned with your highest goals and values. Be willing to delegate or defer to others whenever possible and appropriate.			
9. **Practice** living in the **present**. Learn to savor the unique experience each new moment of living can offer. Quite frequently distress is perpetuated by polluting the present with disturbing ruminations regarding **past or future** concerns. Life is full of simple pleasures that are often overlooked. Strive to see and appreciate the beauty and meaning in each moment of living. By doing so, you can displace stress-producing feelings of worry, guilt and fear.			
10. **Build a social support system**. Nurture the relationships you value by being accepting of others and giving service where you can. Distress is bred in social isolation and from the ensuing sense of alienation from others. For optimal health and personal growth, we all need to be heard, valued and understood — we need each other. This is not a neurotic dependence, but a healthy interdependence.			
11. **Meet** your basic self-care needs when in the midst of high level change and major life transition. Paradoxically, during some of the most stressful times, when it is most critical that we take steps to guard our health, we often unwittingly disregard our self-care needs. Make a concerted and systematic effort to schedule adequate time for rest, relaxation, recreation and physical activity.			

Table 2: *Developing Psychological Hardiness*

	Yes	No
Control. The psychologically hardy have a sense of personal control over the environment.		
1. Are you more inclined to see a full range of options in a given situation rather than focusing on what you can't do?		
2. Do you recognize that you **can't** control everything?		
3. Do you actively focus on what you really can control?		
4. Do you perceive yourself as having personal power?		
5. Do you avoid the feeling of being controlled by other people and circumstances?		
Commitment. Healthy or hardy subjects also rate high on "commitment."		
1. Are you inclined to engage life actively rather than passively let life happen to you?		
2. Are you an active participant in your work, family, and community life?		
3. Do you view your personal activities (such as work, family, and community) as meaningful, purposeful and interesting?		
4. Can you identify and articulate your personal values, goals, and priorities?		
Challenge. This is the attitude that change, even if it is demanding and inconvenient, is the springboard to opportunity.		
1. Do you feel threatened by change and feel a need to cling to the status quo?		
2. Are you willing to take calculated risks when you see the chance for some new success?		
3. Do you attempt to transform events into a personal advantage? For example, a psychologically hardy individual would see the loss of his job as a "challenge" for new experience and an inconvenience that falls within the range of accepted risk. Another person, and one more likely to encounter health problems, might view the loss of a job as a catastrophe and proof of personal inadequacy and low self-worth.		

Remember, our first line of personal defense in dealing with stress lies in our capacity for managing our psychological environment. Accepting full responsibility for our own beliefs, attitudes, values and expectations appears to be the essential ingredient for effective coping.

CORONARY PRONE PERSONALITY

During the past several years investigators such as Drs. C. David Jenkins, Ray Rosenman, Meyer Friedman, and Robert Eliot have explored the association of coronary heart disease and personality traits.[376] These scientists have coined several terms such as "Type A" and "Hot Reactor" to identify individuals who may be "coronary prone" because of their behavioral responses. Although there still remains a fair amount of controversy regarding this topic, the coronary prone personality is typically marked by a compelling sense of time urgency, agressiveness, competitiveness, and chronic hostility or anger.

The behavioral responses described above may actually be fostered by our culture—we are often in a hurry, striving to achieve more success and accumulate more material goods. The positive point is that these personality types are most likely made, not born, and individuals can change their behavior.

(NOTE: Your Health Check Table recommends you remain alert for tendencies that suggest depression, suicide or abnormal bereavement. The information on the following page will assist you to recognize the risk factors for these potential disorders.)

RISK FACTORS FOR DEPRESSION AND SUICIDE

Depression. Depression is a very common problem in medicine. For example, depression occurs in approximately 30 percent of the clients seen by their doctor,[23-30] and one out of three people will suffer from depression.[26]

- Individuals who appear to be at greater risk for depression include:[23]

    a. persons who are young;
    b. persons who are single;
    c. females;
    d. persons who are divorced;
    e. persons who are separated;
    f. persons who are seriously ill;
    g. individuals with a family history of serious depression;
    h. individuals who have recently lost loved ones;
    i. individuals involved with alcohol and drug abuse.

To help you identify whether or not depression may be present in your life, please refer to page 64 of this *Health Check, "How Am I Doing?"* In addition, if you or your loved one is experiencing depression, consider discussing your feelings with your primary-care physician, or a psychotherapist (psychologist, psychiatrist, or social worker specifically trained in psychological counseling).

Suicide. An additional health concern is suicide, ranking third as the leading cause of death among young people. Depression and suicide are often associated. Estimates suggest that of the 50,000 to 70,000 suicides that result each year, 30 to 70 percent of these individuals had previously experienced "major depression."[23, 27, 32]

- Individuals who experience the following conditions are at greater risk for suicide:[31]

    a. psychiatric illness such as schizophrenia;
    b. drug abuse;
    c. divorce or separation;
    d. unemployment;
    e. serious medical illnesses;
    f. living alone;
    g. recent bereavement.

If you, or a loved one, demonstrate serious suicidal intent such as "obtaining a weapon, making a plan, putting affairs in order, giving away prized possessions, or preparing a suicide note"[31] make certain that appropriate counseling is sought. Estimates suggest that as high as one-half the people that commit suicide are intoxicated from alcohol or other drugs.[31, 33, 37] By taking an active role in preventing alcohol and other drug abuse, and by encouraging psychiatric counseling for individuals at risk, you will reduce or prevent the likelihood of suicide.[31, 34-36]

An alternative solution to suicide *always* exists, and individuals who are experiencing suicidal intent must have this true concept of hope reinforced to them.

ABNORMAL BEREAVEMENT

Of the millions who experience the loss of a loved one each year, a large number experience "abnormal bereavement" disorders and prolonged depression.[38-40] If you or a member of your family have recently experienced the death of a close friend or loved one, consider these questions:

1. Do the following risk factors for abnormal bereavement exist?[38, 40]
    - No social support;
    - Living alone;
    - Pre-existing psychiatric or mental health problems;
    - A history of alcohol or drug abuse.
2. Have you sought support from your family, your ecclesiastical leaders, and your primary-care physician? (Physicians should be alert for signs of abnormal bereavement.[38])
3. Have you considered enrolling in a community- or hospital-sponsored class on how to cope with the death of a loved one?

Health Notes

THE RELAXATION RESPONSE

The method outlined below is an adaptation of the technique recommended by Herbert Benson, M.D., in his book *The Relaxation Response.*[41] This method can be learned by virtually anyone. If practiced daily for 10 to 20 minutes, the relaxation response can become a very effective and convenient way of compensating for the stress of everyday living.

For best results follow the steps outlined and practice them daily for four weeks. After that time, it is almost inevitable that you will have become skillful and will be able to put yourself in a state of relaxation at will.

1) Find a place that is quiet, private and as comfortable as possible. Practice during the day is best done sitting or semi-reclining. People who practice lying down often fall asleep and

(continued next page)

lose conscious control. Unless you are using the technique to help yourself go to sleep at night, it is more effective to maintain a wakeful state while practicing.

2) Make yourself physically comfortable and reduce distractions. Close your eyes.

3) Make a mental survey of your muscles starting with your feet and working up to the head. Be sensitive to any muscles that feel tight; consciously command them to relax. Give special attention to the muscles of the face. Consciously let go of any muscle tension around the jaw, mouth, eyes, and forehead. Successfully relaxing facial muscles facilitates the relaxation of other major muscle groups. Your initial conscious efforts at putting yourself in a state of muscular relaxation should take two to three minutes.

4) Breathe through the nose allowing your stomach to rise with each inhalation and fall with each exhalation. Continue this relaxed, rhythmical, diaphragm breathing throughout your relaxation session.

5) With each **exhalation**, consciously repeat in your mind the word "one" (or any other word or sound of your choice such as "peace" or "relax"). This device is designed to occupy your mind and displace stressful thoughts.

6) Do not strive to succeed at relaxation—just let it happen. Distracting thoughts will tend to drift back into your mind. Simply take note of them and deliberately return to the persistent repetition of your word. With continued practice, you will be able to keep your mind clear of distracting and stressful thoughts for more extended periods of time.

7) Continue for 10 to 20 minutes each session. Do not use an alarm that would startle you or detract from the relaxed state you have achieved. When you finish, open your eyes and sit quietly for a minute or two before standing up.

If you follow the above guidelines, you will feel relaxed and refreshed. As a result of developing this relaxation skill, you can have a convenient method of regaining a state of tranquility even in the face of life's inevitable uncertainties.

Daily Health Check #6
WEIGHT CONTROL PROGRAM

RECOMMENDATIONS

Achieve and maintain an optimum body weight by:

1. Avoiding restrictive intake diets;*

2. Changing the **type** of food eaten (rather than the amount) to increase amounts of complex carbohydrates and to decrease fats and sugars (see also, *Daily Health Check #4, Proper Nutrition Program*, page 58);

3. Maintaining a regular physical activity program emphasizing aerobic type exercise. See *Daily Health Check #1, Physical Activity Program*, page 40;

4. Recording your body weight in the daily log (see Appendix C, page 195).

Why Perform

- In adults, excessive weight increases the risk of heart disease, hypertension, blood fat disorders, diabetes, arthritis, and some forms of cancer (colon, rectum, prostate, gallbladder, biliary tract, breast, cervix, endometrium, and ovary).[42-44]
- Overweight individuals may decrease their length of life.
- Obesity, present in approximately 11 million Americans, remains the most significant and widespread nutritional disease in the United States. [18, 19, 42]
- Rapid weight loss may be indicative of disorders such as diabetes, metabolic diseases, or other underlying health problems.

NOTE: For some individuals, excessive obesity poses a potentially serious medical condition. For these high-risk individuals, a prudent recommendation may include their participation in a very-low calorie, medically supervised diet. When carefully monitored by medical and professional staff (such as nutritionist, behavioralists, exercise physiologists), the very-low calorie diet can be an effective means of assisting the high-risk obese patient.

How Performed

THE FAT THERMOSTAT

"Dieting is not effective in controlling weight; it has never worked, and it never will. Admittedly, you can get temporary weight loss with a diet, but each scheme ultimately gives way to weight gain, and subsequent losses become increasingly difficult. You become hungry and more obsessed with food, frequently eating out of control. You get tired and weak, have poor endurance, and generally feel awful about yourself; worst of all you get progressively fatter on less and less food."[45]

This opening statement from a popular weight-loss book summarizes the problems associated with trying to lose weight using the traditional "low calorie" approach to weight control. Although it seems reasonable to suggest that overeating is the major cause of obesity and that restricting the intake of food is therefore the proper treatment, recent research shows little relationship between how much people eat and how fat they are.

The reason low calorie diets don't work may relate to a probable control mechanism in the brain called the "weight regulating mechanism" (WRM) that regulates the amount of fat a person has. This regulator (WRM) probably works much like the thermostat in the house. If the temperature of the house cools below the thermostat setting (setpoint) the furnace is started to maintain the proper temperature.

Research studies exploring the WRM may help us understand how many adults consume more than a million calories a year (equivalent to more than one-half ton of food), and still maintain a stable body weight. Factors which influence, or are influenced by, the WRM are described in Figure 1 (see next page).

According to the "set-point theory," the **body weight** set by the WRM:

- Is influenced by the factors above the dotted line (see Figure 1), such as lack of activity, sugars in the diet, and certain drugs;
- Is maintained by the factors below the line, such as metabolism (energy conservation or wasting) and appetite.

Evidence for the existence of the WRM is compelling. The well-documented tendency for dieters to return to pre-dieting weight strongly suggests that the body strives to retain the weight to which it has become accustomed.

The same pattern has been seen in research studies in which volunteers have undergone either starvation or overfeeding to alter body weight. In both cases, attempts at body weight changes were resisted, and the subjects quickly returned to their initial weight.

One animal study compared the effects of feeding rat chow vs. a typical American diet to two groups of rats. Even when both groups of rats ate the **same number of calories**, the group eating the fatter/sweeter American diet got nearly twice as fat. Apparently, continually eating fats and sweets raises the set-point. Once the set-point is raised, the body stimulates hunger and conserves energy until the new set-point weight is reached.

Since the body's natural tendency is to resist any rapid, substantial change in weight, the important question becomes:

How can the WRM setting be modified so that healthful weight losses can be achieved and maintained?

In the remainder of this section, we will present ideas to help you reprogram the set-point to a lower level. This information is designed to complement the material found in the *Daily Health Check #1, Physical Activity Program* (page 40), *Daily Health Check #4, Proper Nutrition Program* (page 58), and the *11 Nutrition Goal Sheets* (Appendix F, page 206).

CHANGE THE TYPE OF FOOD YOU EAT

The major changes you need to make in your diet are as follows:

- **decreasing fat consumption;**
- **decreasing refined carbohydrates;**
- **increasing complex carbohydrates;**
- **decreasing calorie-containing fluids;**
- **drinking adequate amounts of water.**

The first three guidelines are meal related, and following them will lower your set-point and improve the quality of your diet. The other two guidelines relate to drinking habits. Most overweight people drink too many high-caloric or sweetened drinks and too little water. We will discuss both of these areas in terms of changing the type of food you eat.

We will also discuss the problem of being out of harmony with the eating drives from the weight regulating mechanism and tell you how to help increase the sensitivity to these drives.

Guideline #1: Decreasing Fat Consumption. The average American consumes about 40 percent of his calories in the form of fat. Most nutritionists agree that this level of fat is too high and should be reduced because of the health risks involved.

Figure 1: *Functioning of the Weight Regulating Mechanism (WRM)*

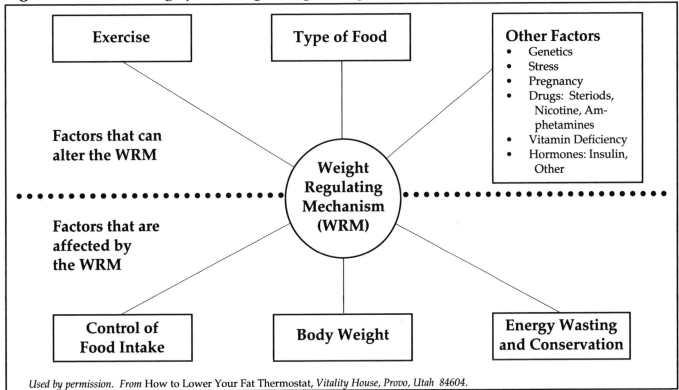

Used by permission. From How to Lower Your Fat Thermostat, *Vitality House, Provo, Utah 84604.*

Because we believe that all dietary suggestions must be practical and livable as well as healthful, we suggest that you reduce your fat intake toward the 20 percent mark. This will cut the fat content of your diet in half but leave the food satisfying and palatable. Besides lowering the set-point so that your weight can normalize more easily, this change will also decrease the caloric density of the food you eat. This means that the same volume of food will contain significantly fewer calories.

To be successful in lowering the fat intake, we suggest you refer to *Daily Health Check #4, Proper Nutrition Program* (page 58), paying particular attention to the *three phase* nutrition approach and the *11 goal sheets* found in Appendix F, page 206.

Guideline #2: Reducing Refined Carbohydrates. Most people have acquired a taste for sugar and white flour. Manufacturers of prepared foods take advantage of this taste by using large quantities of sugar in their products. For instance, most breakfast cereals have sugar as either the first or second major ingredient.

White flour is also a problem since it is used so extensively in foods. Even many whole-wheat breads contain large quantities of white flour. Sometimes the white flour is given a fancy term such as enriched white flour or fortified flour, but it is still a refined carbohydrate and is likely to affect your ability to lose weight.

To accomplish the goal of decreasing the amount of sugar in your diet successfully, we suggest you refer to *Daily Health Check #4, Proper Nutrition Program* (page 58), paying particular attention to the *three phase* nutrition approach. In addition, refer to the *11 goal sheets* found in Appendix F, page 206.

Guideline #3: Increasing Complex Carbohydrates. Many health experts suggest that the majority of our diet should come in the form of complex carbohydrates (60 to 80 percent of our calories). Complex carbohydrates are found in whole grains, vegetables, and fruits, such as whole-grain cereals, brown rice, potatoes, squash, carrots, tomatoes, and apples. These foods should be eaten as they are grown, without processing them to some other form. They are actually composed of sugars that are linked together in such a way that the breakdown process takes much longer than with simple or refined sugars.

Complex carbohydrates do not stimulate the large rise in insulin levels with its attendant rapid fall of blood sugar so typical of refined sugar ingestion.

As suggested for guidelines #1 and #2 above, gradually increase the intake of complex carbohydrates in your diet by following the *Daily Health Check #4, Proper Nutrition Program* (page 58), paying particular attention to the *three phase* nutrition approach. Refer also to the *11 goal sheets* located in Appendix F, page 206.

Guideline #4: Decrease Calorie-Containing Fluids . People commonly take in more calories than their bodies can successfully waste by drinking high calorie fluids. Some people also interpret thirst as hunger and eat when thirsty.

Drinking calorie-containing fluids contributes to obesity in several ways:

- Sugars (or sweeteners) are absorbed quickly and cause a rapid rise in insulin;
- Caffeine drinks (even those without calories) stimulate insulin production;
- Liquids require no chewing and are quickly consumed, leaving the stomach so rapidly that they provide little lasting satiety;
- More calories are ingested than the body can waste, causing excess fat production.

Decreasing the intake of sweet liquids such as soda pop (even if sweetened with artificial sweeteners) is critical. When thirsty, you should drink water; if this fails to satisfy you, eat an appropriate snack.

Guideline #5: Drink Adequate Amounts of Water. Many obese people have become insensitive to their thirst drives and eat when their real need is for water.

To overcome this basic contributor to obesity, you should learn to drink adequate amounts of water (six to eight glasses per day). If uncertain whether a drive represents thirst or hunger, drink a glass of water. If not satisfied with water, you are probably experiencing a hunger drive and should eat some food which requires chewing and will not be digested too quickly. Drinking water may take a while to get used to — be persistent.

You may wish to drink several glasses of water with each meal. This will help distend the stomach and signal satiety. Some people think that drinking water with meals dilutes the digestive juices and is therefore bad for digestion. Unless you have had part of the stomach removed because of ulcers or cancer, or a hiatus hernia, there is no reason to restrict water in any way.

For some people, drinking cold water produces nausea or stomach pain. If this is a problem, try drinking warmer water. Some people have trouble drinking water because they don't like the taste and get more enjoyment out of pop, milk, or juice. In these cases, you may wish to use:

- Bottled water;
- A purification system;
- Ice-chips;
- A few drops of lemon or lime juice.

Guideline #6: Getting in Harmony with the Weight Regulating Mechanism . Being in harmony with your eating drives should become a major factor in your eating behavior.

Chronic dieters are perhaps the best example of people who are out of touch with their weight regulating mechanism. They feel that their weight problem is entirely associated with overeating; that the less they can eat, the better they will lose weight.

With this attitude, they feel that hunger is a sign that they are being "good," that they are succeeding and working toward their goal. This "dieter's mentality" places them in a no-win situation. If they don't eat, they may feel good psychologically, but they will feel weak and miserably physically. If they do eat, they feel guilty, angry at themselves, and in despair that they will never succeed.

When the drives to eat get strong enough, the resolve they once felt breaks down, often resulting in "binge" eating of large quantities of food very quickly, and the food choices are often the very foods the dieter wishes to avoid. Completely out of control, the dieter feels extreme remorse and guilt. The self-image falls further, and the dieter feels the need to diet again.

Practice the following tips:

- "Listen" to your body and pay attention to the feelings it gives you relating to food. Eat when hungry and stop when you receive messages of satisfaction;
- Eat regularly; **at least three times a day**;
- One of your three meals should be a "**full meal**" in which enough food is eaten to produce complete satiety.

Guideline #7: Maintaining A Regular Exercise Program. Exercise is a critical part of the total weight control process. Almost **no one** can successfully maintain proper weight for a lifetime if he fails to participate in regular physical activity.

Discussed below are a number of compelling reasons to exercise for weight loss:

Lowering the Setpoint. Exercise can readjust the setpoint of the weight regulating mechanism.

Increasing Metabolic Rate. Exercise causes the metabolic furnace to burn at a higher level. Even moderate exercise increases the metabolic rate three to eight times. There is even a residual effect from a bout of exercise that keeps the metabolic rate high for several hours after exercise. All of these factors play a role in the basic metabolic activity of the body and make the exerciser a high-calorie consumer whose body is ready and able to "waste" excess energy at any time.

Maintaining Lean Body Mass. Dieting *without* exercise has one serious drawback: you may lose as much lean muscle tissue as you do fat. Of course, this looks good on the scales because the total weight is coming off, but any muscle loss decreases the body's ability to burn fat. Recognize that when exercise is an integral part of your weight loss program, you may not lose weight rapidly early on (muscle mass may actually be increasing). Eventually, however, the weight will decrease and in addition, you will be burning more calories and enjoying all the other positive changes associated with exercise.

Increasing Fat-burning Enzymes. Both fats and carbohydrates are "burned" in the muscles for energy. Fat-burning enzyme levels in endurance athletes are much higher than in untrained persons, and research shows that endurance activity will change those levels so that training causes fat to be burned more effectively.

Changing the Body's Chemistry. Insulin is a hormone that is essential for getting sugar into the cell so it can be burned for energy. However, excess insulin can actually cause increased fat storage. Most obese people have excessive insulin because their cells seem to be resistant to it and the body produces more to overcome this resistance. One of the positive effects of exercise is that it increases the responsiveness of cells to insulin.

Feeling Good. One of the most important aspects of an exercise program is the way it makes you feel. The more you do, the more you will want to do, and this positive cycle will continue as you lose weight and become more fit.

HOW TO EXERCISE FOR WEIGHT CONTROL

The exercise guidelines for weight control are carefully reviewed in *Daily Health Check #1, Physical Activity Program,* page 40. We would encourage you to turn to this section and review the exercise steps.

EVALUATING PROGRESS

The most often asked question about weight control is "How much should I weigh when I have completed my weight loss program?" Another related question is "How will I know when I have reached my ideal weight?"

Because of the basic differences in body build, we suggest you evaluate the amount of fat on the body rather than simply look at body weight. To assist men and women in determining their current body fat percentage and calculating ideal weight, we have included in Appendix G, methods for body fat and ideal weight determination. Please turn to Appendix G, page 215, at this time to learn how to make these calculations.

Daily Health Checks #7 – 11

These *Daily Health Checks* are incorporated into *Lifestyle Counseling* and *Yearly/Periodic Health Checks* sections. Please turn to the page indicated to learn more about these categories.

Monthly Health Checks #1 – 4

These *Monthly Health Checks* are incorporated into *Yearly and Periodic Health Checks* sections. Please turn to the page indicated to learn more about these categories.

Yearly or Periodic Health Checks #1 & #23

PHYSICAL EXAMINATION,
HEALTH HISTORY (INITIAL/INTERIM),
AND HEIGHT AND WEIGHT MEASUREMENT

RECOMMENDATIONS

1. Men and women should have a basic physical examination and health history based on the following schedule:[46]

   a) Ages 19 through 29: every 5 years
   b) Ages 30 through 39: every 4 years
   c) Ages 40 through 49: every 3 years
   d) Ages 50 through 59: every 2 years
   f) Ages 60 and older: every year

2. Use the space provided in your *Health Check Table* to record dates of your physical examinations as well as dates and information (such as blood pressure readings) of health checks performed in conjunction with the physical exam.

3. As part of your physical examination, your height and weight should be measured. In addition, men and women should measure their height and weight at least every two years between ages 19 to 40 and yearly after age 40.

Why Perform

- Represents the foundation of your health maintenance.
- Provides a basis for your physician to understand you as a patient and to help you successfully manage your health needs.
- Facilitates early detection of disease and identification of risk factors.
- Establishes and enhances on-going communication with your doctor. Allows your physician and staff to provide *lifestyle counseling* — a review of current lifestyle habits — and education directed toward health promotion.

Consider the 42-year-old attorney, married and father of three children who had gradually **lost control** of his health. He decided the time had come to make a lifestyle change, and so he scheduled a physical examination.

We found his blood pressure elevated; he had been experiencing recurring headaches and his cholesterol was 257 mg percent. In addition, he was 40 pounds overweight and had a very low fitness level.

He found it very difficult to ever say "no" to the requests of others, and he described his life as "rush, rush, rush." For over two years he had not been on a vacation with his wife or the children. Headaches were more frequent, and he was taking Extra-strength Tylenol® almost daily.

Combining the efforts of the physician and health counselors, lifestyle recommendations were made, and he was encouraged to follow the health maintenance manual.

The results? He exercised regularly, lost weight, improved his nutritional habits, and made priority changes with his wife, family and business. He also found the headaches beginning to lessen. One of the keys to his success was his willingness to form a partnership with his doctor and health counselors in making lifestyle changes.

How Performed

FIVE IMPORTANT STEPS

Follow the five steps below in scheduling your next physical examination.

STEP 1: Review the *Health Check Table* appropriate for your age (*Health Check Tables* begin on page 9), and complete the *Health Questionnaire* (see Appendix A, page 170). Take time in completing this questionnaire, and be as accurate as possible. The questionnaire will be an invaluable component of your maintenance manual, and only a small amount of time will be required to keep the record current.

STEP 2: Record the name of your primary-care physician on the *Health Questionnaire*. If you do not have a doctor, refer to page 142 and review the tips on choosing a primary-care physician; then *select a doctor.*

STEP 3: If you have *not* had a physical examination within the recommended frequency for your age, call and schedule your appointment now!

STEP 4: Take this book with you to the doctor's appointment and review with the doctor your *Health Check Table* and the *Health Questionnaire.* (You may want to photocopy your medical questionnaire to give to your doctor.)

STEP 5: With your *Health Questionnaire* in hand, discuss with your doctor the *High-Risk Health Checks* located in *Section E* of your *Health Check Table.* This process will assist you and your doctor in determining whether additional health checks need to be performed.

INITIAL AND INTERIM HEALTH HISTORY

Initial Health History. The first visit to your doctor should include a physician-patient exchange referred to by physicians as the "health history." Physicians are trained to **listen and observe**, and so hopefully, your doctor will sit-down, unrushed, and "get to know you."

As the basis of the initial visit, your doctor should review with you your *Health Check Table* and your completed *Health Questionnaire.* This material will naturally lead to discussion regarding:

- Personal lifestyle habits;
- General health status (past and present);
- Social environment as pertaining to family, friends, and co-workers;
- Risk factors for heart disease and other illnesses.

To help in the health history process, actively communicate with your physician. Be frank, honest, and open, and feel free to express to your physician your desire to follow your *Health Check Table.*

Interim History. A vitally important component of your on-going health care is the interim history, conducted whenever you visit your doctor after the first visit. The interim history focuses on health-related problems or family illnesses that may have developed since your last physical examination.[46] Be certain you mention these health concerns to your doctor at the time of the interim visit.

HEALTH QUESTIONNAIRE

The health questionnaire allows the physician to learn a great deal about you in a short period of time, and invites further discussion regarding your health. As previously indicated, your health questionnaire is located in **Appendix A**. The questionnaire contains the following sections:

1. General Information
2. Medical History
3. Review of Body Systems
4. Lifestyle History
5. Genetic History

Recognize that although your health questionnaire is lengthy, once completed, the questionnaire will require *little effort* to keep current. **The questionnaire will serve as a basis for your maintenance manual for the remainder of your life.**

Note: If your doctor has mailed you his/her office questionnaire, we would advise you to complete this questionnaire as well.

PHYSICAL EXAMINATION

Concerns. The thought of having a physical examination can generate anxiety or embarrassment; these emotions are normal. Hopefully your physician will be sensitive to your feelings and help alleviate your concerns by performing the physical examination in a very professional manner, respecting your modesty.

Be aware, however, that to perform your physical adequately, your doctor must be very thorough, examining the genital and anal areas and the breasts as carefully as the rest of your body.

The Exam. You will be asked to remove all your clothing, and put on a patient gown. Your physician will then perform the physical exam by carefully inspecting your entire body. The examination will include health checks listed as part of the physical exam in your *Health Check Table*.

To encourage your participation as an active partner in maintaining your health, your doctor should visit with you freely during the exam, discussing what is being done and what the findings are.

In conjunction with your physical, make certain you:

- **Review** with your physician all laboratory tests that are recommended for your age (such as a blood cholesterol screen);
- **Record** the health checks performed (and the results when indicated) in your Health Check Table;
- **Determine** with your doctor whether "High-Risk" health checks need to be performed.

In some instances (because of your personal or family health history), your physician may recommend that a specialist perform certain high-risk health checks such as a colonoscopy.

The Results. Your doctor will generally do one of the following as a follow-up to your physical examination:

- Discuss your exam results the day of your physical and call or write you later with the findings of the laboratory tests;
- Schedule a follow-up visit to review results and make additional lifestyle recommendations;
- Have you visit with a lifestyle counselor (such as a dietician or exercise physiologist) for additional lifestyle counseling.

HEIGHT AND WEIGHT

Height and weight are easily determined, and provide important information in tracking changes in body composition as well as in identifying potential medical problems related to sudden weight loss or significant decreases in height, such as diabetes and osteoporosis. Because obesity remains a major health concern, a periodic assessment of weight can often provide incentive for an individual to initiate healthy lifestyle changes such as a physical

activity program or improved nutritional habits if the weight is gradually increasing.

Height and weight are easily measured in the doctor's office. When your height is measured, you should remove your shoes. Make certain that you stand as tall as possible by stretching your entire body. Ideally, weight should be measured with the patient wearing only a patient gown. If this situation is not practical, the weight should be measured without the shoes and with empty pockets. Most individuals can periodically measure their weight without clothing in the privacy of their home.

Penalty For Neglect

Daily we meet patients who boast that they have not been inside a doctor's office in 15 years — or more! Too often these people find that their chronic illness has become clinically apparent — signs or symptoms have developed — and the illness may be far advanced. Repeatedly we recognize that a simple office visit combined with recommended lifestyle changes could have made all the difference for them a decade earlier.

People generally use the following excuses for not participating in a periodic health examination:

- **Fear.** One patient told us, "I saw my father die of cancer, and if I have it, I don't want to know about it." Unfortunately, the real scenario is, "What you don't know **can** hurt you;"
- **Indifference.** These individuals consider health to be a matter of "luck," hoping fate will deal in their favor;
- **False Confidence.** These people consider their body as indestructible. Their motto is, "It will never happen to me;"
- **Too busy.** Only a brush with disability or death gets the attention of these people;
- **Cost.** Although the average expense to maintain the private automobile generally exceeds the cost of preventive health screening, maintaining the body goes unchecked.

The very fact that you are reading this book is evidence of your interest in following the health maintenance manual. Avoid letting the above excuses get in the way of your positive momentum. *Take charge*, and follow the five steps outlined on page 77.

Yearly or Periodic Health Check #2
and
High-Risk Health Checks #5 and #6

CARDIAC RISK FACTOR SCREENING AND GUIDELINES FOR RESTING AND EXERCISE ELECTROCARDIOGRAM TESTS

RECOMMENDATIONS

1. All individuals should be screened for cardiac risk factors and receive lifestyle counseling regarding risk factor prevention.[47,48] This screening should be performed at least every **one to three years**.

2. All individuals should become familiar with **risk factors** associated with coronary heart disease. Both your doctor and your health questionnaire can help you identify personal risk factors. Risk factors are listed on page 80.

3. Screening for early detection of coronary heart disease by performing resting and exercise electrocardiogram (ECG) tests is **not recommended**, but may be appropriate to perform in defined groups.[47-50, 390, 391] Discuss the guidelines for performing ECG tests (*outlined in Table 1, page 82*) with your doctor.

Why Perform

- Coronary artery disease is the leading cause of death and disability in the U.S.
- Approximately 1.5 million Americans experience a heart attack each year and 520,000 die from coronary heart disease.[51, 52]
- For many, the first heart attack occurs without any previous sign or symptoms.
- Almost half of the individuals who experience their first heart attack die (either suddenly or within a few days of the event).
- Coronary heart disease can be prevented and controlled. Many cardiac risk factors can be modified or eliminated.
- Estimated U.S. cost — $80 billion per year.[52]

Bill's Story. October 17, Bill left for work just as he had for the past 36 years. After lunch, Bill began to feel pressure in the center of his chest. (He later described the pressure as "someone standing on his chest.") He waited for an hour, thinking the discomfort was indigestion. He had had similar discomfort, although not as severe, on two other occasions within the week but the pressure had left with time.

This time, however, the pressure continued. Bill called his wife, and she took him to the Emergency Room of our hospital. The E.R. doctor recommended a coronary angiogram (a procedure used to view the vessels of the heart). The angiogram (performed within a few hours) showed four areas of Bill's coronary arteries were severely blocked, and within an hour of the angiogram, he was undergoing open-heart bypass surgery.

Within three days of the surgery, Bill began a cardiac rehabilitation program by walking our hospital halls and attending classes with his wife on how to modify coronary risk factors. Bill began to listen. During the past 36 years he had slowly reduced his level of physical activity, had given little attention to diet, and had gradually gained over 50 pounds of weight.

Following hospital discharge, Bill continued the rehab program by visiting our hospital three days a week for supervised exercise and additional instruction on nutrition and stress management, and by exercising at home. The results? Here are Bill's words:

"I can't say enough about how good I now feel. I've lost 62 pounds, and I'm walking almost daily (four to five times per week) for a total of about 70 minutes. My whole life has changed, both physically and mentally. I'm also eating the right kinds of food.

"I've discovered that for 36 years I was telling myself I had the world by the tail, but I now realize I wasn't taking care of myself, and my neglect finally caught up with me. I'm not sure how much longer I'll live, but that is no longer my concern. My goal has been to focus on quality of life, not quantity. While enjoying the quality of life, I'll take whatever quantity there is."

Bill's story, multiplied literally thousands of times around the country, illustrates the importance of identifying, and where possible, eliminating heart disease risk factors.

How Performed

FIRST, WHAT IS HEART DISEASE?

The underlying cause of coronary heart disease (**CHD**) is atherosclerosis, a disease of the inner lining of the heart's arteries due to the accumulation of fatty substances such as cholesterol. This buildup can eventually restrict or block the flow of blood to the heart muscle.

CHD is the result of a number of lifestyle and environmental factors superimposed on a genetic tendency. Even though genetic tendencies for coronary artery disease (early heart disease in a parent or sibling) may exist in an individual, the control of environmental and lifestyle influences can significantly slow, halt or even reverse coronary heart disease.

SCREENING FOR CORONARY HEART DISEASE RISK FACTORS

The following CHD risk factors should be screened by your doctor during the periodic health examination or during an office visit for an illness or a scheduled lifestyle counseling session (at least every one to three years):[48,50,373]

A. History of high blood pressure (above 160 mm Hg for the systolic pressure or above 90 mm Hg for the diastolic pressure);
B. Blood cholesterol over 240 mg/dl, LDL-cholesterol over 160 mg/dl or HDL-cholesterol less than 30 mg/dl;
C. Cigarette smoking;
D. Physically inactive;
E. Obesity;
F. Diabetes mellitus;
G. Family history of coronary artery disease (occurring under the age of 55);
H. Abnormal resting ECG, including evidence of an old heart attack, or other abnormalities.

Your health questionnaire found in Appendix A, page 170, includes **all** of the recommendations regarding your personal risk factors, including family history information, personal health practices, and past medical history items. Be certain to take the completed questionnaire with you when you visit your doctor. In addition, be certain to keep the information current.

Once risk factors have been identified, lifestyle counseling can be initiated. In many instances, your physician will have staff members discuss how to improve your lifestyle practices. Your doctor may also refer you to an allied health professional to receive further lifestyle counseling.

Finally, we also encourage you to use this manual as an aid for altering or eliminating risk factors and implementing positive lifestyle practices.

IDENTIFYING MAJOR SIGNS AND SYMPTOMS SUGGESTIVE OF HEART, LUNG OR METABOLIC DISEASES

Any of the following signs or symptoms should be brought to the attention of your physician.[377] Although these signs or symptoms may not represent heart, lung or metabolic disease, your physician can help you interpret them.

A. In the chest or areas surrounding the chest, pain or discomfort that seems to be related to exertion.

B. Unusual shortness of breath or shortness of breath that is brought on by mild exertion.
C. Dizziness or fainting.
D. Ankle swelling.
E. Palpitations or rapid heart rate.
F. Pain in the lower legs, brought on by walking.
G. Known heart murmur.

RESTING AND EXERCISE ECG TESTS
Guidelines for performing resting and exercise ECG tests are outlined in Table 1, page 82.

The electrocardiogram (ECG). The electrocardiogram (ECG) represents the electrical activity of the heart. Just as a stone thrown into a body of water creates a series of concentric circles traveling in an outward direction, the heart's **pacemaker** (a small area of specialized heart tissue located in the upper right area of the heart), generates a small charge of electricity (at rest 60 to 70 times per minute) that spreads over the upper chambers of the heart and triggers the passage of electrical current throughout the lower chambers of the heart. At rest or during exercise, this electrical signal, the **ECG**, can be detected on the surface of the body. The purposes of the ECG test at rest and during exercise are to:

• Uncover "silent" coronary heart disease;
• Determine the safety of beginning a **vigorous** exercise program;
• Determine a person's current fitness level;
• Serve as a basis for an exercise prescription.

We strongly suggest that you and your doctor review the criteria for performing an exercise ECG test, as outlined on page 82.

Exercise ECG Test. To begin the exercise ECG test, sometimes referred to as an "exercise stress test," a technician will place several electrodes (small sticky patches with conductive gel in the center) on your chest area. The electrodes will then be connected to small wires that lead to the ECG machine on which the ECG signal will be monitored by the doctor.

You will then be asked to exercise on a motor-driven treadmill or bicycle ergometer. The speed and grade of the treadmill (or the resistance of the bike) will be increased intermittently until you are unable to continue exercise. Because the doctor will be continuously monitoring the ECG and periodically taking your blood pressure, you should feel confident exercising to your maximal effort.

If potential threatening ECG changes develop, your doctor will discontinue the test. After you complete the exercise portion of your test, the ECG and blood pressure will continue to be monitored during recovery (a period of seven to ten minutes). Following the test, your doctor will interpret the results.

MEASURING FITNESS AND PRESCRIBING EXERCISE

The treadmill or bike test can be used to predict maximal oxygen uptake (VO_2 max). The VO_2 max estimates the amount of oxygen your body consumed during exercise. This value is the best indicator of your current cardiovascular fitness level.

As part of the exercise test, your doctor will record your heart-rate response. The highest heart rate achieved during exercise **or** your predicted VO_2 max can be used to design a safe and suitable exercise program.

Your doctor may also ask you to rate your level of exertion during the exercise test using a "perceived exertion" scale. A perceived exertion rating can be a **very** effective method for determining exercise intensity, or "how hard" you should exercise. We encourage patients to listen to their entire body while performing the exercise ECG test, and communicate freely regarding their perceived exertion level.

Remember, *you are in charge* during the exercise test. Your physician will not encourage you to exercise longer than you are able.

NOTE: In our laboratory we encourage people not to hold onto the railings of the treadmill while the test is in progress. Holding on may reduce the accuracy of predicting your VO_2 max as you are able to lift a portion of your weight off the treadmill and thereby increase the amount of exercise time. If you must use the railing for balancing yourself, we encourage you to use just one finger or to hold very lightly.

Penalty For Neglect

So predictable are the consequences of risk factors for heart disease that *risk ratios* can be calculated to assess a person's probability of suffering from heart disease. We use the risk ratio almost daily as a teaching tool to help people identify how personal health practices (cigarette smoking, obesity, lack of exercise) coupled with other factors (cholesterol and blood pressure values) are contributing to their overall risk for developing heart disease.

We remember a gentleman who visited our facility for a periodic physical exam and lifestyle counseling. His risk

Table 1: Guidelines for Having a Resting or Exercise ECG Test

Resting Electrocardiogram (ECG)

Routine electrocardiogram screening in individuals without symptoms is not recommended. It may be prudent to perform resting electrocardiograms for males over age 40 who have two or more cardiac risk factors (see page 80) or who participate in special occupations (pilots, firemen, police officers, bus or truck drivers, and railroad engineers). [47]

Exercise ECG Stress Test[48, 50, 51, 377, 378]

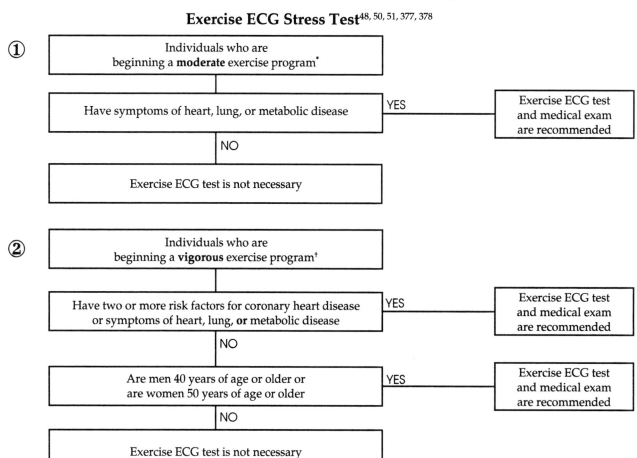

① | Individuals who are beginning a **moderate** exercise program*

Have symptoms of heart, lung, or metabolic disease — **YES** → Exercise ECG test and medical exam are recommended

NO

Exercise ECG test is not necessary

② | Individuals who are beginning a **vigorous** exercise program†

Have two or more risk factors for coronary heart disease or symptoms of heart, lung, **or** metabolic disease — **YES** → Exercise ECG test and medical exam are recommended

NO

Are men 40 years of age or older or are women 50 years of age or older — **YES** → Exercise ECG test and medical exam are recommended

NO

Exercise ECG test is not necessary

③ Individuals with known heart, lung, or metabolic disease should have an exercise stress test and medical exam prior to beginning an exercise program or before markedly increasing the amount of exercise. [50]

④ It may be prudent for men over the age of 40 who have at least two or more cardiac risk factors to consider undergoing a maximal exercise ECG stress test, or for individuals who participate in special occupations (pilots, firemen, police officers, bus or truck drivers, and railroad engineers) to consider a maximal exercise ECG stress test beginning at age 40. [50]

* A **moderate** exercise program is defined as physical activities such as walking or increasing daily activities. It is also described as activities that can be performed "well within the individual's current capacity" — activities that can be carried out "comfortably for a prolonged period" such as 60 minutes. [53, 377]

† A vigorous exercise routine is described as activitiy "intense enough to represent a substantial challenge" resulting in a significant rise in heart rate and breathing rate. Vigorous activity (intensity greater than 60 percent VO_2 max) such as "training for a marathon or participating in vigorous competitive sports" can generally be sustained by untrained individuals for a period of only 15 to 20 minutes. [53, 377]

The frequency of performing the resting and the maximal exercise ECG stress test for the above guidelines will vary based upon the severity of risk factors and the discretion of your physician.

factors for heart disease were identified:

- 54-year-old male;
- Cigarette smoker;
- Total cholesterol of 292 mg/dl;
- HDL-cholesterol of 34 mg/dl;
- Systolic blood pressure reading of 154 mm Hg.

His risk ratio (calculated from the Framingham Heart Study data) indicated that within the next five years he had a **19 percent chance** of having clinical heart disease, or symptoms that could possibly result in a heart attack.[371]

To help motivate this patient, we calculated his risk ratio if he were to make the following changes:

- Lower cholesterol to 220 mg/dl (by eliminating his high-fat diet);
- Raise HDL-cholesterol to 40 mg/dl (by regular exercise and weight reduction);
- Quit smoking;
- Reduce systolic blood pressure to 130 mm Hg (by regular exercise and improved nutrition).

Using the assumed improved values, his new risk ratio for developing significant heart disease in the next five years was close to **six percent**, an astounding **68 percent decrease** in his cardiac disease risk.[371]

Within a week this gentleman had quit smoking, started walking and had complied with our recommendation to begin seeing our nutritionist for dietary recommendations.

We should indicate that some individuals who make all the right lifestyle changes may still require pharmacologic treatment (drug therapy) for the treatment of certain coronary risk factors such as high blood pressure and high cholesterol.

You are *never* too late to identify risk factors and initiate preventive measures to reduce your risk ratio. To neglect to do so will ultimately bring poor health.

EARLY PREVENTION PAYS OFF

This health check would not be complete without mention of the importance for children and adolescents to begin the practice of good nutrition, regular physical activity and positive health maintenance practices. Heart disease can begin at a very early age. Parents and older siblings who practice healthy lifestyles can assist children by simply being positive "role models."

Children should be screened for coronary heart disease risk factors if their parents have a history of early coronary heart disease or significant coronary risk factors such as very high cholesterol.

Health Notes

PERIPHERAL VASCULAR DISEASE

Peripheral vascular disease (PVD) refers to atherosclerotic changes (fatty deposits) that may occur in the arteries and the veins that are away from the heart. With advancing age there is an increased likelihood for individuals to develop PVD. Symptoms for PVD often appear in the lower extremities. You should be alert to the following symptoms which may suggest the presence of PVD:[379]

- An ache, pain, cramp or tightness in the buttocks, hips, thighs or calves that is brought on with walking and is relieved within minutes by rest (this is often call claudication);
- Pain that occurs at nighttime or during rest and that is only relieved when the leg is placed on a footstool or left to hang over the edge of the bed;
- Impotence in men;
- Skin sores (such as ulcers) or dead tissue (gangrene);
- Sudden onset of pain, paleness or whiteness, no pulse, numbness or tingling, coolness in one leg while the other leg is warm, or paralysis (resulting from a blocked artery);
- a throbbing mass in the abdominal area (this may suggest the presence of an abdominal aneurysm).

Discuss any of these symptoms with your physician.

(Source: "Coping with Your Circulatory Problems: Getting Back in Circulation," by Abbott Laboratories.)

Yearly or Periodic Health Check #3

BLOOD PRESSURE SCREENING

RECOMMENDATIONS

1. All adults should have their blood pressure measured at every visit with a health care professional and at least every two years during ages 19–39 and yearly after age 40.[46,54,385] Record your blood pressure reading in your Health Check Table.

2. The guidelines used for classifying blood pressure and the suggested follow-up for blood pressure measurement is listed below:[54]

A. CLASSIFICATION OF BLOOD PRESSURE
Range, mm Hg   Category

Diastolic Blood Pressure, DBP

Range	Category
< 85	Normal blood pressure
85-89	High normal blood pressure
90-104	Mild hypertension
105-114	Moderate hypertension
>115	Severe hypertension

Systolic Blood Pressure, SBP*

Range	Category
<140	Normal blood pressure
140-159	Borderline isolated systolic hypertension
>160	Isolated systolic hypertension

*assuming diastolic <90

B. FOLLOW-UP OF BLOOD PRESSURE
Range, mm Hg   Recommended Follow-Up

Diastolic

Range	Recommended Follow-Up
<85	Recheck within two years
85-89	Recheck within one year
90-104	Confirm within two months
105-114	Evaluate or refer promptly to source of care within two weeks
>115	Evaluate or refer immediately to source of care

Systolic, when diastolic blood pressure is <90

Range	Recommended Follow-Up
<140	Recheck within two years
140-199	Confirm within two months
>200	Evaluate or refer promptly to source of care within two weeks

(If recommendations for follow-up of diastolic and systolic blood pressure are different, the shorter recommended time for recheck and referral should take precedence.)

NOTE: These classifications are based on the average of two or more readings on two or more occasions. A classification of borderline isolated systolic hypertension (SBP 140 to 159 mm Hg) or isolated systolic hypertension (SBP > 160 mm Hg) takes precedence over high normal blood pressure (diastolic blood pressure, 85 to 89 mm Hg) when both occur in the same person. High normal blood pressure (DBP 85 to 89 mm Hg) takes precedence over a classification of normal blood pressure (SBP < 140 mm Hg) when both occur in the same person. Classifications are taken from the Joint National Committee on Detection, Evaluation, and Treatment of High Blood Pressure, 1988.

Why Perform

- Approximately 58 million Americans have hypertension (elevated blood pressure).[54]
- High blood pressure increases the risk for heart disease, stroke and kidney disease. Early detection and treatment of high blood pressure can greatly reduce the risk for these diseases.
- Early detection is especially important for the following high risk groups:[54]

  Offspring of individuals with hypertension;
  Blacks;
  Obese individuals;
  Persons with high normal blood pressure;
  Pregnant women;
  Elderly people;
  Individuals with diabetes.

- The higher one's blood pressure, the greater the risk.

THE SILENT DISEASE

One of our colleagues, a cardiologist, first discovered he had hypertension while attending a medical conference in Seattle. During the conference he stopped to have his blood pressure taken at one of the exhibits. Although our friend was taking the blood pressure of several patients each day, he had not bothered to have his own measured for a few years. To his surprise the blood pressure was elevated — 160/110!

As is the case with most people who are found to have high blood pressure, no cause was determined for our friend's hypertension. Although his quickly initiated life-style changes (exercise, salt restriction and weight loss) helped reduce his blood pressure somewhat, they did not lower it sufficiently and he began taking medication. Now, with medication his blood pressure remains normal.

Because blood pressure (the force exerted by the blood on the walls of your arteries) is a silent pressure, people are not aware if their blood pressure is high. In fact, like our cardiologist friend many people have high blood pressure for years without being aware of the problem. The only way to determine if it is normal is to have it checked. For this reason, we strongly urge people to follow the health check guidelines for measurement of blood pressure.

How Performed

WHAT BLOOD PRESSURE MEANS

The aortic valve, located at the top of the left ventricle (the chamber of the heart that pumps oxygenated blood to the body) opens and closes with the pressure changes of the heart. The blood pressure is highest when the heart contracts or beats. This is the systolic pressure. As the heart builds pressure in its chamber, the aortic valve eventually opens and a surge of blood causes a momentary rise in the pressure on the walls of your arteries. Typical resting systolic pressure ranges from 100 to 140 mm Hg.

After the rise in pressure has passed, the heart reduces its pressure; the aortic valve closes and during this relaxed phase of the heart the pressure within the arteries is called the diastolic pressure. The diastolic pressure is the minimal pressure in the arteries at all times. A normal diastolic pressure reading falls between 65 to 90 mm Hg.

Too high a blood pressure can eventually result in harm to the body. If the systolic pressure (measured at rest) reaches 160 or greater, there is an increased danger of damaging the kidneys and clogging the blood vessels. An elevated diastolic pressure can be as dangerous as a high systolic reading. If the diastolic pressure is elevated, the heart must work harder to push the blood from its chambers. A high diastolic pressure, uncontrolled over a long period of time, can lead to heart failure.

HOW BLOOD PRESSURE IS MEASURED

Blood pressure can be measured in your doctor's office, at home, or in a store. Recognize that blood pressure is variable and can be affected by many extraneous factors. For this reason, hypertension should not be diagnosed on the basis of a single measurement. Elevated readings should be confirmed on **at least two or more** subsequent office visits, with average systolic and diastolic values above 140 and/or 90 mm Hg, respectively.

Be advised that many people have what is called "white coat hypertension" in which their blood pressure rises when taken in the doctor's office, only to return to the normal range following the visit.[55]

The Joint National Committee on Detection, Evaluation, and Treatment of High Blood Pressure has recommended the following techniques for accurate measurement:[54]

1. Sit with your arm bared, supported and positioned at heart level;

2. Do not smoke or ingest caffeine within 30 minutes prior to measurement;

3. Rest quietly for 5 minutes before measurement;

4. Use an appropriate cuff size. The rubber bladder should encircle at least two-thirds of your arm;

5. Take measurements with a mercury sphygmomanometer, a recently-calibrated aneroid manometer, or a validated electronic device;

6. Record both systolic and diastolic measurements. Use the disappearance of sound (Phase V) for the diastolic reading;

7. Take the average of two or more readings. If the first two readings differ by more than 5 mm Hg, obtain additional readings.

Your doctor or medical assistant should inform you of your blood pressure reading and should advise you of the need for periodic remeasurement.

REDUCING THE RISK

Hypertension is controllable. Since 1972, the number of strokes occurring in the U.S. has dropped an amazing **50 percent**. If you are found to have high blood pressure, the following options can be taken to reduce your hypertension:[54]

- **Weight control;**
- **Restriction of alcohol;**
- **Restriction of sodium;**
- **Avoidance of tobacco;**
- **Biofeedback and relaxation;**
- **Regular exercise;**
- **Modification (reduced intake) of dietary fat;**
- *Possibly* **increased potassium and calcium;**
- **Antihypertensive drugs.**

Yearly or Periodic Health Checks #4, #10, and #11

and

High-Risk Health Checks #4 and #27

RECTAL EXAM, BLOOD STOOL TEST, SIGMOIDOSCOPY EXAM, COLONOSCOPY EXAM, AND PROSTATE SPECIFIC ANTIGEN (PSA) TEST
(SCREENING FOR COLORECTAL AND PROSTATE CANCER)

RECOMMENDATIONS

1. Digital rectal exam should be performed:[46, 56, 57, 388]
   A) Every year on men and women ages 40 and older;
   B) As part of the periodic physical examination.

2. Blood stool testing should be performed yearly on men and women ages 50 and older.[46, 56, 57, 388]

3. A proctosigmoidoscopy examination should be performed on men and women beginning at age 50. If this initial exam is normal, repeat the procedure every three to five years.[57, 388]
   The American College of Physicians (ACP) has recommended that colorectal cancer screening include the sigmoidoscopy test (performed every three to five years) or an air-contrast barium enema test (performed every five years) for individuals age 50 and older. The ACP also suggests that individuals age 40 and older who are at risk for colon cancer have a colonoscopy or an air-contrast barium enema every three to five years.

4. Individuals who are identified as high risk for colon-rectal cancer should have special surveillance by their physician. This may include blood stool testing, digital rectal exams, sigmoidoscopy and/or colonoscopy exams at ages earlier than the normally recommended age and at more frequent intervals.[57, 58] High risk persons may include those people with a: [57, 58]
   - Strong family history of colorectal cancer;
   - History of familial polyposis coli (high number of polyps in the large intestine);
   - Personal history of polyps, colon cancer or inflammatory bowel disease like colitis;
   - Women with a history of endometrial, ovarian or breast cancer.

5. Become familiar with the following warning signs or symptoms of colorectal cancer:
   - **A major change in bowel habits (persistent diarrhea or constipation, or change in the frequency, size or shape of the stool);**
   - **Blood in the stool;**
   - **Rectal bleeding.**
   Cancer expert Dr. Jerome DeCosse has suggested "abdominal bloating, pain in the lower back, or bladder" also as possible symptoms if these problems do not subside. If any of these symptoms occur, **contact your physician.**[56] The symptoms mentioned do not necessarily indicate you have colon cancer. Hemorrhoids, for example, are a major cause of blood in the stool. The key is to check with your doctor.

6. The following men over age 50 should consult with their physician to determine whether or not

(continued)

they should have a prostate specific antigen (PSA) test.[374, 375] Men who:
- Have a family history of prostate cancer;
- Have symptoms or test or physical exam results suggestive of prostate cancer;
- Are scheduled to have a prostate resection (TURP);
- Are undergoing treatment for prostate cancer (surgery, radiation, or hormone therapy).

7. Be certain to record in your *Health Check Table* when you participate in colorectal and prostate screening health checks.

Why Perform

"The president has cancer," was the announcement of Dr. Steven Rosenberg, head of surgery at the National Cancer Institute, as he reported to the world the results of Ronald Reagan's colon biopsy.

Fourteen months earlier, a small noncancerous polyp had been detected in the President's lower colon during a routine sigmoidoscopy examination, and one year later (again during a routine sigmoidoscopy exam), a second polyp was discovered and in addition, the routine blood stool test was positive. These results prompted another test, a colonoscopy in which a two-inch polyp was discovered. The polyp and a two-foot section of colon were surgically removed.[59]

We all know this story had a good ending. Because the president's cancer was detected and treated early, he recovered and completed his term of office.

Early detection is the *key* for successful treatment of colorectal cancer. In fact, screening for colorectal cancer can save thousands of lives each year.[56]

COLORECTAL CANCER

- Colorectal cancer (cancer of the colon and rectum) is the second leading cause of death from cancer.[57]
- Early testing of patients without symptoms results in the detection of polyps, the detection of increased numbers of early stage cancers and the detection of fewer advanced stage cancers.[57, 71, 74, 75]
- Detection and diagnosis of an early stage cancer with follow-up treatment leads to better survival.[57]
- National trends toward earlier detection and treatment of colorectal cancer are associated with decreasing death rates.[57, 63, 72, 73]

- The removal of premalignant tissue (such as some polyps) whose history leads to cancer will reduce the incidence and eventual death of individuals.[57]
- More men are diagnosed with colorectal cancer than women (62.1 vs. 44.8 percent)[60], and almost all cases are diagnosed after age 50.

Because colorectal cancer develops over a period of time (sometimes even years), screening for cancer of the large bowel (rectum and colon) can detect cancer ahead of the symptom stage, and precancerous polyps can be removed without major surgery.[61] In fact, if diagnosis is made when the cancer is still in its early stages (before signs and symptoms occur) and treated, the survival rate for the first five years is approximately 90 percent.[60]

In the past 10 years the five-year survival rate for colorectal cancer has been increasing — partly a result of improved early detection techniques.[57, 60] Another reason for the increase in colon cancer survival is that approximately 50 percent of the colon cancer occurs within the first 25 cm. of the large bowel, a distance that can be reached with modern sigmoidoscopes.[63, 64]

PROSTATE CANCER

- Prostate cancer is a significant health problem for men as it relates to both disability and death, and is the third leading cause of death from cancer in men.[65, 66]
- In light of the advancing age of the U.S. population, the overall impact of prostate cancer on national health will increase.[67]
- The routine digital rectal examination appears to be the most reasonable screening test for prostate cancer with regard to the overall efficiency, noninvasiveness, risk of injury, availability and cost.[67]
- The National Cancer Institute reports prostate cancer is the most common cancer in men over the age of 50 with increasing incidence every decade after age 50.[67]
- Black males have a higher incidence of prostate cancer.

The reason a periodic digital rectal examination is important is because men with prostate cancer are generally unaware of their disease (there are usually no symptoms). Estimates suggest that about 50 percent of the prostate problems detected with the digital rectal exam are cancerous.[68] If cancer detection is early, the treatment is generally very successful, allowing one to continue to lead a normal and productive life.

For some men over age 50, physicians are now recommending the prostate specific antigen (PSA) test (see "Recommendations," page 87, for criteria in recommending this test).[375]

Problem Signs. If any of the following symptoms begin to occur, consult your physician. They may be indicative of a prostate problem.[68]

- Urinary disorders such as urinating frequently (especially at night), painful burning sensation on urination, urine flow not easily stopped.
- Blood in your urine.
- Pain in your lower back, pelvis or upper thighs that continues.

How Performed

SCREENING PROCEDURES FOR COLORECTAL AND PROSTATE CANCER

Listed below are the procedures used to screen for colorectal and prostate cancer.

1. *Digital rectal examination.* The digital rectal examination is simple and painless. By inserting a gloved, lubricated finger (or digit) inside the rectum, your physician can check for growths in the rectal area and examine the male prostate gland.

2. *Sigmoidoscopy examination.* Using a rigid or flexible scope, your physician can carefully examine 10 to 24 inches of the lower colon, depending on what type and length of scope is used.[76-79]

3. *Colonoscopy examination.* This examination permits the physician to examine the entire length of the colon, using a much longer colonoscope. This test is now being recommended as the exam of choice for individuals with a family history of familial polyposis coli or cancer family syndrome.

4. *Blood stool test* (or stool guaiac test). This test is used to check for occult (hidden) blood in the stool. The test is inexpensive, painless and relatively simple to perform.

5. *Prostate Specific Antigen (PSA) Test.* This test screens for prostate cancer and is used to follow the course of prostate cancer. All that is required for this test is a blood sample.

To learn more about how these procedures are performed, refer to the information below.

Digital Rectal, Sigmoidoscopy and Colonoscopy Exams. The large bowel or large intestine is illustrated in Figure 1. The large bowel is approximately three to five

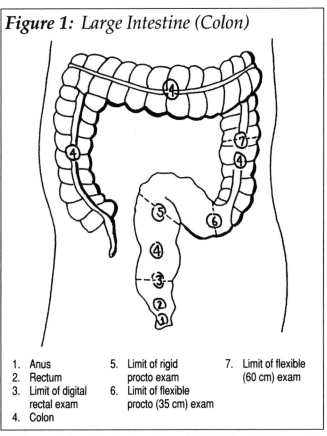

Figure 1: Large Intestine (Colon)

1. Anus
2. Rectum
3. Limit of digital rectal exam
4. Colon
5. Limit of rigid procto exam
6. Limit of flexible procto (35 cm) exam
7. Limit of flexible (60 cm) exam

Used by permission of the American Cancer Society; Colorectal Cancer: Go For Early Detection

feet in length and consists of the colon and rectum (this is why the assessment is sometimes referred to as a colorectal screening).

As illustrated in Figure 1, there are varying lengths of the rectum and colon that can be examined based upon the instrument used:

- **Area #3**: Limit of digital rectal exam;
- **Area #4**: Colonoscopy exam length (whole colon);
- **Area #5**: Limit of rigid procto exam;
- **Area #6**: Limit of flexible procto (35 cm) exam;
- **Area #7**: Limit of flexible procto (60 cm) exam.

Digital Rectal Exam. Inserting a gloved, lubricated finger inside the rectum, your physician can check for growths in the rectal area or on the male prostate gland.

Your doctor will feel for irregularities in the prostate (for size, shape, texture, and nodules). Let your doctor know if it is tender when he examines your prostate. You can help your doctor in performing the test if you try to relax the muscles around the anal area and to take slow deep breaths during the exam.

Five to ten percent of all colon tumors can be detected using the digital rectal examination.[69] At this time, the physician may also take a stool sample for occult blood.

Scope Exams. To perform this exam, your doctor will ask you to either kneel on a patient table with your elbows supporting your upper body or to lie on your side. If the procedure is performed in the kneeling position, your doctor may also slightly tilt your body (head down).[70]

Prior to the scope being inserted into the rectum, the doctor will apply a clear lubricant (this may initially be cold). The sigmoidoscope is then gently inserted and advanced. To assist in the visualization of the large intestine, the physician may occasionally introduce air into the colon. The air tends to expand the intestinal wall to permit easier advancement of the scope.

If a suspicious area of tissue is viewed, the physician may choose to biopsy the intestine for further tests, or if a polyp is discovered, the doctor may remove it with the appropriate instrument. This may cause a small but negligible amount of bleeding, but the procedure will not be painful.[70]

This procedure is not as uncomfortable as it sounds. If your physician is gentle and sensitive, and addresses your concerns, you will find this potentially embarrassing screening to be quite acceptable.

Scope Lengths. Four different kinds of scopes are used to examine the colon.

- The **rigid sigmoidoscope** is a hollow, lighted tube (10 to 12 inches), used to examine the entire rectum and the lower part of the colon. See Figure 1.
- Two **flexible sigmoidoscopes** have been developed using flexible fiber optics. These scopes flex around the curves in the colon, allowing a greater area of visualization. The lengths of the flexible sigmoidoscopes are *24 inches* and *14 inches*. To visualize the area of the colon that the scopes can inspect, refer to Figure 1, previous page.

According to the National Cancer Institute, estimates of polyp discovery for these scopes include:

- **25-30 percent for the rigid scope;**
- **50-55 percent for the 35 cm. scope;**
- **65-75 percent for the 60 cm. scope.**[57]

Dr. Massimo Crespi and his colleagues suggest that "since the yield is greater with the 60 cm. scope, this should be the instrument of choice in experienced hands and for use in centers. The 35 cm. scope is a step forward compared to rigid sigmoidoscopy used by family practitioners."[63] Discuss this information with your doctor.

- The **colonoscope** is recommended for use in patients with a family history of colon cancer or a family history of polyposis coli (the presence of numerous polyps in the large intestine). This scope examines the entire length of the colon.[80]

If you need to have a colonoscopy exam, you will need to clear your entire colon of stool. This will require you to make additional preparation as it relates to diet and laxatives. A possibility also exists for you to have an intravenous line (IV) placed in the arm so you can receive a pain reliever like Demerol and/or a sedative such as Valium.[80]

Be certain to talk to your physician if you have a strong family history of colon cancer or intestinal polyp disease to decide whether or not this test should be performed.

Blood Stool Test. In the early stages of colon cancer, the only symptoms may be bleeding. Unfortunately, the blood may be mixed with the stool and undetectable. The blood stool test, often referred to as an occult blood stool test, can be used to identify **"occult"** or concealed blood.

Be advised that there are many causes for blood in the stool other than colorectal cancer (i.e., hemorrhoids). If the blood stool test reveals hidden blood, your primary-care physician will help you determine what additional tests, if any, will need to be performed. The blood stool test remains the first-line screening method for bowel cancer.

To perform the blood stool test, your physician should supply you with three specimen cards and three small sticks. You can also purchase testing kits from your local pharmacy. Each card has an area for two stool specimens to be placed. Instructions for performing the blood stool test are located on the cards. Your doctor's office will chemically treat the stool specimens to determine if any occult blood is present.

Prior to your taking this test, the following preparation should be followed:[80]

1. Your diet should consist of plenty of high fiber foods (fruits, vegetables and bran) three days prior to and during the testing. These foods may increase bleeding of possible cancers.
2. Avoid red meats. This food may result in a false positive test. Also suggested is the avoidance of eating turnips, radishes or horseradish.
3. Also avoid taking aspirin, anti-inflammatory medication, vitamin C supplements and iron pills. These items may also increase the likelihood of a false positive test.
4. Individuals with active hemorrhoidal or menstrual bleeding should avoid the blood stool test. You may want to discuss this item with your personal physician.

POSSIBLE CAUSES OF COLON CANCER

Factors that have been identified as potential causes of colorectal cancer are:

- **Diet;**
- **Genetics;**
- **Colon Disorders;**
- **Age.**

Diet. Most research scientists studying large population trends feel that colon cancer increases as a result of a high-fat, high-protein and low-fiber, low-complex carbohydrate diet.[56]

Some experts have suggested that dietary fiber may reduce the risk of colon cancer by: 1) decreasing the time the stool is in the large bowel (reducing the amount of time for intestinal irritation by the stool); and 2) increasing the absorption of water by the stool, resulting in a diluting effect upon the possible cancer-causing agents and other bowel irritants. These cancer prevention benefits have led experts to recommend people reduce their intake of fat and protein and at the same time increase the consumption of fiber and complex carbohydrates.[56]

Genetics. Cancer expert, Dr. Jerome DeCosse, has reported:[56]

1) Approximately one in 100 patients who develop bowel cancer have a family background of polyps (familial polyposis) of the large intestine.
2) Approximately 10 to 15 percent of the individuals that develop colorectal cancer will be without polyposis but the family history will show that one or more close relatives will have reported cancer of the colon or rectum.

Colon Disorders. Individuals with a history of ulcerative colitis, Crohn's disease or polyposis are at increased risk for developing colon cancer.

(*NOTE:* Individuals with colon disorders or with a family history of colon cancer, should carefully review with their primary-care physician whether or not a more rigorous screening schedule should be undertaken and at an earlier age. High-risk individuals should consider a colonoscopy procedure for colorectal screening.[56-58, 62])

Age. Finally, the risk of colorectal cancer increases with age, especially after the age of 40 or 50. For this reason the American Cancer Society and the National Cancer Institute have established the guidelines for digital rectal screening to begin at age 40, and the proctosigmoidoscopy screening and occult blood tests to commence at age 50.

Penalty For Neglect

Unfortunately, each of us as authors knows of patients who have neglected periodic colorectal or prostate cancer screening or they have **waited too long** to report troublesome symptoms such as rectal bleeding. Their neglect has often been tragic.

Although in 1987 there were approximately 145,000 new cases of colon cancer and 60,000 deaths, Dr. DeCrosse has estimated that half of the patients diagnosed with colorectal cancer can expect to be cured, a statistic that **could be improved** if more individuals would follow the screening guidelines for bowel cancer.[56] Practice smart medicine and follow the guidelines.

Health Notes

The American College of Physicians has recommended that screening for colorectal cancer should include a sigmoidoscopy for individuals 50 years and older. They have also said that the *air-contrast barium enema* can be used for colorectal cancer screening every five years beginning at age 50 in place of a sigmoidoscopy.

The air-contrast barium enema is an X-ray examination of the colon (large intestine). As part of the procedure, liquid barium sulfate is introduced into the colon through the anus. Once the colon is coated with the barium, the colon is then filled with air and X-rays are taken to detect polyps, tumors, or inflamation that might be present in the colon.

The entire colon must be free of stool and gas prior to the air-contrast barium enema test. Cleaning of the colon often involves eating a clear-liquid diet for a day or two prior to the test, drinking large amounts of water, and ingesting laxative-type medications. The test can be somewhat uncomfortable; individuals who are participating in this test should visit with their physician about the test procedure. Pregnant women should inform the doctor of their condition.[395]

The American College of Physicians have recommended individuals who are 40 and older and who have familial polyposis coli, inflammatory bowel disease, or a history of colon cancer in a parent or sibling should have an air-contrast barium enema or colonoscopy (in addition to annual fecal occult blood tests), every three to five years.[387]

Yearly or Periodic Health Check #5
Monthly Health Check #2
and
Daily Health Check #11

CLINICAL SKIN EXAMINATION,
SKIN SELF-EXAMINATION AND SKIN CANCER PREVENTION

RECOMMENDATIONS

1. As part of the periodic physical examination, your physician should perform a complete skin examination, especially on individuals at risk for developing skin cancer.

2. All adults should perform monthly skin self-examinations. This recommendation is **especially** important for individuals at risk for developing skin cancer. Use your Health Check Table to record your participation in this health check.

3. Individuals at high-risk for skin cancer may require more frequent clinical skin cancer screening as directed by their physician. High risk individuals include those who:[81-83]

   - **Have a personal or family history of skin cancer (including malignant melanoma);**
   - **Have increased occupational or recreational exposure to sunlight;**
   - **Have clinical evidence of suspicious moles.**

4. Individuals should take preventive steps to reduce the risk for skin cancer by using sunscreen preparations, wearing protective clothing including hats, and avoiding excessive exposure to ultraviolet rays.[81, 84]

Why Perform

- Melanoma cancer has increased in the U.S. more than any other cancer.[85]
- More than 500,000 people are diagnosed each year with skin cancer.[86]
- Over 8,000 persons die each year of skin cancer (6,000 from malignant melanoma and 2,000 from squamous or basal cell cancer).[66]
- Examination of the skin is the principal screening technique for detecting skin cancer, and the survival from malignant melanoma is directly related to the stage of the cancer.[81, 84, 85]
- The likelihood of basal or squamous cell skin cancer causing disfiguration or disability is less likely if diagnosed and treated early.[81]
- The clinical skin exam and the skin self-exam are easily performed and are entirely painless.

The suntan has become a modern day symbol of attractiveness. Unfortunately, new cases of skin cancer are increasing at alarming rates and **sun exposure** remains the number one risk-factor for developing skin cancer. Cancer of the skin is now recognized as the most common form of all human cancers.

As a young man of 19, one author of this book spent two years in Australia (several months of which were in Queensland where the highest incidence in the world for melanoma skin cancer exists).[85] Fair complected and with reddish-brown hair (secondary risk-factors for developing skin cancer), the author was exposed every day for several hours to the sun, but took no precautions to avoid its damaging rays. Now, years later, the effects of the sun's exposure are beginning to emerge with several darkish colored "liver spots" appearing on the face. In addition a dermatologist has had to freeze-burn several areas of pre-cancerous skin.

The author now takes every precaution to reduce the risk of further skin damage by using sun-screen and **always** wearing a hat. In addition, the author performs regular skin self-exams and follows the recommended health checks for physician skin examinations.

How Performed

TYPES OF SKIN CANCER

There are three types of skin cancer:

1. BASAL CELL: Skin cancers that appear on the face, scalp, neck, and hands.

2. SQUAMOUS CELL: Less common than basal cell cancer, squamous appear on the cheek, ear, neck, temple, forehead, and hand.

3. MALIGNANT MELANOMA: The least common of the skin cancers, but the most deadly if not treated early. Melanoma generally occurs in areas that are exposed to the sun — in women the primary areas of occurrence are the back, the face and the lower legs; and in men the torso is the most common.

CLINICAL SKIN EXAMINATION

Your physician should perform a complete skin examination at the time of your periodic physical, especially if you are at increased risk for skin cancer. Because malignant melanoma may appear anywhere in the skin, a total body skin examination is recommended. Although this exam may be somewhat embarrassing to individuals, your physician can easily perform this screening procedure in a very professional manner using a paper or cloth sheet.

In addition to the periodic clinical skin examination, you should alert your physician to any of the following:[84]

1. **Any ulcer of the skin that does not heal in six weeks;**
2. **Any lump or growth that bleeds persistently;**
3. **Any lump or growth that enlarges, especially those that are hard or firm to the touch;**

4. **Any pigmented "mole" that is splotchy, brown, black or has irregular indented borders like a maple leaf;**
5. **Any growth or mole that is changing in size or shape;**
6. **Any mole that itches or is tender.**

SKIN SELF-EXAMINATION

Regular self-inspection of skin areas is the best method for early detection and successful treatment of skin cancer. Early recognition of melanoma, for example, is **not** difficult, and it is estimated that over 90 percent of the melanomas that arise on the skin's surface can be detected with the naked eye.[85]

To assist you in performing a complete skin self-exam, The American Cancer Society has devised a **"Ten-Step"** plan. These ten steps are illustrated and described on the following pages.[87]

In addition to the ten-step self-examination, some skin specialists have suggested you make a "body-map" of your skin, identifying on a piece of paper the approximate location of moles and "birthmarks." Using this map may help you determine if a change in your skin has occurred.

Finally, a simple **ABCD** rule outlined by the American Cancer Society to help you remember the important signs of melanoma is listed below.

A. **ASYMMETRY.** One-half does not match the other half.
B. **BORDER IRREGULARITY.** The edges are ragged, notched or blurred.
C. **COLOR.** The pigmentation is not uniform — shades of tan, brown and black are present. Red, white, and blue may add to the mottled appearance.
D. **DIAMETER GREATER THAN SIX MILLIMETERS.** Any sudden or continuing increase in size should be of special concern.

SKIN CANCER PREVENTION

Individuals should practice measures listed below to prevent skin cancer:[81]

- **Stay out of the sun from 10 a.m. to 2 p.m.;**
- **Cover up with hats, shirts and pants;**
- **Use a sunscreen preparation (at least a #15 SPF number) to cover the area of the body that will be exposed to the sun;**
- **Tan gradually;**
- **Do not use sunlamps or tanning booths/centers.**

Figure 1: *Ten-Step Skin Self-Examination*

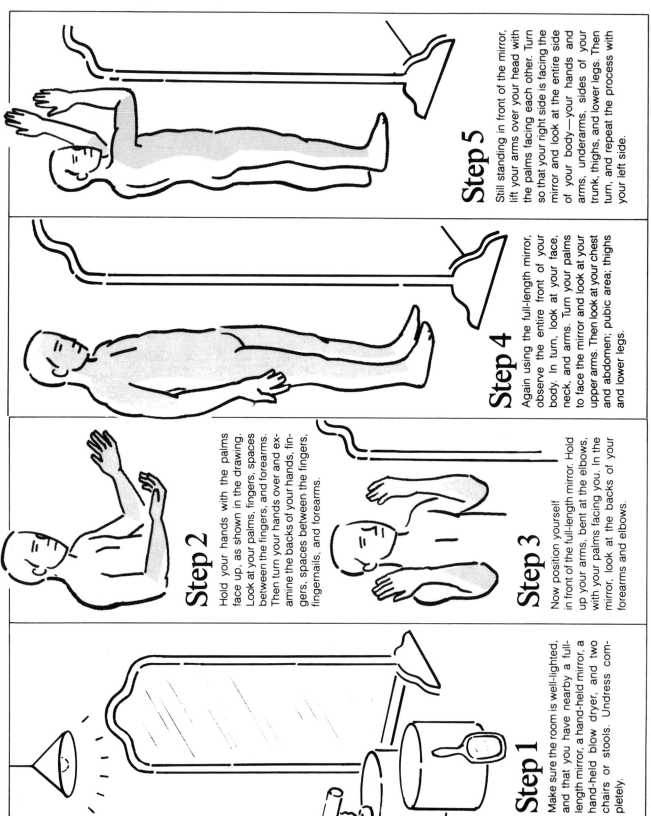

Step 1

Make sure the room is well-lighted, and that you have nearby a full-length mirror, a hand-held mirror, a hand-held blow dryer, and two chairs or stools. Undress completely.

Step 2

Hold your hands with the palms face up, as shown in the drawing. Look at your palms, fingers, spaces between the fingers, and forearms. Then turn your hands over and examine the backs of your hands, fingers, spaces between the fingers, fingernails, and forearms.

Step 3

Now position yourself in front of the full-length mirror. Hold up your arms, bent at the elbows, with your palms facing you. In the mirror, look at the backs of your forearms and elbows.

Step 4

Again using the full-length mirror, observe the entire front of your body. In turn, look at your face, neck, and arms. Turn your palms to face the mirror and look at your upper arms. Then look at your chest and abdomen; pubic area; thighs and lower legs.

Step 5

Still standing in front of the mirror, lift your arms over your head with the palms facing each other. Turn so that your right side is facing the mirror and look at the entire side of your body—your hands and arms, underarms, sides of your trunk, thighs, and lower legs. Then turn, and repeat the process with your left side.

© 1985, American Cancer Society, Inc., New York, N.Y.

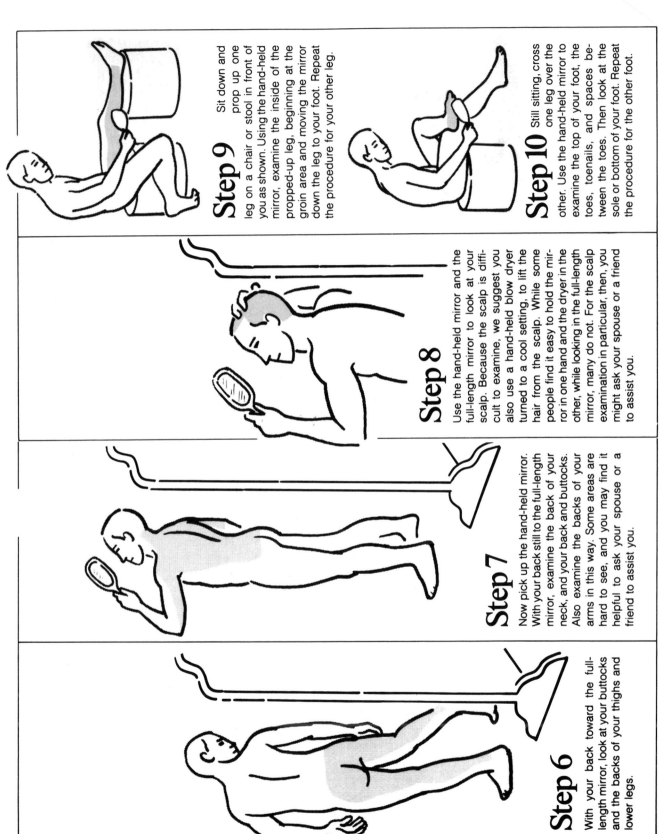

Step 9   Sit down and prop up one leg on a chair or stool in front of you as shown. Using the hand-held mirror, examine the inside of the propped-up leg, beginning at the groin area and moving the mirror down the leg to your foot. Repeat the procedure for your other leg.

Step 10   Still sitting, cross one leg over the other. Use the hand-held mirror to examine the top of your foot, the toes, toenails, and spaces between the toes. Then look at the sole or bottom of your foot. Repeat the procedure for the other foot.

Step 8   Use the hand-held mirror and the full-length mirror to look at your scalp. Because the scalp is difficult to examine, we suggest you also use a hand-held blow dryer turned to a cool setting, to lift the hair from the scalp. While some people find it easy to hold the mirror in one hand and the dryer in the other, while looking in the full-length mirror, many do not. For the scalp examination in particular, then, you might ask your spouse or a friend to assist you.

Step 7   Now pick up the hand-held mirror. With your back still to the full-length mirror, examine the back of your neck, and your back and buttocks. Also examine the backs of your arms in this way. Some areas are hard to see, and you may find it helpful to ask your spouse or a friend to assist you.

Step 6   With your back toward the full-length mirror, look at your buttocks and the backs of your thighs and lower legs.

© 1985, American Cancer Society, Inc., New York, N.Y.

Penalty For Neglect

Early detection and treatment is the key to survival for the 27,000 individuals who are diagnosed with malignant melanoma each year. In fact, melanoma can be 100 percent curable.[66, 85]

When malignant melanoma is detected at an early stage (Stage I), the five-year survival rate is greater than 80 to 90 percent, but if the cancer has progressed to Stage II disease, the survival rate drops to 27 to 57 percent.[81, 88] One study showed that patients with melanoma waited an average of **11 to 18 months** from the time they detected the potential problem to the time of report to their doctor.[81, 89]

We recommend individuals also be aware of squamous and basal cell skin cancers. If left untreated, these cancers can cause serious disfigurement, disability or even death.

Health Notes

The following information includes a more detailed description of the three kinds of skin cancer.

BASAL CELL: Generally, the skin cancers that appear on the face, scalp, neck, hands and arms (areas that are most exposed to the sun) are *basal cell* skin cancers. Basal cell cancer is the most common form of skin cancer and also the least fatal.

This type of skin cancer is very slow growing, taking months or even years to reach a size that would appear as an abnormality. Generally, basal cell cancers are without pain, and no symptoms exist unless small ulcers form (occasionally the small ulcers will bleed).[84] Cancer specialist Dr. Fitzpatrick further suggests the basal cell "tumors are usually, unless long neglected, small and single, with a round or oval shape. They may be pink or red and scaly, although they are usually white, wax-like or pearly, and hard rather than firm. Basal cell carcinomas rarely, if ever, spread to other parts of the body. Yet, they can invade and slowly destroy nearby bone and cartilage if not properly treated."[84]

SQUAMOUS CELL: *Squamous cell* skin cancer does not occur as frequently as basal cell but is much more common than melanoma cancer. Dr. Fitzpatrick describes squamous cell cancers as "more variable in appearance than basal cell cancers and tend to grow more rapidly. They can develop sores in their centers that do not heal. These sores, or lesions, are small,

rough, crusty, and reddish but the best underlying feature is their hardness. They may be attached to body structures beneath the skin."[84]

They occur on the cheek, ear, neck, temple, forehead, and hand; for a definite diagnosis a biopsy is required. Squamous cell cancers can spread more rapidly than basal cell and can even infiltrate the lymph system if left untreated. Surgery to remove cancerous growth and surrounding tissue, sometimes followed by radiation therapy, is commonly used in treating squamous cell cancers.[84]

MALIGNANT MELANOMA: The third type of skin cancer is *malignant melanoma* — the least common of the skin cancers, but the most deadly if not treated early. The death rate from malignant melanoma is increasing faster than any other type of cancer with the exception of lung cancer.[85] This type of skin cancer also spreads very quickly.

Within our skin are pigment cells, referred to as melanocytes. These pigment cells are responsible for producing a pigment called "melanin" that causes us to tan in response to ultraviolet light - a process designed to protect the skin from eventual burning. Occasionally, the melanocyte cell transforms into a cancer cell and the uncontrollable growth of these cancer cells is referred to as "melanoma."

The chief cause for the normal pigment cell changing into malignant melanoma is thought to be the result of sun exposure. How much sun is "excessive" varies from person to person. No one is immune to the damaging effects of the sun, and everyone should avoid unnecessary sun exposure.[84] Individuals living near the equator and in Australia have much higher rates of melanoma, and in the U.S., the greatest occurrence of malignant melanoma is in the Southeast and Southwest. Often individuals who develop melanoma have fair skin that burns and freckles easily, light eyes and either red or blond hair.[84]

Melanoma generally occurs in areas that are exposed to the sun — in women the primary areas of occurrence are the back, the face and the lower legs; and in men the torso is the most common. Melanoma occurs most frequently among black people on the palms, the soles, and under the nails (these occurrence sites are less common among white people).[84] Melanoma can also occur on other areas of the body. If this skin cancer does travel to distant sites, the chances of survival from this cancer are greatly reduced. Again, early detection is essential.

Twenty to 30 percent of melanomas begin in the pigment cells of moles. Because everyone has moles, please do not be alarmed with every mole — most moles are harmless. The key is to learn to recognize normal moles from "abnormal" looking moles.

A normal mole is an evenly-colored brown, tan, or black spot in the skin. Normal moles are also flat or raised, and their shape is round or oval and with sharply defined borders. Moles are generally less than six millimeters in diameter (about the size of a pencil eraser). A mole may be present at birth or may appear spontaneously, usually in the first few decades of life. Sometimes several moles appear at about the same time, especially in sun-exposed areas of the skin. Once a mole has fully developed, the size, shape, or color normally remains the same for many years. Most moles eventually fade away in older persons.

A sudden or continuous change in a mole's appearance is a sign that you should see your physician.[87] Sometimes these are atypical moles that run in the family. These moles themselves may turn into melanomas or they may serve as markers which identify the individual at higher risk for melanoma developing elsewhere in the skin.

Some "birthmarks," otherwise called congenital moles, may also carry an increased risk of melanoma. Sometimes these moles should be removed before malignant changes can take place.[84]

People who have many moles or certain types of atypical moles and those with relatives who have had melanoma are more likely to develop this kind of cancer. Aside from these factors, melanoma most often occurs among people who work or spend a great deal of recreational time in the sun, especially if they have been severely sunburned in their teens or twenties.

Researchers recommend the removal of all moles that meet any of the following criteria:[84,87]

- Present at birth, no matter what the size;
- Larger than one-centimeter in diameter;
- In hidden places (like the scalp, mouth, vagina, or anus) that cannot be easily observed for changes in color or shape.

Yearly or Periodic Health Check #6
and
Monthly Health Check #3

CLINICAL TESTICULAR EXAMINATION
AND TESTICULAR SELF-EXAMINATION

Why Perform

- Testicular cancer is the most common form of cancer in men ages 20 to 34 years, and the second most common for men 35 to 39.[91]
- Although testicular cancer is uncommon, this form of cancer results in significant degree of disability and death among young men.[91]
- If caught early, this is one of the most curable cancers; if not, it is one of the most deadly.[91]
- The testicle is an organ that is readily accessible to examination by the individual. Also, most testicular cancers are first discovered by men themselves.[91]
- Because testicular cancer often develops without symptoms, an important practice is for men to perform the simple testicular self-examination.[91]

Approximately 5,100 new cases of testicular cancer are diagnosed each year. Testicular cancer is **highly** curable, if detected **early**. (The five-year survival rate of early diagnosed testicular cancer [Stage I] is now 91 to 99 percent).[90]

Men who have the following conditions are at increased risk for testicular cancer.

- **Failure of a testicle to descend into the scrotum (cryptorchidism).**
- **Suturing of an undescended testicle to the scrotum (orchiopexy).**
- **Reduction in size of a testicle (or testicular atrophy).**
- **Also, white males have a 4.5 times higher risk than black males.**[91]

How Performed

CLINICAL EXAMINATION

Following puberty, the testicles, part of the male reproductive system, produce the male hormone, testosterone, and sperm. To determine whether the testicles are normal, the physician palpates the testicles and the surrounding structures as part of a periodic physical examination. This painless procedure only takes a few minutes to perform. While having your clinical testicular exam, ask your doctor to further instruct you on how to perform the testicular self exam.

In many patients, testicular tumors are first detected by the doctor as part of a routine physical examination. For this reason, the testicular self examination cannot be substituted for a physician testicular exam.

TESTICULAR SELF-EXAMINATION

The routine testicular screening self-examination helps familiarize men with what feels "normal" pertaining to their testicular anatomy, making detection of any abnormal characteristics such as a lump or swelling in one of the testicles easier. The examination should be done once a month. Choose the same day of each month to help you remember when to perform the self-exam. Preferably, the exam should be performed after a warm bath or shower when the scrotal skin is most relaxed.

To perform the testicular self-exam, refer to the four steps outlined below by the U.S. Public Health Service.

1. Stand naked in front of a mirror. Look for any swelling on the skin of the scrotum. One testicle may hang lower or be larger than the other; this is normal.
2. Examine each testicle gently with both hands. The index and middle fingers should be placed underneath the testicle while the thumbs are placed on the top. Roll each testicle gently between the thumbs and the fingers (see Figure 1).
3. Find the epididymis (a cord-like structure on the top back of the testicle that stores and transports sperm). Do not confuse the epididymis with an abnormal lump.
4. Feel for any small lumps — about the size of a pea — on the front or the side of the testicle. These lumps are usually painless. If any hard lumps are found, see your doctor as soon as possible.

Figure 1: Testicular Self -Exam

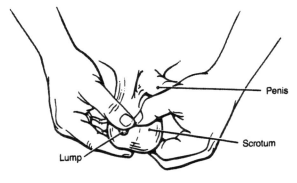

Used by permission. The American Cancer Society: Cancer Book; *Doubleday and Company, Inc., New York.*

In addition to the testicular self-examination, please be advised of the following conditions that should be brought to the attention of your doctor. If you:

*   Cannot find one or both testicles;
*   Feel a soft collection of thin tubes above the testicle, (this may be a varicocele, which is a collection of dilated veins in the scrotum);
*   If you notice the rapid onset of pain, swelling, or heaviness in the scrotum, lower abdomen or groin. (These symptoms are rarely caused by testicular cancer, but may represent an infection or blockage of blood flow to the testicle which requires prompt medical attention);
*   Have painless swelling, or a change in the consistency of the testicles.

Please place a check in your Health Check Table for the first few times you perform this exam and before long the practice will be a habit.

TREATMENT

Just a word about treatment. A suspected testicular tumor may require surgical exploration and biopsy through an incision above the groin to verify the diagnosis. If a mass within the testicle is discovered, the entire testicle is usually removed surgically. The malignancy is almost always confined to one testicle. For cosmetic purposes, an artificial testicle made of medical plastic can often be inserted at the time of surgery, or at a later date. Virility and fertility are not affected, since one testicle is adequate for maintaining sexual and reproductive function.[92, 93]

After surgical removal of the affected testicle, treatment is determined by the type of cancer involved and whether the cancer has spread. In some instances, the surgical removal of lymph nodes and chemotherapy or radiation therapy may be necessary.

Penalty For Neglect

The main reason men don't perform testicular self-exams is because they simply forget. Men also put off seeing their physician about concerns they may have regarding their testicles because the early symptoms of testicular cancer are generally mild, or they may be fearful of having cancer.[93] These untimely delays can result in the spread of the testicular cancer to the lymph nodes and other areas of the body, reducing the likelihood of successful treatment.

Yearly or Periodic Health Check #7

SCREENING FOR THYROID DISEASE

RECOMMENDATIONS

1. As part of your periodic physical examination, your physician should palpate the thyroid gland, checking for nodules or enlargement.[46]

2. A prudent approach for individuals at high-risk for thyroid disease is to have thyroid screening tests such as a serum T4 test. Women age 60 and older should consider periodic thyroid function tests (after consulting with their primary-care physician).[94, 389]

Individuals at increased risk for thyroid disease include:[94]

- **Persons with symptoms such as neck mass or hoarseness;**
- **Women over age 60;**
- **Individuals who have received low-dose upper-body irradiation during infancy, childhood, or adolescence;**
- **Persons with a family history of multiple endocrine tumors.**

Why Perform

- About two to three percent of the U.S. population have hypo- or hyperthyroid disease, conditions especially common in women and older adults.[94, 95]
- The estimates for thyroid cancer include: Approximately 11,000 people in the U.S. will be diagnosed each year, and approximately 1,000 people will die from this cancer.[66, 94]
- The five-year survival rate for thyroid cancer is now over 90 percent.[66]
- Palpation of the thyroid gland is easily performed as part of the periodic physical examination.[46]

The word thyroid is derived from the Greek word *thyreos*, meaning "shield," and the word *eidos*, meaning "form." The thyroid gland partially forms around the neck's thyroid cartilage and the upper rings of the trachea, and has a shield-like appearance. Although the thyroid is a rather small gland, symptoms resulting from thyroid disease are great.

Hyperthyroidism can result in:[94]

restlessness	emotional instability
insomnia	heat intolerance
shortness of breath	heart palpitations
eye disease	diarrhea
muscle wasting	weakness
tremors	rapid heart rate

Hypothyroidism can cause:[94]

lethargy	confusion
poor memory	cold intolerance
weight gain	constipation
loss of hair	shortness of breath
muscle tenderness	increased sensation such as numbness, prickling, and tingling

Individuals, whose physicians detect thyroid problems, feel a great relief to determine a "reason" for the "nonspecific and insidious symptoms attributed mistakenly to other medical or psychiatric causes."[94]

One group of people who should especially be aware of the need for early detection of thyroid cancer is the approximately one million Americans who underwent low-dose upper-body irradiation as children or adolescents. Perhaps as many as 90,000 of these individuals have irradiated-related cancers.[94-96]

The good news is that through early detection of thyroid disease or thyroid cancer, successful treatment is possible.

How Performed

During your routine physical examination, your doctor will simply examine the thyroid gland by moving his or her fingers around the entire area of the thyroid gland. Your doctor will be feeling for lumps or anything that feels "abnormal" as it pertains to size and consistency. The test is quickly performed and does not cause any discomfort. Whether or not your doctor will be able to detect any abnormality is not always certain, but minimal time spent palpating the gland is well worth the check.[46]

For individuals at high risk for developing thyroid disease, the doctor may order a thyroid blood screening test. When "stimulated" by a pituitary hormone called "thyroid-stimulating hormone" (TSH), the thyroid gland produces two types of hormones that help to regulate the metabolism of the body. The two thyroid-produced hormones are called thyroxine (T4) and triiodothyronine (T3). When your doctor orders a thyroid blood test, these two hormones are measured.

In addition, the laboratory will calculate an index referred to as *free thyroxine index* (FTI). This index is calculated by multiplying the T4 value by the T3 value.[97] Greater values may be indicative of hyperthyroidism and lower than normal values, hypothyroidism.

With your medical history, and the blood test results, your doctor can make a decision as to whether or not further thyroid testing is needed.

Yearly or Periodic Health Check #8
and
Monthly Health Check #4

CLINICAL ORAL CAVITY EXAMINATION
AND ORAL CAVITY SELF-EXAMINATION

RECOMMENDATIONS

1. As part of your periodic physical examination and your regular dental check-up, your physician and dentist should inspect your oral cavity, screening for oral cancer. These clinical exams should especially be performed on all individuals at increased risk for oral cancer.

2. All adults ages 40 and older should perform regular oral cavity self-examinations.[98] This recommendation is **especially** important for individuals who are at increased risk for developing oral cancer. See your *Health Check Table* for keeping record of your participation with this health check.

    Individuals who are high risk for oral cancer include:[99]

    - **Persons who smoke cigarettes, pipes or cigars;**
    - **Persons who use snuff and chewing tobacco;**
    - **Persons who drink alcohol excessively;**
    - **Persons over the age of 45 years.**

3. All adults should be counseled to:[99]

    - Receive regular dental check-ups (see *Lifestyle Counseling Health Check #3, Dental Health*, page 132);
    - Discontinue the use of all forms of tobacco and limit the use of alcohol consumption (see *Lifestyle Counseling Health Check #1, Substance Use*, page 123);
    - Take protective measures to protect lips and skin from prolonged exposure to ultraviolet rays (see *Daily Health Check #11, Skin Cancer Prevention*, page 92).

Why Perform

- Oral cancer accounts for about six percent of all cancers.[100]
- Estimates indicated that in 1989 alone approximately 30,000 newly diagnosed cases and 8,600 deaths would occur due to oral cancer.[66, 98]
- If detected early, oral cancers are highly curable, but if the cancer has spread to other sites, then the outlook is quite grim.

The primary tool for screening and detecting oral cancer is through clinical inspection of the oral cavity by your doctor and/or dentist and through self-inspection. The risk of developing oral cancer is very low in individuals who do not smoke cigars, pipes or cigarettes or use tobacco products such as snuff and chewless tobacco, and who do not drink alcohol in excess.[98-100] Occasionally oral cancer occurs in persons without these risk factors.

Many sores can and do occur in the mouth that are not cancerous in nature, such as a cold sore. Other harmless ulcerations may occur as a result of the foods we eat or due to rough teeth. However, any sore or ulcer that develops in the mouth or throat and doesn't appear to be healing or seems to bleed easily, should be immediately evaluated by your doctor.[100]

Other oral cavity concerns to discuss with your doctor include:

- **A lump or thickening;**
- **A whitish patch;**
- **A persistent sore throat;**
- **Difficulty in swallowing or chewing food;**
- **A feeling that you have something present in your throat.**[100]

Keep in mind that pain is most often **not** a symptom of oral cancer.

How Performed

CLINICAL EXAM BY DOCTOR AND DENTIST

The oral cavity examination, performed by your doctor and dentist, includes a detailed inspection of your entire mouth cavity. Your doctor will use his gloved hand and a small gauze sponge to grasp your tongue. The tongue will then be moved about to allow closer inspection of the mouth. To examine certain parts of your oral cavity, a mirror will be required.

Your doctor should also palpate the tongue, the floor of the mouth, the salivary glands, and check the lymph nodes of your neck.[46, 98]

ORAL CAVITY SELF-EXAMINATION

Your tongue is a great detective when it comes to discovering potential oral cavity problems. As previously indicated, be certain to report to your doctor any new ulcers or troublesome areas (such as a whitish patch or a lump or thickening) that appear in your oral cavity and do not resolve themselves within a week or two. You may choose also to use a mirror in a well-lighted room to inspect your oral cavity for any suspicious areas. Be certain to move your tongue up, down and to the sides so you can better see the mouth.

PREVENTION

As important as the oral cavity clinical and self-exam are, perhaps even **more** important are the preventive measures you should take to **avoid** oral cancer, such as avoiding the use of tobacco products and drinking excessively. Estimates suggest that over 90 percent of all oropharyngeal cancer (cancer of the back portion of the mouth) is a result of cigarette smoking.[99, 101]

Yearly or Periodic Health Check #9

BLOOD CHOLESTEROL SCREENING

RECOMMENDATIONS

1. All adults age 20 years and older should be tested to determine their blood cholesterol level.[102] Record the date of your test and your cholesterol value in your *Health Check Table*.

2. Individuals with a "desirable cholesterol" (levels below 200 mg/dl) should have their cholesterol measured at least once **every five years**.[102, 383]

3. Individuals with a total cholesterol greater than 200 mg/dl should consult with their primary-care physician to:

   - Determine if lipoproteins (HDL and LDL) and triglycerides should be measured;
   - Review other risk factors for coronary heart disease;
   - Review follow-up guidelines established by the National Cholesterol Education Program Committee.

4. Clinically accepted classification of blood cholesterol is depicted below:[102]

   TOTAL CHOLESTEROL

< 200 mg/dl	Desirable Blood Cholesterol
200-239 mg/dl	Borderline High-Risk Blood Cholesterol
> 240 mg/dl	High-Risk Blood Cholesterol

   LDL-CHOLESTEROL

<130 mg/dl	Desirable LDL-cholesterol
130-159 mg/dl	Borderline High-Risk LDL-cholesterol
> 160 mg/dl	High-Risk LDL-cholesterol

5. Individuals with a family history of early heart disease (family members under age 55 with diagnosed heart disease) should consult with their physician to determine if lipoproteins (HDL and LDL) should be measured.

Why Perform

- A major cause of coronary heart disease – resulting in more than 1.5 million heart attacks and 520,000 deaths each year in the U.S. – is increased levels of blood cholesterol.[52, 103, 104]
- Cholesterol levels predict future occurrence of death and disability from coronary heart disease.[102]
- For every one percent reduction in blood cholesterol there is a two percent reduction in the risk for developing coronary heart disease (CHD).[102, 105]
- Once identified through screening, high blood cholesterol levels can be lowered by following established guidelines.[102]

Atherosclerosis. "Man is only as old as his arteries." This statement made centuries ago by Leonardo da Vinci has major relevance in our society today. Atherosclerosis, the build up of cholesterol, fat and other substances in the walls of the arteries, represents the number one cause of death and disability among most industrialized nations.[104]

The National Cholesterol Education Program (NCEP) Committee has summarized the conclusive evidence demonstrating the direct association between high blood cholesterol and CHD. These findings support the high-priority need for physicians and every American adult to detect, evaluate and treat high blood cholesterol. In fact, the NCEP panel has concluded that medical research proves "beyond a reasonable doubt" that by reducing total blood cholesterol and LDL-cholesterol, you can reduce your risk for heart disease.[102]

Population Studies. Perhaps the most popular evidence associating CHD with high cholesterol is found in studies in which large populations of the world are compared. Countries in which the blood cholesterol levels of the people are high have a corresponding increase in CHD.[102] And individuals who move from a country where CHD is low to a country with a high incidence of CHD, eventually increase their level of blood cholesterol and acquire a higher risk for CHD.

Animal Studies. Studies involving monkeys and baboons have also contributed to the understanding of the relationship between CHD and high blood cholesterol. Given a typical American diet, high in fat and cholesterol, these animals have increases in blood cholesterol levels and develop atherosclerosis. When the animals are then given a diet low in cholesterol, there is an accompanying decrease in the degree of atherosclerosis.[102]

Human Studies. A popular study, the Coronary Primary Prevention Trial, involved 3,800 men (previously identified to have elevated blood cholesterol) who underwent drug and dietary therapy to reduce the cholesterol level. The results showed that for every **one percent** reduction in cholesterol there was a **two percent** reduction in the risk for coronary heart disease. In addition, those subjects that received dietary instruction coupled with cholesterol lowering medication, had a reduction in the expected rate of fatal heart attacks by 24 percent![105]

Another study by Dr. Blankenhorn showed men who had undergone coronary bypass graft surgery and had then participated in diet and drug therapy to lower their cholesterol had "slowed progression and produced regression of coronary atherosclerosis."[106, 107]

Genetics. Cardiovascular geneticist Dr. Roger R. Williams and many other investigators have also shown a genetic interaction with the association of high blood cholesterol and the incidence of CHD. Studies involving families with genetically caused blood cholesterol disorders have helped substantiate the conclusion that high cholesterol levels can lead to early or premature heart disease.

In fact, the incidence of CHD is even more pronounced in individuals with very high cholesterol levels — with the top 10 percent of people with high cholesterol having a fourfold increase in the rate of death due to CHD.[102, 106, 108]

In conclusion, Dr. Antonio Gotto, past president of the American Heart Association, has stated: *"Tens of thousands of lives could be saved each year if Americans were tested for high levels of blood cholesterol at doctors offices, clinics, schools and the work place, and those at risk were identified and treated."*

How Performed

HOW CHOLESTEROL IS MEASURED AND WHAT THE RESULTS MEAN

Blood serum cholesterol is generally measured by having a health-care worker draw blood from your arm using a small needle. You needn't be fasting and the sample can be taken any time of the day. Preferably, you should have the sample taken while in a sitting position.

Also available on the market are automated blood cholesterol machines designed to measure your cholesterol by examining a small droplet of blood obtained by a finger prick. In some instances, your doctor may suggest you have a blood cholesterol test that identifies the HDL-cholesterol (the "good" cholesterol) and the LDL-cholesterol (the "bad" cholesterol). The results of your cholesterol test is expressed in mg/dl.

NATIONAL CHOLESTEROL EDUCATION PROGRAM GUIDELINES

How to proceed after a blood cholesterol check has been carefully outlined by the National Cholesterol Education Program (NCEP) and endorsed by the American Heart Association (AHA).[102, 106] Individuals with a "desirable cholesterol level" (levels below 200 mg/dl) should have their cholesterol measured at least once **every five years**. For individuals with a total cholesterol level greater than 200 mg/dl should consult with their doctor about:

- Having LDL-cholesterol, HDL-cholesterol and triglycerides measured;
- Appropriate follow-up procedures;
- Coronary risk factors (see *Yearly or Periodic Health Check #2, Cardiac Risk Factor Screening*, page 79).

HDL-CHOLESTEROL, TOTAL CHOLESTEROL/HDL-CHOLESTEROL RATIO, AND TRIGLYCERIDES

HDL-Cholesterol. Although the NCEP committee has not made specific recommendations regarding the appropriate levels of HDL-cholesterol and triglycerides, individuals should be aware of how their values compare to the American adult population. Some cholesterol authorities have suggested the HDL-cholesterol should not be below 35 mg/dl. HDL-cholesterol, the "good-guy" lipoprotein, tends to protect one against heart disease — the higher the HDL value, the better. The NCEP has listed the following as major causes for **reduced** HDL-cholesterol:

- Cigarette smoking;
- Obesity;
- Lack of exercise;
- Use of steroids;
- Beta-blocking agents;
- Very high triglyceride values;
- Genetic factors.

Cholesterol/HDL ratio. Many primary-care doctors find the ratio of total cholesterol/HDL-cholesterol (simply divide your total cholesterol by your HDL-cholesterol) as a good indicator of one's risk for CAD. The lower the ratio of total cholesterol/HDL-cholesterol, the lower the risk for heart disease. The average risk for heart disease based upon the ratio of total cholesterol/HDL-cholesterol is:

	Men	Women
1/2 average	3.43	3.27
Average	4.97	4.44
Two times average	9.55	7.05
Three times average	22.39	11.04

William P. Castelli, HDL in Assessing Risk of Coronary Heart Disease.

Because some individuals who have a very low total cholesterol may also have a relative low HDL-cholesterol, the ratio is an important aid in determining whether or not the HDL-cholesterol is too low in comparison to the total cholesterol value.

For example, if a man's HDL-cholesterol is not very high (let's say 40 mg percent), but his total cholesterol is 160 mg percent, then the ratio of total cholesterol/HDL-cholesterol will be 4.0 (a less than average risk for heart disease).

Triglyceride. Triglyceride levels are generally used by your primary-care physician to help determine what kind of blood lipid problem a person may have. Studies have shown regular exercise, reducing the intake of simple sugars and alcohol consumption and decreasing body fat all lower the triglyceride level.

DIETARY GOALS FOR LOWERING BLOOD CHOLESTEROL

Many individuals with elevated blood cholesterol will be able to achieve the goal of lowering their cholesterol with dietary intervention. For this reason, the NCEP committee and the AHA have recommended that diet be considered as the **first line** of treatment for persons at high risk for blood cholesterol.

Table 1 makes reference to two dietary approaches recommended by the NCEP and the AHA. These two diets, Step I and Step II, are briefly outlined below:

Table 1. *Dietary Therapy of High Blood Cholesterol*

Step I Diet	
Nutrient	**Recommended Intake**
Total Fat	Less than 30% of total calories
Saturated Fatty Acids	Less than 10% of total calories
Polyunsaturated Fatty Acids	Up to 10% of total calories
Monounsaturated Fatty Acids	10 to 15% of total calories
Carbohydrates	50 to 60% of total calories
Protein	10 to 20% of total calories
Cholesterol	Less than 300 mg/day
Total Calories	To achieve and maintain desirable weight

Step II Diet	
Nutrient	**Recommended Intake**
Total Fat	Less than 30% of total calories
Saturated Fatty Acids	Less than 7% of total calories
Polyunsaturated Fatty Acids	Up to 10% of total calories
Monounsaturated Fatty Acids	10 to 15% of total calories
Carbohydrates	50 to 60% of total calories
Protein	10 to 20% of total calories
Cholesterol	Less than 200 mg/day
Total Calories	To achieve and maintain desirable weight

To assist you with the recommended dietary change, we suggest you refer to the *Daily Health Check #4, Proper Nutrition Program*, page 58.

Some individuals may also need the help of a dietician to assist them in implementing the Step 1 and Step 2 Diets into their daily eating behavior. If your primary-care physician and staff are not aware of a registered dietician in your area, you may want to consider writing the American Dietetic Association (216 W. Jackson Blvd., Suite 800, Chicago, IL, 60606) for help in locating such a person in your particular area.

Remember, a substantial reduction in one's cholesterol **can** be achieved through gradual modifications in the diet.

DRUG THERAPY FOR LOWERING CHOLESTEROL

Steps for lowering high LDL-cholesterol with drug therapy should be carefully reviewed with your primary-care physician. Generally, only after at least six months of dietary intervention are cholesterol-lowering drugs to be introduced for treatment.

Health Notes

The word *lipid* describes the various types of fats in the body. The two lipids carried through the blood are cholesterol and triglyceride. Fats and proteins are combined to form molecules called lipoproteins. The three lipoproteins that circulate in the blood are high-density lipoprotein (HDL), low-density lipoprotein (LDL), and very-low-density lipoprotein (VLDL). Illustrated below is the approximate percentage of fat and proteins carried by these lipoproteins.

The LDL contains less protein and more triglyceride than the HDL. VLDL contain primarily triglycerides as well as some cholesterol. All three contain cholesterol. The LDL carry the cholesterol that may enter the walls of the arteries, promoting atherosclerosis. The HDL removes the cholesterol that otherwise would remain as plaque in the arteries. Therefore, the HDL may help protect people from atherosclerosis.

Table 2. Approximate Composition of Lipoproteins

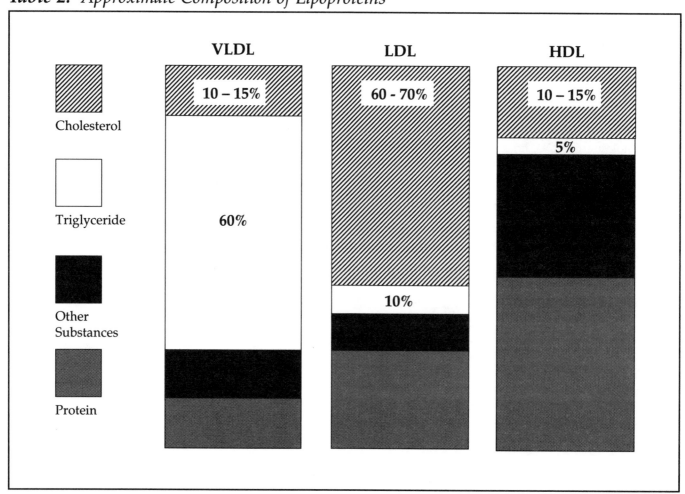

Yearly or Periodic Health Check #12

PAP TEST AND PELVIC EXAMINATION
(SCREENING FOR CERVICAL CANCER)

RECOMMENDATIONS

1. All women who are, or have been, sexually active or have reached age 18 years, should have *annual* pap tests and pelvic examinations. After a woman has had *three or more consecutive* satisfactory normal annual examinations, a Pap test may be performed at the discretion of your physician. However, a prudent recommendation for women age 20 to 65 is to have a Pap test at least every three years.[46, 109, 110, 388]

2. Record participation in this health check in your *Health Check Table*.

3. The U.S. Preventive Services Task Force has suggested that Pap smears can be discontinued after age 65, but only in conditions in which your physician can document a previous history of Pap tests that have been *consistently* normal.[111] The American College of Physicians recommend a screening Pap smear every three years for women age 65 to 75 who have not been screened within 10 years prior to age 66.[388] We would suggest you visit with your physician about this recommendation if you are 65 years or older.

Why Perform

- Cervical cancer is one of the most common cancers — two percent of all women are affected by this cancer by age 80, with approximately 7,000 deaths per year in the United States.[109]
- The number of deaths from cervical cancer has decreased by about 50 percent since 1950, due largely to screening for early detection.[110, 111]
- Cervical cancer, when detected and treated in the earliest stages is almost 100 percent curable, but if diagnosis and treatment are delayed, the cure rate is only 50 percent.[109]
- The pelvic examination may reveal other reproductive organ problems.

Female cancer is **highly curable** if detected and treated early. Unfortunately, only *half* of the women with invasive cervical cancer are cured because the disease has not been found soon enough.[109]

A recent study designed to assess the effects of cervical cancer screening among women in the Scandinavian countries confirmed the positive benefit of the Pap test in reducing death and disability from cervical cancer. The lead investigator, Dr. N. E. Day, indicated the data showed that "...mass screening scheduled every two to five years can reduce the incidence of invasive cervical cancer by **80 percent**," and that "...the more negative smears a woman has had, the less risk there is of her developing an invasive tumor."[110, 112]

Generally, women who are at high-risk for developing cervical cancer will require closer surveillance such as a yearly Pap smear. The risk factors that have been identified to increase a woman's chance of certain gynecological cancers include:[109-111]

- Over age 40;
- First intercourse at an early age;
- Diabetes;
- Mothers took DES while pregnant;
- Strong family history of gynecological cancer;
- History of infertility, abnormal uterine bleeding, obesity, failure to ovulate, and abnormal Pap tests;
- Multiple sexual partners.

In conclusion, early detection through regular screening — before symptoms appear — is the key to preventing cervical cancer.

How Performed

FEMALE REPRODUCTIVE ANATOMY

The female reproductive sites are illustrated below:

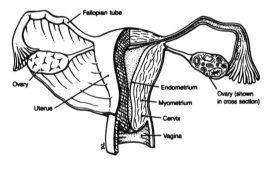

Figure 1: *View of Female Reproductive Organs (from Back)*
Used by permission. The American Cancer Society: Cancer Book; Doubleday and Company, Inc., New York

Cancer can develop in any of the female reproductive sites shown in Figure 1. The greatest incidence of cancer occurs in the cervix and the endometrium, followed by the ovaries. Less frequent is cancer of the vulva and vagina, and cancer of the fallopian tubes is quite rare.[111]

PELVIC EXAMINATION AND PAP SMEAR

The pelvic examination should take place in a comfortable well-lighted room. You will be asked to undress and cover-up with a clinical gown. Your doctor will ask you to lie on your back on the examining table. The table will most likely have stirrups attached to either side and near the end of the table. You will be asked to bring your knees towards your chest and to then place your feet in the stirrups.

To help your doctor keep the vagina open and to improve visualization, a speculum — an instrument shaped like a duck's beak — will be used. The speculum may initially feel cold, but the examination should not hurt. If you do feel pain, you should tell your physician. Deep slow breaths can help you relax.

Once the speculum is in place, your doctor will use a cotton swab and/or a spatula to scrape cells from the opening of the cervix and the wall of the vagina near the cervix. The specimen will be placed on a glass slide and then stained for observation. This procedure is called the Pap test.[111, 113]

The Pap test, named after the late Dr. George Papanicolaou, is without pain; it is relatively simple to perform, and is 90 percent accurate.[109] To prevent disturbing the cells of the vagina and the cervix, women should avoid the use of "tampons, birth-control foams or jellies, or douches" for a few days prior to the Pap test.[109]

In addition to the Pap test, your doctor will examine the vagina, cervix, uterus and rectum for growths or other abnormalities. The physician will gently press on the abdomen with one hand to feel for any unusual growths in the uterus or ovaries. There may be a slight discharge following the exam, so it is advisable to bring a thin sanitary napkin to the examination room.[109] Your physician should report any findings to you as the examination progresses. Don't hesitate to ask questions.

Finally, the U.S. Task Force recommends that your physician be certain to submit your Pap test specimen to a laboratory that has been shown to have appropriate quality control measures to further guarantee that your results are accurate.[111]

Penalty For Neglect

Dr. S. C. Gusberg of the Mount Sinai School of Medicine (New York City) states:

"Many women delay seeking a diagnosis through fear: fear of cancer itself, fear of loss of pelvic organs, fear of surgery or of anesthesia, fear of loss of childbearing or of sexual ability, fear of invalidism or of aging brought about by loss of the sexual organs."

His reassurance for women who share in these fears is that early detection of cancer — prior to symptoms — permits treatment without the loss of sexual function, pelvic organs, or "femininity."[109]

Yearly or Periodic Health Check #13 and #14
Monthly Health Check #1
and
High-Risk Health Check #7

PHYSICIAN BREAST EXAMINATION, MAMMOGRAPHY, AND BREAST SELF-EXAM

(SCREENING FOR BREAST CANCER)

RECOMMENDATIONS

1. Women should have a breast examination performed by their physician or professional staff member at least:
   - **Every year after age 40; and/or**
   - **Whenever a physical examination occurs.**[114]

2. Beginning at age 40, women should have a mammogram every **one to two years** until the age of 50. (This frequency is recommended by the National Cancer Institute and the American Cancer Society. The American College of Physicians and the USPSTF recommend yearly mammograms for women in their 40s if they have a family history of breast cancer or if they are otherwise at increased risk.) After age 50, the mammogram should be performed **each year.**[114,]

3. Women who have a personal history of breast cancer should have a mammogram yearly.[114, 383]

4. Woman should practice breast self-examination on a monthly basis (see page 114 for details).[114]

5. Women should become familiar with the primary and secondary risk factors for developing breast cancer. These risk factors, compiled by the American Cancer Society, are listed below:

PRIMARY RISK FACTORS
- Advancing age — In 1987, about 45 percent of breast cancers occurred in women over age 65.
- Personal history — Previous breast cancer.
- Family history — Breast cancer that developed before menopause in a woman's mother or sister.

These three factors account for 85 to 90 percent of the risk for developing breast cancer. **But**, 70 percent of women who are diagnosed with breast cancer do not have **primary** risk factors.

SECONDARY RISK FACTORS
- Family history — Breast cancer in maternal grandmother or aunts.
- Obesity.
- Pregnancy history — No pregnancies, or first birth after age 30.
- Menstrual periods — Onset of menstruation before age 10 and menopause after age 55.
- Previous cancer — Cancer previously identified anywhere else in your body and especially uterus, ovary, and colon.
- Exposure to radiation — Excessive and prolonged exposure to ionizing radiation, primarily in certain occupations, will increase your risk.
- Alcohol consumption — New research indicates excessive alcohol consumption over sustained periods increases the risk of breast cancer.

These minor risk factors account for 10-15 percent of the risk for developing breast cancer.

Why Perform

- Breast cancer is the most frequent cancer in females. Approximately **one out of every ten women** will develop breast cancer during her lifetime.[114]
- Breast cancer is second only to lung cancer as the leading cause of death from cancer.[114]
- When breast cancer is detected in the early stages, the survival rate is excellent (**90 percent**).[114]
- The physician breast examination and the mammogram are proven methods for detecting early breast cancer and significantly lowering death rates.[114]

Perhaps the most dramatic illustration of why early detection practices save lives is illustrated in Figure 1.

Figure 1: Sizes of Breast Lumps
Used by permission of the American Cancer Society

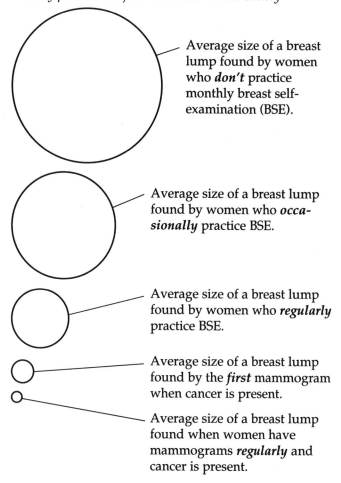

Average size of a breast lump found by women who *don't* practice monthly breast self-examination (BSE).

Average size of a breast lump found by women who *occasionally* practice BSE.

Average size of a breast lump found by women who *regularly* practice BSE.

Average size of a breast lump found by the *first* mammogram when cancer is present.

Average size of a breast lump found when women have mammograms *regularly* and cancer is present.

Early Detection Pays Off. Women who are following the breast cancer screening health checks have an **85 to 90 percent** chance of finding and treating breast cancer suc-

cessfully.

One study involving 62,000 women had one-half of the women receive a professional breast examination and two-view mammography and the remaining half follow their usual practices in receiving medical care. Eighteen years of follow-up showed a **30 percent reduction** in death due to breast cancer in the women receiving the professional breast exam and mammography.[69, 114, 115]

Mammogram Only? Some women feel assured to have a mammogram **only**, and they neglect having the physician breast examination. This is a **false assurance**! From five to 10 percent of the cancerous breast tumors are detected by the physician breast exam but **not** by mammography.[69]

These facts aren't meant to frighten you, but to incite you to action.

In conclusion, we like the poster of The American Cancer Society in which a normal mammogram of a breast is shown and beneath the x-ray is the statement, "Now breast cancer has virtually nowhere to hide."

How Performed

PHYSICIAN (PROFESSIONAL) BREAST EXAMINATION

To perform the breast exam, your doctor will give you a patient gown and ask you to remove any clothing above your waist. Your doctor will visually inspect your breasts, looking for changes in shape or size; skin dimpling, scaling, or puckering; secretion from the nipples; or any other changes from the usual.

Your doctor will then examine your breasts, chest and armpits, feeling the tissue for lumps and attempting to distinguish any unusual findings from the "lumps and bumps" that can normally arise within the breast.[116]

Pay special attention to the way the examination is performed—the procedure can serve as an excellent guide for your breast self-exam. You may want to demonstrate to your doctor how you are performing breast self-exams and invite your physician to offer constructive criticism.

Mention to your doctor any discomfort or unusual feeling that isn't like your normal premenstrual breast tenderness. **One-third** of breast cancers manifest themselves by a change in the way your breast feels rather than by a lump large enough to be felt by you or your care provider.

Consider asking your doctor the following questions:

- What should I look for when I do breast self-examinations?
- How can I distinguish lumps from other parts of my breast?
- Do you have a rubber breast model that I can use to increase my skills for detecting a breast lump?
- Based upon my personal history do my risk factors suggest I have a physician breast examination and/or mammogram on a more regular interval?

MAMMOGRAM

A mammogram is a low-dose X-ray of the breast used to detect abnormalities and identify tumors up to *two years* before they can be felt by you or your physician. Experts agree that the monthly breast self-exam and periodic physician exam must be combined with mammography.[116]

Schedule your mammogram appointment for a time when your breasts are not swollen or tender — between five and 10 days after your menstrual period. The do's and don'ts for this test include:

- **Don't** wear deodorant, perfume or powder;
- **Do** wear two-piece clothing to the appointment;
- **Do** tell your doctor if you are breast feeding;
- **Do** tell your doctor if there is any chance you might be pregnant;
- **Do** tell your doctor if you have breast implants.

To perform the exam you will be asked to disrobe from the waist up, to put on a gown, and to remove any jewelry around your neck. Depending upon the type of X-ray equipment used, you will be asked to stand or sit. Your breast will be positioned on a resting plate (this contains the X-ray film) and a compressor devise will be lowered onto your breast to further flatten the breast tissue. The pressure on your breasts may cause some slight discomfort. Generally, two pictures are taken of each breast, a top view and a side view. This procedure usually takes about 15 minutes. Feel free to visit with the technician about any questions or concerns you have.

Many women have the notion that mammography isn't necessary unless there are breast cancer symptoms present. *This is not the case!* A screening mammogram can detect breast problems well before any noticeable physical symptoms present themselves, and for this reason the screening mammogram is **especially** intended for women who have no symptoms.

If the mammogram is used for women who have symptoms, then the procedure is referred to as a *diagnostic mammogram*; generally more X-ray views are taken than would be taken for a screening mammogram.

Finally, women who have had breast implants sometimes feel that a mammogram is no longer necessary. *This also is not the case.*

BREAST SELF-EXAMINATION

Breasts vary in size, shape, and texture. Because of this varied anatomy, it is normal for the breasts to feel lumpy or uneven. In fact, about 70 percent of women have breasts that are nodular, lumpy by nature.

Most breast cancers are discovered by women performing breast self-examinations (**BSE**). BSE should be done *each month* approximately five to seven days after your menstrual cycle when the breasts are least likely to be swollen or tender. If you no longer menstruate, check your breasts on an easy-to-remember date each month.

Don't panic if you find a lump! Always have a new lump checked by your physician, but remember: **four out of five** breast lumps are not cancerous.[116] Be aware that the non-cancerous lump may also swell or become painful with hormone changes associated with the menstrual cycle. (These lumps are not generally considered a greater risk of breast cancer.)

One way to keep track of the noncancerous (benign) lumps unique to your breast is to make a "map" of your breasts (see Figure 2). Using the diagram below, make a dot, circle, or x where you find a lump the first month. Do it again the next month. Within two to three months you'll have an accurate map of where your lumps are.

Figure 2: Breast Map

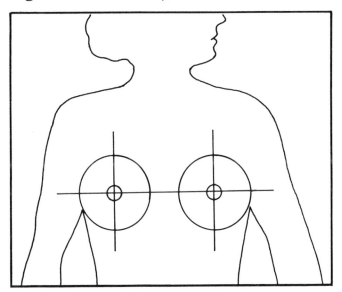

We suggest you refer to Figure 3 and its accompanying description when performing your BSE:[116]

Figure 3. *How to Do Breast Self-Exam*

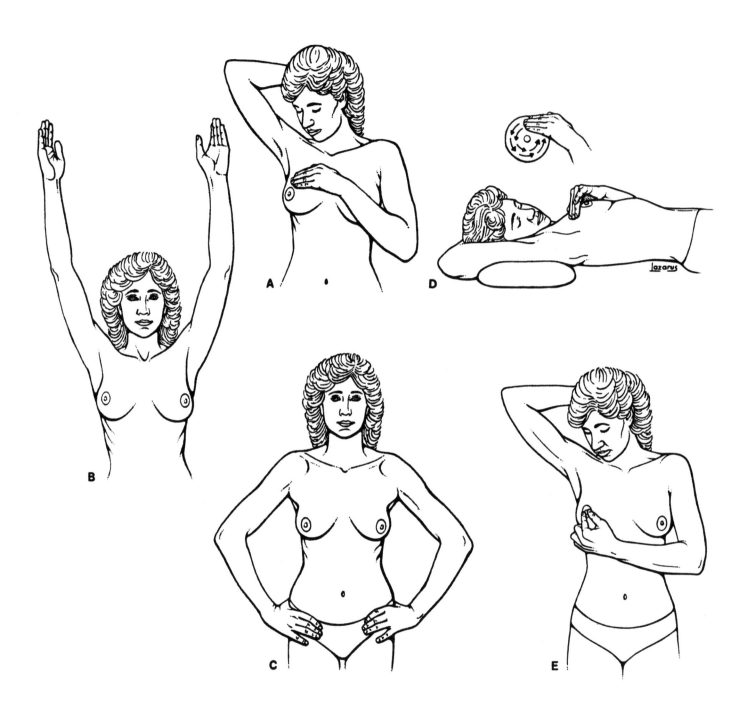

All women should examine their breasts each month. For menstruating women, this should be done in midcycle; for others, at a specific time each month. The three-step examination starts in the shower or tub, by carefully feeling each breast for any thickening or lumps (A). Then stand before a mirror, first with arms overhead and then lowered; look for any changes, such as puckering of the skin (B and C). Next, lie down and place one arm under your head. Using the other hand, examine the entire breast, moving clockwise and from the outer portion toward the nipple (D). Repeat this procedure on the second breast, placing the opposite arm under your head. Finally, squeeze each nipple to see if there is a discharge (E). Any lump, change, discharge or other unusual finding should be checked by a doctor.

Used by permission. The American Cancer Society: Cancer Book; *Doubleday and Company, Inc., New York.*

Yearly or Periodic Health Check #15
and
High-Risk Health Check #3

HEARING TEST
(SCREENING FOR HEARING LOSS)

Why Perform

- Estimates suggest that over 17 million Americans have some type of hearing problem.[117, 118]

- There are approximately five million Americans who are at high-risk for hearing loss due to their occupational exposure to excessive noise (such as factory, maintenance, and farm workers).[117, 119]

- The type of hearing loss that generally occurs with aging "becomes increasingly common after age 50."[117,120]

- The U.S. Preventive Services Task Force reports the following incidence of hearing impairment in older adults:

  - **23 percent of persons aged 65 to 74;**
  - **33 percent of those aged 75 to 84;**
  - **48 percent of persons aged 85 and older.**[117]

Hearing impairment, if left undetected and uncorrected, can not only be very frustrating, but in the elderly this problem can lead to "social isolation, depression, reduced mobility, and an exacerbation of coexisting psychiatric conditions."[117, 121, 122]

Unfortunately, as hearing impairment progresses with age, many people fail to take advantage of screening believing there is little that can be done to correct the problem.[117, 123, 124] In truth, **many** people benefit from the detection and treatment of hearing loss as diagnosed by a hearing test.

How Performed

As part of your periodic health examination, your doctor will inspect your ear canal. In some instances, a hearing problem may be due to a build-up of wax in the ear canal — this wax can easily be removed by the doctor. Let your doctor know if you have a history of hearing impairment. If you have had hearing problems, your doctor should:

- **Determine if additional hearing tests are necessary;**
- **Determine if you should see an ear, nose and throat (ENT) physician.**

For individuals who have evidence of hearing loss, an otoscopic examination should be performed by a physician, and audiometry testing should be conducted by a trained audiologist. These hearing tests are designed to test for:

- *Degree:* This refers to the volume above normal that is necessary to be able to hear.
- *Configuration:* This "describes the range of pitches (or frequencies) at which the loss has occurred."
- *Type:* This refers to the probable cause of the hearing loss — when the auditory system has a problem.[125]

The physician will be primarily involved in determining the type of hearing loss and the audiologist will assist individuals by determining the degree and configuration of hearing loss.

Audiology tests are not painful and are easily performed. The test may be conducted in a soundproof room, and the person being examined may be required to wear earphones. During the examination, various words and tones will be heard and the audiologist will ask the patient to identify these sounds. Using this information, the physician and audiologist can determine the best course of treatment, including the fitting of a hearing aid.

Yearly or Periodic Health Check #16
and
High Risk Health Check #26

TONOMETRY

(SCREENING FOR GLAUCOMA)

AND VISUAL ACUITY

RECOMMENDATIONS

1. Individuals age 40 to 64 should be screened for increased eye pressure approximately every two to four years.[126, 394] Individuals age 65 or older should be screened every one to two years.[126, 394] Record in your *Health Check Table* when you participate in this health check.

2. People at high risk for glaucoma may require testing at an earlier age than 40. More frequent examinations may also be necessary.[127, 128]

   Individuals at risk for developing glaucoma include:[126-129]

   - **family history of glaucoma;**
   - **diabetic;**
   - **black race;***
   - **previous eye injury;**
   - **previous eye surgery;**
   - **taking cortisone medication;**
   - **elderly (occurrence is two to four percent in people over 75).**

3. Individuals with existing eye problems should follow the recommendations of their eye doctor regarding frequency of eye examinations.

* (Blacks should be screened every three to five years between ages 20 to 39.[394])

Why Perform

- Glaucoma is the second leading cause of new cases of blindness in the U.S. — affecting nearly two million people.[126, 128]
- Estimates suggest that there are a million people with *undetected glaucoma*, and that over 8.5 million individuals suffer from visual impairment.[126, 130, 131]
- Although glaucoma cannot be prevented, early detection and treatment can prevent blindness from this disease.[126]
- Vision problems, especially in the elderly, may be closely associated with "injuries due to falls and motor vehicle accidents, diminished productivity, and loss of independence."[123, 130]
- Many older adults are not aware of their visual changes and up to **25 percent** of these people may be using an improper lens prescription.[123, 130]

Why A Glaucoma Check? One of the leading causes of blindness in people over 40 is glaucoma, a disease that affects nearly 300,000 new people each year in the United States.[126] The good news is that treatment for preventing blindness from glaucoma is most effective. Glaucoma doesn't generally warn its victims with obvious symptoms until the disease is far advanced.[132] For this reason, we recommend tonometry (a procedure to check for unusually high eye pressure) be periodically performed.

Why A Visual Acuity Test? In addition to preventing blindness through periodic tonometry screens, we recommend that individuals maintain a reasonable surveillance of their personal vision, and that older adults have eye examinations every year or two.

Age is the greatest predictor of vision impairment. For older individuals, visual deficits can be a major disability, often interfering with normal daily activities. Maintaining normal visual acuity can greatly assist in preventing injuries in the elderly such as falls and motor vehicle crashes. In addition, corrective lenses can also improve the independence of these individuals with vision impairments.[130]

How Performed

The human eye is filled with a jelly-like fluid that gives the eye its oval shape. Although the cause of glaucoma is not exactly known, in the early stages of this disease the pressure of the eye's fluid begins to increase in the front of the eye. This increased pressure eventually causes a rise in pressure at the back of the eye where the retina is located (the retina transfers light signals to the brain).

If left untreated, the pressure eventually pushes against the retina restricting its normal blood supply. Initially, the effects of the blood restriction is a reduction in peripheral vision (the ability to see to the side). Eventually, the disease can cause the loss of central vision or total blindness.[133]

If your family members have had glaucoma, be certain to mention this to your doctor during your periodic physical examination. In addition, tell your doctor if you have had an eye injury or eye operation and whether or not you have noticed any vague problems with your vision.

GLAUCOMA SCREENING — TONOMETRY

The most common screening test for glaucoma is called tonometry. There are three different types of tonometry tests; all are designed to test the amount of pressure in the eye. If the pressure measurement is greater than 21 mm Hg in **either** eye, or if there is a difference in pressure between the eyes of more than 6 mm Hg, then you should be encouraged to see an eye specialist: an ophthalmologist.

The test is relatively simple and only takes a couple of minutes to perform. Two of the three types of tonometry tests require a few drops of anesthetic to be placed on the surface of your eye. This is not painful, however.

ASSESSING VISUAL ACUITY

In addition to the testing for glaucoma, your eye doctor will most likely perform a series of additional tests designed to check the eyes for:

- Refractiveness;
- Conditions such as cataracts or corneal problems;
- Retinal problems.

These examinations are painless and the only possible bothersome part of the exam is having the eyes dilated. Simply wearing dark glasses (until the medicine used for dilating the eyes wears off) will easily take care of the possible discomfort.

PROTECTING YOUR EYES FROM INJURY

In addition to recommending screening for glaucoma, the National Society to Prevent Blindness encourages people of all ages to maintain a lifetime of good vision through professional eye care and by practicing eye safety. Eye safety includes:

- Appropriate use of safety glasses at work, in school labs, or in sports like racquetball;
- Being very careful with sharp objects (especially important for children and youth);
- Avoiding sunlight without tinted (ultra-violet blocking) glasses;
- Knowing the appropriate first-aid tips for eye accidents.

Eye Health Checklist

If you have any of the symptoms listed below, contact your ophthalmologist.

- ❏ Blurry vision uncorrectable by lenses
- ❏ Double vision
- ❏ Dimming of vision that comes and goes, or sudden loss of vision
- ❏ Red eye
- ❏ Eye pain
- ❏ Loss of side vision
- ❏ Haloes (colored rays or circles around lights)
- ❏ Crossed, turned, or wandering eye
- ❏ Twitching or shaking eye
- ❏ Flashes or streaks of light
- ❏ New floaters (spots, strings, or shadows)
- ❏ Discharge, crusting, or excessive tearing
- ❏ Swelling of any part of the eye
- ❏ Bulging of one or both eyes
- ❏ Difference in the size of the eyes
- ❏ Diabetes

Used by permission, American Academy of Ophthalmology.

Yearly or Periodic Health Check #17 and #18

URINE AND BLOOD SCREENING
(URINALYSIS, COMPLETE BLOOD COUNT (CBC) AND SMAC–20)

RECOMMENDATIONS

1. Certain studies suggest that the routine urinalysis and biochemical blood profile (CBC and SMAC-20) in the healthy (non-symptomatic) population is not recommended.[72, 134-140] Because many primary-care physicians still recommend periodic urinalysis and other blood tests, we suggest the following:

   A. The periodic urinalysis, CBC and SMAC-20 should be considered an *optional* health check;

   B. The frequency of performing this health check is left to the discretion of you and your physician.

2. Detailed information regarding the parameters tested as part of the urine and blood tests is found in Appendix H, page 220.

Why Perform

Most physicians (and patients) continue to have interest in the results of routine urine and blood tests. We have concluded that participation in this health check should be optional. Future medical research may discover more revealing blood and urine tests, but until this advancement occurs, the need for routine urine and blood tests in nonsymptomatic patients remains minimal.

How Performed

URINALYSIS

To perform this test, you will be requested to void a few ounces of urine (one-half cup) into a specimen container. Your urine sample will then be analyzed using a small plastic strip ("dipstick") with chemically treated pads. The various body chemicals present in the urine react with the pads on the dipstick revealing various shades of color. When an abnormal color appears, your doctor can assess whether the deviation represents a potential problem.

The urine sample can give your physician details about the health of your kidneys, bladder, and other organs of the body. Listed in Appendix H, page 220, are the parameters that are tested as part of the routine urinalysis.

In addition the following information is discussed in Appendix H:[141]

- **Why these parameters are tested;**
- **What the normal values are;**
- **What the results mean.**

CBC AND SMAC-20 BLOOD TESTS

To obtain your blood sample, a small needle will be introduced into one of your veins (generally a vein on the front of the arm). This procedure, a venipuncture, will be performed by a nurse or blood technician, and one to three tubes of blood will be obtained (this represents a **very** small amount of your total blood supply). Typically your blood undergoes the following tests:

- Complete Blood Count (CBC);
- SMAC-20.

The **complete blood count** (CBC) is a traditional blood test designed to analyze the types of cells in your blood (red blood cells, white blood cells and platelets), and to measure components of the blood cells, like hemoglobin. Because there are different types of white blood cells, occasionally these cells are differentiated as part of the CBC test.

The **SMAC-20** test stands for "Sequential Multiple Analyzer–Computerized," which essentially means 20 different substances within the blood sample are analyzed in a sequence using an automated, computerized machine. The test looks at such items as kidney and liver-related chemicals, electrolytes (like sodium and potassium), and glucose (blood sugar).

Listed in Appendix H[141] (page 220) are the parameters that are tested as part of the CBC and the SMAC-20. In addition the following information is discussed in Appendix H:

- **Why these parameters are tested;**
- **What the normal values are;**
- **What the results mean.**

URINE AND BLOOD REPORT

Most laboratories generate a printed report of the urine and blood test results. This report should also include a listing of **"normal values."** For example, the printed report should include the blood glucose value with a normal range (most labs report the normal range for glucose to be 70 to 115 mg/dl). You doctor should discuss any values that are outside the listed normal range.

If your doctor doesn't share a copy of your urine and blood results, request a copy. This information can easily be kept with your maintenance manual for future reference.

Yearly or Periodic Health Checks
#20, #21, and #22
and
High-Risk Health Checks #19 and #20

TETANUS/DIPHTHERIA VACCINATION
INFLUENZA VACCINATION
PNEUMOCOCCAL VACCINATION

RECOMMENDATIONS

1. *Tetanus/diphtheria:* All adults should have a tetanus-diphtheria booster every **ten years** *after* a primary immunization series.[142]

2. *Influenza:* Individuals aged 65 and older and persons at increased risk* should receive **yearly** influenza vaccinations.[142]

   * High-risk persons for influenza include people:[142]
   - With chronic heart/lung disorders;
   - With metabolic diseases such as diabetes;
   - With hemoglobinopathies;
   - With kidney dysfunction;
   - On immunosuppressants;
   - Who are health-care providers for high-risk groups;
   - Who reside in chronic care facilities.

3. *Pneumococcal disease:* Individuals aged 65 and older and persons at increased risk for pneumococcal infection† should receive a pneumococcal vaccination **at least once**. (*Note:* Although revaccination is not recommended, revaccination of high-risk groups after six or more years following the initial vaccination may be a prudent practice.)[142]

   † High-risk groups for pneumococcal infection include persons with:[142]
   - Chronic heart or lung disease;
   - Sickle cell disease;
   - Nephrotic syndrome;
   - Hodgkin's disease;
   - Cirrhosis – liver disease;
   - Multiple myeloma;
   - Conditions associated with immunosuppression;
   - Living quarters in places with identified increased risk for pneumococcal infection.

4. Other immunizations and vaccinations such as tuberculosis, hepatitis B vaccine, and rubella immunization are discussed in the *High-Risk Health Checks* section of your maintenance manual, see pages 156, 162, 163.

5. When you receive an immunization or a vaccination, be certain to record the date you participated in this health check in your *Health Check Table*.

Why Perform

- Pneumococcal disease and influenza are major causes of death and disability in the United States.[142]
- Pneumococcal disease accounts for approximately 40,000 deaths per year, and about five percent of the patients with pneumococcal pneumonia die.[143]
- One study has estimated the pneumococcal vaccine to

be 60 to 70 percent effective in preventing pneumococcal infection.[144-147]

- Influenza vaccine has also been demonstrated to be 70 to 80 percent effective.[148]

Tetanus. Due to immunizations, tetanus is now an uncommon disease.[142] The tetanus bacteria, however, is present everywhere in the environment and is a serious threat to persons inadequately immunized.[149]

In fact, of the individuals contracting tetanus, 26 to 31 percent die from the serious infection.[150] The majority of tetanus cases are among the elderly, over the age of 60, and it is felt that much of the elderly population are without the proper level of tetanus antibodies.[149]

Most people believe that tetanus is only caused from an injury such as stepping on a rusty nail. Actually, only a third of the tetanus cases are related to an injury or wound. Therefore, having a routine tetanus vaccination (every 10 years) is preferable to waiting until an injury occurs.[149-151]

Diphtheria. Similar to tetanus, diphtheria has become a very uncommon disease. The spread of diphtheria is generally the result of personal contact with an infected person or carrier. Most diphtheria cases occur in younger people, younger than 15 years of age.[149, 152]

Influenza. Influenza is now recognized as one of the major problems facing our public health.[153, 154] Estimates suggest that during epidemic years, the influenza virus can cause in excess of 80 hospitalizations and approximately 12 deaths per 100,000 people.[149] Yearly vaccination is recommended because of the fact that the strains of influenza vary from year to year. High-risk groups should especially participate in receiving a routine influenza vaccination.

Pneumococcal Disease. Pneumococcal disease represents a major cause of death, especially in the elderly, although the disease occurs among all age groups. The incidence of pneumococcal infection increases gradually at age 40 and doubles among people over age 60.[155] Like influenza, pneumococcal disease has greater deleterious effects on the high-risk groups.

SUMMARY

Planned immunization/vaccination programs have played a major part in improving health care in the world. We salute the current efforts by Rotary International and other organizations to remove the threat of polio from off our planet.

Unfortunately, complacency is a major obstacle to immunization programs: the idea that modern-day medicine may cure "everything" has reduced in people's minds the importance of periodic vaccinations.

Most adults have **not** been immunized in agreement with the standard immunization guidelines.[142, 154] Studies have shown that immunizations with pneumococcal and influenza vaccines are very cost effective (especially for individuals over age 65) and may significantly reduce suffering and death.[142, 155]

Make certain to follow the immunization and vaccination recommendations given in this health check; you will be practicing smart medicine. By taking the **time** to be vaccinated against diseases such as pneumococcal pneumonia or influenza, you can save personal suffering or even your life.

How Performed

Immunization involves an injection from a small needle into the muscle of the arm. The immunization can be given at your doctor's office or at a county or state health department. You may want to compare costs when considering where to receive your immunization.

The tetanus-diphtheria booster often causes muscle soreness around the injection site. To reduce soreness, move your arm for a period of time following the injection.

Studies have shown that fever, sore or achy muscles, and severe reactions to the pneumococcal disease vaccine occur in fewer than one percent of patients.[142, 156, 157]

Remember, please be certain to record your immunization and vaccination dates in the space provided in your *Health Check Table.*

Lifestyle Counseling Health Check #1
and
Daily Health Check #7
SUBSTANCE USE

Why Perform

Every member of today's society has been affected in one way or another by chemical abuse. Substance abuse looms as perhaps the **major** health and social problem of the decade. This section discusses the use of alcohol and other drugs and tobacco, and includes additional reference material for your use.

ALCOHOL USE

- ALCOHOL IS A DRUG!
- In America, over 11 million people abuse or have a dependence on alcohol.[159]
- Estimates suggest that in the U.S. over half of the adult population use alcohol and that:[160, 161]
  - **Eleven percent use alcohol daily;**
  - **Ten percent report losing control while drinking or admit to a dependence;**
  - **Eight percent admit to binge drinking (five or more drinks in one sitting).**
- In 1980, there were 69,000 deaths that were a direct result of alcohol, and each year an estimated 300,000 alcohol-related disabilities occur.[159, 162]
- **Fifty percent** of "all deaths from motor vehicle crashes, fires, drownings, homicides, and suicides are the result of alcohol intoxication."[163]
- Cirrhosis of the liver, a leading complication from alcohol dependence, was the *ninth* leading cause of death in the United States in 1986.[164]

- Alcohol is a "gateway drug." A majority of those who abuse illicit drugs such as marijuana, cocaine and heroin, have first abused the drug alcohol.[372]

Is Alcohol Use A Problem? Three sets of simple questions are included below to help individuals determine if alcohol use is a problem in their lives or the lives of their loved ones.

A. Set #1

What is the approximate intake of alcoholic beverages?

beer: ❑ none ❑ occasional ❑ often:_____drinks/week
wine: ❑ none ❑ occasional ❑ often:_____drinks/week
liquor: ❑ none ❑ occasional ❑ often:_____drinks/week

Moderate alcohol intake is defined as **fewer** than two drinks per day. One drink is equal to:

- 12 ounces of beer;
- 5-ounce glass of wine;
- 1.5 fluid ounces (one jigger) of distilled spirits.[158]

Anything greater than the **moderate** intake (more than 14 drinks per week) is defined as "**excessive**," and you should seriously evaluate how to reduce or eliminate your alcohol consumption.

B. Set #2

1. Are you drinking out of habit, or do you choose when to drink?
2. Why do you drink alcohol?
3. Do you have close family members who are alcoholics?

Question #1. This question helps assess whether or not drinking is becoming a habit. If you are **not** making a conscious choice of **when** to drink, then this may be a warning sign of substance abuse.

Question #2. This is designed to get you thinking about why you drink alcohol. If your answer is: "Alcohol takes the edge off after a stressful day," or "It helps me relax and unwind," be advised that these responses are danger signals. Consider substituting for alcohol a lifestyle activity that actually has positive pay-offs such as regular exercise, the kind of practice that can result in a beneficial addiction. **Remember**, when compared to the risk of alcohol use, there are no health benefits to consuming alcohol.

Question #3. People whose parents or other close family members (first-degree relatives) have a history of alcohol dependence must realize that the risk of their developing a similar problem is increased.[162]

C. Set #3

The final set of questions is referred to as the CAGE screening instrument. An affirmative answer to at least *two of the four* questions may suggest there is a probable alcohol abuse problem.[158] The questions are listed below:

C: Have you ever felt you ought to **C**ut down on drinking?
A: Have people **A**nnoyed you by criticizing your drinking?
G: Have you ever felt bad or **G**uilty about your drinking?
E: Have you ever had a drink first thing in the morning to steady your nerves or get rid of a hang-over (**E**ye-opener)?

If An Alcohol Problem Exists. If you suspect an alcohol problem exists (based upon the above sets of questions) there are several agencies and organizations whose sole existence is to assist the chemically dependent person and loved ones. These agencies include:

Alcoholics Anonymous (AA): This self-help organization helps the person abusing alcohol to regain a healthy lifestyle. Anyone is welcome to the meetings; only first names are used for identification. Members will be happy to serve as an escort for individuals attending their first meeting.

Professional Help: Inpatient care at a hospital or an alcohol recovery center may be required for medical detoxification and treatment. This care is generally provided by physicians and a professional support team. Long-term after-care is generally a strong component of these programs. Many insurance companies will now assist in the payment of professional treatment programs.

Al-Anon (for adults) and Alateen (for teenagers) Family Groups: This self-help organization is designed to assist the family members and friends of the alcoholic. This organization provides a group support system and assistance in helping the victim of chemical abuse regain perspective and hope. Confidentiality is maintained, and there is no cost.

Adult Children of Alcoholics (ACA): This group assists adults who, as children, were raised in a home where alcohol abuse was present. The organization is designed to help victims overcome self-defeating thinking and behavior patterns.

Information and Referral: The National Council on Alcoholism and the National Clearinghouse for Alcohol Information provide counseling literature and referrals for problem drinkers and their families.

Women's Resources: Women's Centers, Battered Women's Shelters, Women's Health Collectives, and State Commissions on Woman are potential sources of assistance for women who are suffering as victims from a family member who is abusing alcohol.

In conclusion, we salute individuals, community groups and various companies that are devoting time and money to educate our **young people** about the serious consequences of drinking alcohol. We hope that alcohol use and abuse among our youth will decrease steadily during this decade and beyond.

TOBACCO USE

- **One out of six** deaths that occur in the United States is the result of cigarette smoking.[165, 166]
- "Cigarette smoking is the *most important* modifiable cause of death."[165-167]
- Each year in the United States an unbelievable 390,000 people die as a result of cigarette smoking — or over 1,000 people per day.[167]
- Consider the correlation between smoking and death by cancer (over 130,000 deaths) as detailed by the U.S. Preventive Services Task Force:[165, 167] *"In adult men, smoking accounts for 90 percent of all deaths from cancer of the lung, trachea and bronchus; 92 percent of deaths from cancers of the lip, oral cavity, and pharynx; 80 percent of deaths from cancer of the larynx; 78 percent of deaths from esophageal cancer; 48 percent of deaths from cancer of the kidney; 47 percent of deaths from bladder cancer; 29 percent of deaths from pancreatic cancer; and 17 percent of deaths from stomach cancer."*
- Innocent victims of smoking include the approximate 4,000 *nonsmoking* people who die from the affects of breathing the smoke of others, and the low-birth rate children whose mothers smoke during pregnancy.[165, 166, 168]

We all remember the catastrophic industrial accident in Bhopal, India, in which approximately 3,500 men, women and children died unnecessarily as a result of a toxic gas leak. The whole world was outraged. Yet, in this country 3,500 premature deaths occur *every 3.5 days* as a result of the effects of cigarette smoking. In other words, a Bhopal-like catastrophe takes place **100 times** each year in the U.S.. Where is the outrage? In addition to the tragic loss of lives, the smoking related-illnesses cost the U.S. approximately $200 billion each year, and one-third of all adults continue to smoke.[169]

How to Quit —And The Benefits. A smoker who has stopped for a period of 15 to 20 years reduces the risk of developing lung cancer to the same risk as a person who has never smoked.[165, 170, 171] A "rule-of-thumb" is that for every year after a person has quit smoking, five to six years of the effects of smoking are erased.

Once you have decided to "kick the habit," we suggest the following tips:

- Sign a written **contract** that includes a *deadline* or a *date* for quitting.
- Encourage others to lend their **support**. Many smokers continue because their spouse or co-worker(s) smoke.
- A "**smoke-free**" environment can persuade you to quit. There are now a number of companies that are smoke free.
- If you have tried stopping smoking several times, take hope. Recent statistics suggest that people who have made **repeated** efforts to quit actually increase the likelihood of finally quitting.[172]
- Consider the **avoidance of alcohol or caffeine** use. Studies suggest that those people who use substances such as alcohol or caffeine have a more difficult time quitting smoking.[172]
- Consider having your doctor prescribe **nicotine chewing gum** during your initial efforts to quit.
- Consider the stop smoking **resources**, listed below:
  - "Step-by-Step Quit Kit" can be obtained by writing the School of Public Health, Department of Health Behavior/Health Education, University of Michigan, 109 South Observatory Street, Ann Arbor, MI 48109.
  - "Calling It Quits," "Quit It, A Guide to Help You Stop Smoking," and "For Good, A Guide to Living as a Non-Smoker" can be obtained from the Office of Cancer Communication (Room 10-A-18), National Cancer Institute, Bethesda, MD 20205.
  - "Fresh Start" can be obtained from the American Cancer Society within your state (contact local representatives).
  - "Clearing the Air – How to Quit Smoking and Quit for Keeps," can be obtained from the U.S. Department of Health and Human Services, Public Health Service, NIH, National Cancer Institute (NIH publication # 89-1647).

Stopping smoking is possible. Do the very best thing you ever did for yourself, set a contract with a deadline to "kick the habit."

DRUG USE

- Estimates suggest that one to three million Americans are using cocaine on a regular basis; 500,000 are addicted to heroin and over two million are using the drug; and over 10 million are using marijuana.[158, 173-175]
- Use of cocaine can cause sudden death due to stroke, heart attack and other medical complications, and approximately 10 in every 1,000 heroin addicts die as a result of "overdose, suicide, violence," and other medical complications.[173, 174]
- Addiction to "crack," the smokable form of cocaine, can cause addiction from the *first* use of the drug.[176]
- Dependence on these drugs leads to serious negative behavioral changes, often crippling potential personal and professional growth for the young adult population.[177]
- Intravenous use of these drugs is "an important risk factor" for contracting AIDS — 25 percent of all AIDS cases result from intravenous drug usage. Of the estimated 900,000 intravenous drug users in the U.S., statistics suggest that in some cities up to **half** of these users are infected with the AIDS virus.[178]
- Babies born to mothers who are chemically dependent suffer withdrawal effects and long-term physical and psychological effects.[179]

In the wonderful fantasy movie, *The Princess Bride*, the hero, strapped to a torture-machine that sucks out life, is killed. The hero's body is taken to the village miracle worker, Miracle Max, and to everyone's relief, Max declares the victim only "part way dead." With a magic pill from Max, the hero is revived.

Drug abuse, like the torture-machine, literally sucks life from its users. The abuser becomes tightly strapped against his will and eventually even the user's agency to resist the chemical substance is lost. Unfortunately, restoration to a healthy, happy and productive life is not as easy as swallowing a pill from Miracle Max. **We wish it were!**

Is Drug Use A Problem? We strongly suggest that individuals visit with their physicians about drug use habits or patterns. This discussion should also include the use pattern of prescribed medications. The problem of "invisible overdosing" is a real issue for those people who are taking multiple medications, both prescribed and over-the-counter.[180]

Listed in the next column are questions to help you recognize whether or not drugs are becoming a problem in your life or the lives of your loved ones. The more questions that you answer **yes** to, the more likely there is a problem. Discuss the questions answered "yes" with your doctor.

Have you or your loved one:

YES	NO	
		Shown a pattern of withdrawal from other family members, friends, or co-workers, or demonstrated a decreased interest in school, career, or possessions?
		Altered or abandoned normal drives or non-drug-related pleasurable activities?
		Demonstrated a significant change in personality or an unwillingness to communicate?
		Been spending large amounts of money, selling household items, or suspected stealing from friends or family members?
		Noticed any of the following symptoms: weight loss?
		loss of interest in physical appearance?
		chronic runny nose?
		frequent upper-respiratory infections?
		feeling depressed?
		repetitious, compulsive acts such as tapping of fingers or playing with hair?

Information taken from DHHS Publication No. (ADM) 89-1559. From the Office for Substance Abuse Prevention; distributed by the National Clearinghouse for Alcohol and Drug Information.

If A Drug Problem Exists. If you, your physician or your family determine that a drug problem exists, your physician can recommend appropriate counseling or a drug treatment program. These programs include the concerted efforts of physicians, counselors, and therapists, and the program encourages the additional support of family, friends, and clergy.

In addition, an excellent source for drug prevention, recognition, and treatment for youth with drug problems is: *Not My Kid: A Parents' Guide to Kids and Drugs*, by Bev Polson and Dr. Miller Newton (published by Avon Books, 1790 Broadway, New York, NY 10019).

In conclusion, the surest advise for eliminating the risk of a drug abuse problem (including the drug alcohol) is to never be a user!

Lifestyle Counseling Health Check #2
High Risk Health Checks #14 and #15
and
Daily Health Check #8

INJURY PREVENTION
(MOTOR VEHICLE, HOUSEHOLD, AND ENVIRONMENTAL)

AND PREVENTING VIOLENT INJURIES

RECOMMENDATIONS

The following adapted guidelines relating to injury prevention are suggested by the U.S. Preventive Services Task Force.[181, 182] *Note*: Review these guidelines from time to time and record your participation in this health check in your *Health Check Table*.

1. Individuals should *always* use safety belts and child safety belts when riding in motor vehicles. Individuals riding motorcycles should *always* wear safety helmets.

2. Individuals who are under the influence of alcohol or other intoxicating drugs should not drive a motor vehicle. (These individuals should also avoid potentially dangerous activities such as swimming, boating, handling of firearms, and bicycling.) Persons should avoid riding in a vehicle in which the driver is under the influence of alcohol or other intoxicating drugs.

3. To prevent injury and death from fire, the very young and the elderly should wear fireproof sleep wear. Alcohol and smoking should be avoided late at night, and individuals who cannot quit the use of tobacco should avoid smoking while near bedding or upholstery. Smoke detectors should be located on every floor of homes and apartments and should be tested regularly. Gasoline and other flammable products should be stored in safety cans out of doors.

4. Pertaining to **household injuries**:
   A. Hot water heaters should be set at 120°F.
   B. Firearms should be locked in a compartment and kept *unloaded*.
   C. Parents, grandparents or guardians who have children in the home should:
      - Keep a one-ounce bottle of Syrup of Ipecac for inducing vomiting;
      - Display the telephone number of the local poison control center;
      - Place all medications, toxic substances, matches, and firearms in child-resistant cabinets.
   D. To prevent children from falling:
      - Collapsible gates or other barriers should be placed across stairway entrances;
      - Four-foot latch gates should be installed around swimming pools;
      - Window guards should be installed in high-rise buildings or homes with multiple stories.
   E. To prevent injuries in the homes of elderly persons:
      - Inspect the home or living quarters for proper lighting;
      - Remove or repair loose rugs, electrical cords and toys;
      - Install handrails and traction strips in stairways and bathtubs;

- Inspect for unstable appliances and furniture;
- Where possible, replace low beds and toilets;
- Make certain stairs are clear of articles or potential obstacles.

5. Adults and children riding bicycles should wear helmets and avoid riding bicycles in motor vehicle traffic.

6. Other recommendations pertaining to the *elderly*:
   A. Elderly persons should avoid climbing ladders and walking on ice.
   B. Elderly persons should schedule periodic eye examinations to determine visual acuity.
   C. To avoid falls, elderly persons and individuals caring for older people should inquire about possible side effects of medications as it pertains to coordination and mobility.
   D. When practical, elderly persons should learn the proper techniques of cushioning a fall.
   E. With the okay of the personal physician, elderly persons should get involved in physical activity programs designed to increase flexibility, strength and mobility (please see *Daily Health Check #1, Physical Activity Program*, page 40).

7. Pertaining to violent injuries:
   A. Individuals who are at high risk of becoming either "victims or perpetuators" of violence should seek counseling or be referred to appropriate counseling by their physician or allied health care worker. Young adult males should especially be instructed regarding the risk of violent injury associated with the easy access of firearms and intoxication from alcohol and other drugs.[183]
   B. Physicians who encounter patients (children and adults) with unusual injuries should carefully examine and interview the patient with attention to possible abuse or neglect. Every effort should be made to help prevent further injury.[183]

Why Perform

Injuries (motor vehicle and other injuries) are the leading cause of death in the U.S. among individuals aged one to 44.[181-184] In addition to the high incidence of death from injuries, each year there are 60 million nonfatal injuries,[185] and literally millions of violent crimes are being reported (and/or unreported) each year in the U.S.[183]

Injury prevention should be a high priority at home, on the road, at recreational outings and at the work place. This section focuses on motor vehicle and fall injury prevention and the need to prevent drownings, fires, poisonings, and firearm and violent injuries.

MOTOR VEHICLE INJURY

- 48,000 deaths (approximately one-half of all deaths caused by injuries) are due to motor vehicle crashes.[181, 186-188]
- Motor vehicle injuries are the leading cause of death in people under age 45, and they represent the *fourth* leading cause of all deaths in the U.S.[181]
- In 1986, motor vehicle injuries resulted in **3,100** children's deaths and 38 percent of *all* deaths in young people ages 15 to 24.[186]
- Approximately **50 percent** of all motor vehicle deaths are alcohol related, and in 1986 there were 1.7 million people arrested for driving while under the influence of alcohol.[181, 189]
- Proper use of lap and shoulder belts can reduce the risk of "moderate to serious" injury or death from a vehicle crash by 40 to 50 percent.[190]

Seat Belt Usage. "Do you *always* wear your seat belts?" This question is asked of all our patients. For individuals and families less committed to wearing safety belts (including child safety seats for small children), we've wished we could arrange a visit to our emergency room to view the victims who have failed to buckle up.

In our homes, the rule-of-thumb is: Seat belts buckled before car engine is engaged. Remember, your chances of dying in a vehicle accident or having a serious injury is automatically reduced by **50 percent** the moment you buckle your safety belts.

Consider also that children who are **not** restrained in a motor vehicle are more than *"ten times* **as likely to die"** if involved in a motor vehicle crash as compared to children who are properly restrained.[181,191,192] In contrast, children who are properly restrained in safety belts reduce the likelihood of **"serious injury by 67 percent"** and death by **71 percent.**[187]

Driving Under the Influence. The second major preventive action individuals can take to reduce death and serious injury on the roads is to **not** drink alcohol and drive, and to **not** drive while under the influence of other intoxicating drugs such as marijuana. This strong caution is particularly important for young people (ages 15 to 24).

We have been impressed with the efforts of adult community citizens to contract with the youth — pledging to pick up the young people that have been drinking (no questions asked) and drive them home. Of course, our hope is that in the future the need for such service will decline because youth will naturally be abstaining from alcohol intake.

Safety Helmets. Individuals who wear safety helmets while driving a motorcycle can decrease the chances of a head injury by **75 percent** and reduce the risk of death by **30 percent**.[181, 193] **Always** wear a safety helmet when driving a motorcycle or riding as a passenger.

ACCIDENTS FROM FALLS

- Falls are the number one cause of non-fatal injuries in the U.S.[182, 184]
- The majority of the falls that result in death are among older adults.[183]
- Hip fractures, a common result of falls in the elderly, result in significant pain, disability and a reduction in "functional independence."[196]
- Of the elderly population admitted to a hospital for a fall, only about *50 percent* are alive a year following the accident.[197]
- Measures to prevent falls *reduce* the incidence of injury, short- and long-term disability, and death.

Falls and the Elderly. Because of the weakness of the bones and muscles the elderly are often unable to sustain even a minor fall without escaping injury. The elderly are also prone to have more accidental falls because of:

Gait problems   Medicine interactions
Periodic dizziness   Blood pressure changes
Legs giving out   Other physiologic problems

If a fall occurs among a family member, every effort should be made to determine the cause of the fall so additional falls can be avoided. In addition, doctors and pharmacists should take every precaution to inform individuals of medications that may cause dizziness or that may interact with other medicines.

Safety in the Home. One potential danger area of many homes is the stairway. Make certain that all family members are instructed *not* to leave items on the stairs. As a small boy, one of the authors remembers opening a door at his uncle's home, thinking it was the bathroom entrance. Unfortunately, the door was to the basement and with one step forward the rest of the trip was downhill. This story suggests that all doors leading to a stairway should be *labelled* with a *warning sign*.

In addition, remember to make certain that the water heater temperature is set at 120° Fahrenheit.

In conclusion, the following "Home Safety Checklist" has been prepared by Drs. Rubenstein and Robbins.[197]

Table 1. Home Safety Checklist: Summary of the Most Important Items from Several Published Lists.

AREA	RECOMMENDATION
Living spaces	Remove throw rugs
	Secure carpet edges
	Remove low-lying furniture and objects on floor
	Reduce clutter
	Remove cords and wires on floor
	Check lighting for adequate illumination at night (especially bathroom pathway)
	Secure carpet or treads on stairs
	Eliminate low furniture for sitting
	Avoid waxing floors
	Ensure that telephone is reachable from floor
Bathroom	Install grab bars in tub and shower
	Use rubber mats in tub and shower
	Remove floor mats when not using tub and shower
	Install raised toilet seat if seat is low
Outside	Repair cracked sidewalks
	Install handrails on stairs and steps
	Keep shrubbery trimmed back on access path to house
	Install adequate lighting outside doors and in walkways leading to doors

Reprinted by permission from "Evaluation of Falls in Elderly Persons," (LZ Rubenstein and AS Robbins) in Practical Care of the Ambulatory Patient, *eds. BM Stults and WH Dere, W.B. Saunders Company, Philadelphia, 1989.*

ACCIDENTS FROM DROWNINGS

Individuals who are at greatest risk for drowning are small children (aged one through three) and young males (aged 15 to 24).[182, 194] Precaution should be taken by owners of swimming pools to install fences and latched gates around the pool. Care should also be taken among all children and adults to use proper flotation devices while swimming in lakes, ponds, and at ocean beaches.

Important to note is the fact that approximately half of all drownings resulting from swimming and boating accidents are associated with alcohol or other intoxicating drugs.[182, 198, 199] The preventive measures in this situation are obvious.

ACCIDENTS FROM FIRES

Educational efforts have successfully informed the public of the need for home smoke detectors. A few years ago we learned of a family that had actually purchased a smoke detector as a Christmas present, installed the battery, wrapped the present and placed it under the tree. Prior to Christmas the house caught fire, and the wrapped smoke devise sounded the alarm, alerting the sleeping family. There were no fatalities or injuries. Keep these facts and tips in mind:

- A home fire occurring *without* a smoke detector is **two to three** times as likely to result in deaths of family members than the home with an installed detector;[182, 183, 195, 200, 201]
- Purchase the kind of detector that will alert you when the battery is low;
- Follow the guidelines regarding cigarette smoking and fires:
  - Flame-resistant clothing should be used for the very young and old;
  - Avoid smoking late at night and/or when near bedding or upholstery.

ACCIDENTS FROM POISONING AND FIREARMS

Injury and death from poisoning and firearms can be prevented by:

- Using child-resistant containers and keeping all medicines and other household agents such as cleaning solutions in locked cabinets;
- Keeping firearms unloaded **and** keeping them in a locked cabinet can prevent death due to firearms among children;
- Following gun safety rules and regulations.

PREVENTING VIOLENT INJURIES

Violent injuries remain a very serious health problem. Consider the following statistics regarding violent injuries:

- There were 530,000 reported cases of aggravated assault in 1986;[183, 202]
- Victims who experience violent crimes suffer from physical injuries, disability, fear, anxiety, isolation and sometimes death;[183, 203]
- About 90,000 rapes are reported yearly;[183, 202-207]
- Estimates are that two to four million women are abused each year by their spouses;[183, 202-207]
- Estimates also indicate that "battering" may occur in as much as 25 percent of couples (accounting for up to six percent of the total number of visits that women make to emergency rooms);[183, 208]
- Statistics reveal that an alarming one to two million cases of child abuse are reported each year, and that as many as *5,000 children* die each year from physical abuse;[183, 206, 209, 210]
- Finally, in 1986, over 20,000 Americans were murdered.[183, 202] Those individuals at greatest risk are:
  - Young males;
  - Minorities;
  - Blacks (**One in 21 black males dies from murder**).

The physician is generally in an excellent position to examine patients for signs of abuse and to interview patients regarding their involvement in personal violence.[183] Studies have shown that people are more likely to talk to their doctor than to any other professional about potential abuse problems.[183, 211]

Efforts should be made by doctors to direct individuals who have been identified as a victim or perpetrator of abuse to appropriate community services such as group and individual counseling.

In addition, every effort should be made by doctors or clergy who are aware of child-abuse situations to remove the abuser from the child's environment until such time as the threat of future abuse is resolved.

Those individuals who have a history of violent behavior should be encouraged to seek counseling regarding how to resolve conflict peacefully and what the consequences are of participating in violent behavior.[183] Individuals (especially young adult males) who have easy access to firearms and who become intoxicated with alcohol or other drugs are at a significantly increased risk for committing a violent crime.[183]

Finally, we should each be aware of those around us — family members, friends and neighbors — who display signs of abuse. We should also encourage victims of abuse to contact protective services and persuade perpetrators of abuse to seek appropriate counseling.

Lifestyle Counseling Health Check #3
Daily Health Check #10
and
Yearly or Periodic Health Check #19
DENTAL HEALTH

RECOMMENDATIONS

1. All adults should have a dental examination at least yearly. Some individuals may require more frequent dental visits based upon personal dental history and recommendations of the dentist. Participation in this health check should be recorded in your *Health Check Table*.

2. During regular dental examinations, dental personnel should be alert for signs of oral cavity disease.

3. In addition to regular dental visits, individuals should learn proper techniques for brushing and flossing teeth and should perform these activities on a daily basis. Individuals should also be aware of the recommended use of fluoridation and of avoiding food high in sugar and starch content for protection against dental caries.

4. Record the name(s) of your dentists in your *Health Questionnaire* located in Appendix A, page 170.

5. Individuals who are generally at increased risk for dental disease include:[212]

   - The elderly population;
   - Pregnant women;
   - Individuals who smoke and/or abuse alcohol;

   - Individuals with a high rate of tartar accumulation;
   - Individuals whose medical history includes diabetes, AIDS virus, or xerostomia (excessive dryness of the mouth);
   - Individuals with active periodontal disease and a history of the same.

Why Perform

- Periodontal diseases (diseases that are the result of bacterial infections that attack the gums, bone, and ligaments that secure the teeth in the jaw) can be *prevented* by *daily* brushing and flossing and by periodic professional cleaning of the teeth.[213]
- Without regular dental checkups, an individual may not know that they have a periodontal disease and if the disease is left untreated it can damage the gums and bone to a point where loss of the tooth is inevitable.[213]
- Periodontal diseases can occur at any age — even in young children. More than 50 percent of individuals over the age of 18 have at least *early stages* of some form of periodontal diseases, and of the adults over the age of 35, estimates are that *three out of four* have some type of periodontal disease.[213]

RECOGNITION OF DENTAL PROBLEMS

The dental industry has been a pioneer in preaching prevention. Many dentists now suggest that the current preventive efforts should not only focus on tooth caries but emphasize also the prevention of periodontal disease through periodic check-ups and dental health education.

Periodontal Disease. Early warning signs for periodontal disease are listed below. You are encouraged to see your dentist if you notice any of these signs.[214]

1. Gums that bleed while brushing your teeth.
2. Gums that are red, swollen, or tender.
3. Gums that have separated from your teeth.
4. Persistent bad breath.
5. The appearance of pus between teeth and gums.
6. Teeth that are loose or separating.
7. A change in the way your teeth match together when you bite.
8. A change in the fit of partial dentures.

Endodontic Disease. In addition to the warning signs for periodontal disease, you should be aware of the symptoms for possible endodontic disease (disorders of the soft tissues inside the root canal system):

1. Increased tooth sensitivity to hot or cold exposure with associated pain lingering for an extended period of time.
2. Unexplained pain in areas such as the ear or jaw — this may represent referred pain from a tooth.
3. Headaches that have no apparent cause and that are sometimes accentuated by food or drinks that are cold.
4. Avoiding chewing on one side of your mouth because biting is painful.

If you recognize any of these signs or symptoms, be certain to discuss them with your dentist.

PREVENTING DENTAL DISEASE

There is excellent documentation that regular brushing and flossing can prevent dental caries and retard the progression of periodontitis.[212, 215-217] Preventive activities can be preformed by dentists and dental hygienists such as cleaning, scaling, root planning of teeth, and careful oral and dental examination for the early detection of dental disease.[212] In addition, other preventive measures can include the use of fluoride and sealants,[212, 218-220] dental appliances for proper tooth spacing and inspection for oral cavity cancer.[212]

Studies have also demonstrated that regular tooth cleaning by your dentist and dental hygienists will reduce tooth decay. Also, between professional tooth cleaning, individuals must practice daily brushing and flossing to prevent periodontal disease effectively.[212, 213, 215]

To assist individuals with proper techniques for effective brushing and flossing, the following techniques are suggested:[214]

BRUSHING TECHNIQUE

- A soft-bristled toothbrush and the use of fluoride toothpaste is generally recommended.
- Begin by placing the head of your toothbrush against your teeth, with the bristle tips angled at about 45° against your gumline.
- Gently "scrub" the teeth by moving the brush back and forth in short (half-a-tooth-wide) strokes several times.
- Carefully brush the outer surfaces of each tooth, keeping the bristles angled against the gumline.
- Then transfer to the inside surfaces of all the teeth, still using short back-and-forth strokes.
- Next, brush the chewing surfaces of the teeth.
- Clean the inside surfaces of the front teeth by tilting the brush vertically and making several gentle up-and-down strokes with the "toe" (the front part) of the brush.
- Brushing your tongue will freshen your breath and clean your mouth by removing bacteria.

FLOSSING TECHNIQUE

- Pull off about 18 inches of floss and wind most of it around one middle finger.
- Wind the remaining floss around the same finger on your opposite hand, and use it to "take up" the floss as it becomes soiled.
- Holding the floss firmly between thumbs and forefingers with about an inch of floss between them, gently "saw" or guide the floss between your teeth. Never "snap" the floss into the gums.
- As you reach the gumline, curve the floss into a C-shape against one tooth and carefully slide the floss into the space between the gum and the tooth until you feel resistance.
- Holding the floss tightly against the tooth, carefully scrape the side of the tooth, moving the floss away from the gum.
- Repeat this method on the rest of your teeth. Don't forget the back side of your last tooth.

Finally, a well-balanced diet with a reduction in foods high in refined sugar can reduce dental caries. Avoiding high sugar and starch snacks between meals is an additional means toward reducing dental decay.[212] See *Daily Health Check #4, Proper Nutrition Program*, page 58.

Lifestyle Counseling Health Check #4

PREVENTION OF HIV VIRUS (AIDS) AND
OTHER SEXUALLY TRANSMITTED DISEASES

RECOMMENDATIONS

1. Individuals (adolescents and adults) should visit with their physician about personal sexual practices. Record your participation in this health check in your *Health Check Table*.

2. Sexually active persons should strongly be advised that abstaining from sex or maintaining a mutually faithful monogamous sexual relationship with a partner known to be uninfected with sexually transmitted diseases are the *most effective* strategies to prevent infection with human immunodeficiency virus (AIDS virus) or other sexually transmitted diseases.[221]

3. Individuals at high-risk for sexually transmitted diseases should follow the screening recommendations given for syphilis, gonorrhea, chlamydia, genital herpes, hepatitis B, and infection with human immunodeficiency virus (AIDS virus). These recommendations are outlined in the section *High-Risk Health Checks*, pages 162 and 165– 167.

4. Individuals should be advised about the indications and proper methods for using condoms and spermicides in sexual intercourse and about the health risks associated with anal intercourse.[221]

5. Intravenous (IV) drug users should be encouraged to enroll in a drug treatment program (see *Lifestyle Counseling Health Check #1, Substance Use*, page 123) and should be sternly warned against the extreme dangers in sharing drug equipment or using unsterilized needles and syringes.[221]

Why Perform

For the first time ever, AIDS is now reported as the sixth leading cause of death among men aged 25 to 44 years. Estimates are that one to 1.5 million people have been infected with the human immunodeficiency virus (HIV) or the virus that can lead to AIDS.[221-223]

In addition to the enormous human suffering, the estimated cost of sexually transmitted disease in the U.S. is around $4 billion per year with an estimated cost for AIDS alone to reach $13 billion by 1992.[221, 223–225]

SEXUALLY TRANSMITTED DISEASES (STD)

The U.S. Preventive Services Task Force has vividly outlined the tremendous burden of suffering from sexually transmitted diseases (STD).

Consider the facts associated with different kinds of STD:

Syphilis. A bacteria-caused disease, primary and secondary syphilis is diagnosed in approximately 35,000 people each year in the U.S.[237] This disease produces ulcers of the genitalia, pharynx, and rectum, and may progress to skin sores and cardiovascular and nervous system illnesses.[238] From an epidemiological standpoint, syphilis may also be associated with infection with AIDS.[228, 229]

Gonorrhea and Chlamydia. Two million cases of gonorrhea and two to four million cases of chlamydia infection are diagnosed each year in the U.S.[221, 230–232, 239, 240] Chlamydia and gonorrhea can produce urethritis, epididymitis, and proctitis in men and pelvic inflammatory disease (PID) in women.[224, 239, 241] PID is a major risk factor leading to ectopic pregnancy and infertility among women—approximately one million cases of PID are reported each year in the U.S.[221, 224, 242]

Genital Herpes. This viral infection is very widespread and no cure for the malady has been discovered. Each year in the U.S. there are approximately 270,000 cases, and it is estimated that about 20 million people "are already infected and suffering recurrent episodes."[233, 234] The virus causes painful ulcerative lesions.[221, 244]

Human Immunodeficiency Virus (HIV - AIDS Virus) and AIDS. In addition to the one to 1.5 million people in the U.S. who are infected with the AIDS virus, there are now a reported 82,000 cases of AIDS (end of 1988).[235] This disease can be transmitted through:

- **Sexual contact;**
- **Exchange of blood or blood products.**

AIDS is now the "**seventh** leading cause of years of potential life lost in the United States, and is the leading cause of death in intravenous (IV) drug abusers and hemophiliacs."[221, 246, 247] AIDS contributes to the development of several kinds of diseases and the general outcome from AIDS is death (there are no current medical treatments to prevent death). By the year 1992, there will be approximately 365,000 cases of diagnosed AIDS and it is thought that 260,000 Americans will have died from this disease.[221, 223]

Hepatitis B. A sexually transmitted disease that can also be transmitted through the use of blood and blood products, hepatitis B virus (HBV) has been estimated to affect 500,000 to one million people in the U.S.[221, 236, 248] Individuals who have been infected with this virus are at increased risk for contracting hepatitis, liver disease and liver cancer, and it is estimated that each year over 5,000 people die from these medical disorders.[221, 248]

STD AMONG INFANTS

The human cost of sexually transmitted diseases can be easily seen in the children born to mothers who are infected. Consider the following facts, again compiled by the U.S. Preventive Services Task Force.[221]

- Congenital syphilis *often* results in fetal death or serious neonatal complications.[237]
- Active infections of gonorrhea or chlamydia can result in complications with the pregnancy and infections in the newborn.[241]
- Of the infants infected with genital herpes, 65 percent will die if left untreated, and **less than 10 percent** of the infants with central nervous system infection develop normally.[244]
- Approximately 30 to 35 percent of the infants born to women with AIDS will be infected with the AIDS virus.

INDIVIDUALS AT RISK

The individuals who are at greatest risk to be infected with sexually transmitted diseases include:

- Young people;
- Those who have multiple sexual contacts;
- Prostitutes;
- Homosexual and bisexual men;
- Individuals whose sexual partners are already infected with an STD;[221, 241, 242, 249]
- Individuals who underwent a blood transfusion between the years of 1978 and 1985 (these people are at increased risk for hepatitis virus [HBV] or AIDS virus [HIV]);
- Individuals who are intravenous drug users (these people are at increased risk for HBV and HIV viruses).[221, 250, 251]

PREVENTING SEXUALLY TRANSMITTED DISEASES

If you and your partner are the only individuals who have had sex together, and you each are uninfected, then there is virtually zero risk of contacting a sexually transmitted disease. (The only risk would be through blood or blood products as it pertains to AIDS virus and hepatitis B virus.) The risk for contacting a sexually transmitted disease increases significantly as individuals begin to increase the number of sexual contacts; especially is the risk increased if a person engages in sexual contact with a partner he or she knows little about.

One of our colleagues stated that if you choose to have sex with a person who has been promiscuous, you are in a sense accepting the risk of having sex with all of your partner's "unknown" sexual contacts.

The U.S. Public Health Service has stated the following sexual counseling recommendations:

- **Abstain from sex or maintain a mutually faithful monogamous sexual relationship.**
- **Abstain from engaging in sex with individuals who are not known with certainty to have a negative blood test for any sexually transmitted diseases and who have not been the sole partner for six months prior to or any time after the test.**
- **Do not practice anal intercourse.**
- **Do not use unsterilized needles or syringes.**
- **Intravenous drug users should enroll in a drug treatment program.**
- **Always use a condom if there are doubts about the status of the sexual partner.**

We believe physicians should visit with their patients about sexual activities and when appropriate, discuss the risks of developing sexually transmitted diseases. Because the young adult population continues to have problems with the spread of sexually transmitted diseases, we believe it especially important that *parents, physicians, clergy, and where appropriate, schools* get involved in educating children on the tremendous suffering that inappropriate sexual activity can cause to them and to others. Physicians should also counsel young people about the potential hazardous association of alcohol use leading to inappropriate sexual activity.

In addition to physician counseling and education by other concerned persons regarding sexual activities, the Center for Disease Control (CDC) and the Federal Drug Administration (FDA) have recently published detailed instructions for people on the proper use of condoms.[252, 253] These guidelines include caution that condoms do not provide complete protection against infection and that condoms *must* be used by following their recommended instructions to be effective.[221, 252, 253]

Instructions on how to properly use condoms can be obtained from *Condoms and Sexually Transmitted Disease...Especially AIDs* (Food and Drug Administration, DHHS Publication No. [FDA] 90-4239, Rockville, MD, U.S. Department of Health and Human Services 1990), or the National AIDS Hotline: 1-800-342-AIDS.

Lifestyle Counseling Health Check #5

PREVENTING LOW-BACK INJURIES

RECOMMENDATIONS

1. All individuals should review educational instruction for preventing low-back injury. Proper body mechanics to prevent low-back injuries should be an integral component of the education process. Participation in this health check should be recorded in your *Health Check Table*.

2. All individuals should be encouraged to participate in a consistent physical activity program (*Daily Health Check #1, Physical Activity Programs*, page 40), and practice stretching and strengthening activities designed to increase the stability of the back (*Daily Health Check #2, Body Strength Program*, page 47 and *Daily Health Check #3, Body Flexibility Program*, page 53). Finally, preventive measures should be taken to maintain ideal body weight (*Daily Health Check #6, Weight Control Program*, page 69) and to follow a healthy diet (*Daily Health Check #4, Proper Nutrition Program*, page 58).[254]

2. Individuals who are at high-risk for low-back injury should consider participation in a "back school" education and conditioning program. Many "back school" programs are designed to address the back-care needs of specific industries with reference to the type of labor involved.

3. Risk factors for low-back injury include:[254-260]

   - Occupations that require frequent and repetitive lifting (especially when the lifting is performed in a forward bending and twisting position);
   - Cigarette smoking;
   - Exposure to vibration caused by vehicles or machinery.

4. Companies whose work procedures naturally increase the risk of employees having low-back injury may benefit from pre-employment screening and selective placement. The screening procedure should be appropriately matched with the likelihood of risk for low-back injury while on the job. Spinal X-rays are not recommended for use in screening for back injury risk.[254]

Why Perform

Consider the enormous impact that low-back injury has upon our society today:

- Estimates suggest that between 60 and 90 percent of the people living in industrialized nations will

Note: Back School, *a booklet produced by Cottonwood Hospital Medical Center, a facility of Intermountain Health Care, was used as source material for this section.*

experience serious low-back pain sometime during their life;[254, 258-260]

- Close to 70 percent of individuals suffering from an event of serious low-back pain will have a reoccurrence within one year of the initial pain;[255]
- One of nine back problems is the result of an accident;[255]
- Low-back pain disables approximately 5.4 million Americans and the estimated cost for low-back injuries is $16 billion per year.[254, 256]

The **good news** is that most back complaints are short lived and only a very small percentage of back problems require corrective surgery.[255, 261] Generally, the time required for individuals to recover from back pain is:[255]

- 50 percent recover within one month;
- 75 percent recover within three months;
- 95 percent recover within six months;
- 96 percent recover within one year.

TREATMENT OF LOW-BACK INJURY

Most medical experts involved in research regarding back pain treatment suggest that only three treatments have been shown to alter the course of an existing back problem. These three treatments are:

Surgery of the back. Only *one to three percent* of individuals with back problems require surgery.

Physical Activity. A physical activity program reduces the likelihood of experiencing low-back pain by *ten times*, and the physically active lifestyle decreases the chances of repeated occurrence of back pain.[255, 262]

Back Education. Proper body mechanics can improve the quality of your life when suffering from chronic low-back pain and help you get back to work in a shorter period of time.[255, 263]

*Note: Other treatments **may** help a person with low-back pain get some short-term relief, but these methods have not been proven effective in altering the long-term course of low-back pain. They include: spinal manipulation;[264] heat, ultrasound, and massage;[265, 266] hot tubs; ice; traction;[267] corsets; TENS (transcutaneous electrical nerve stimulator);[268] and acupuncture/acupressure.*

Preventing and Improving Low-Back Pain

PHYSICAL ACTIVITY

To learn more about pursuing a physical activity program, refer to the section *Daily Health Check #1, Physical Activity Programs,* page 40. Participating in regular physical activity is the greatest favor you can afford your back.

In addition, various stretching and strengthening activities for the back, abdomen and legs are found within these sections: *Daily Health Check #3, Body Flexibility Program,* page 53; and *Daily Health Check #2, Body Strength Program,* page 47.

BODY MECHANICS

The remainder of this section discusses body mechanic techniques that if practiced, can reduce the likelihood of being bothered with an "aching back."[255] Practicing these simple but very practical techniques should become "second nature" as they are performed on a daily basis.

Keep close to your work. Lifting or handling objects away from your center of gravity (naval) can increase the stress on your spine by as much 1,000 percent.[255]

Don't twist while lifting. Twisting adds pressure to the spine and may cause added disc damage and excessive strain to other back structures.

Never jerk. Sudden maneuvers may also injure the structures of the spine. Grasp the object firmly and lift slowly. If the object is too heavy, get help.

Let other muscles help. Sliding objects close to your body with your arms, lifting objects with your legs, and holding your pelvis stable with your stomach and buttocks, can shift stress from your back to other parts of your body to make activities more comfortable.

Stabilize the pelvis. Roll your pelvis upward (pelvic tilt) to flatten your back, then roll downward so that your back is slightly arched. Next tighten your stomach and buttock muscles and lock your back into a stable position. While holding this position, try standing up from a chair or squatting down to pick up an object. If this technique helps, use the same technique while getting out of your car, vacuuming or pushing a grocery cart. Use it to do any activity that may cause pain or that you feel unsure about.

To summarize, when you lift an object:

- Stabilize the pelvis;
- Keep the weight as close as possible;
- Lift slowly, don't jerk;
- If you must turn, turn with your feet, not your body;
- Maintain a wide base of support.

TIPS FOR SITTING

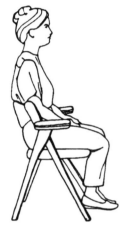

Sitting doubles the amount of pressure on the disc. Try not to sit for prolonged periods of time without getting up. To sit properly:

- Concentrate on keeping both shoulders comfortably back and down;
- Keep your lower back near the back of your chair and your abdominal muscles tightened;
- Avoid slumping, or sitting in a chair that is too high or low or too far from the work area.

Selecting a Chair

- The chair should be firm enough to prevent slouching.
- The chair should provide support for the lower back at least four to six inches above the bottom seat position.
- The chair should allow the knees to be comfortably bent with both feet touching the floor.

Getting in or Out of a Chair

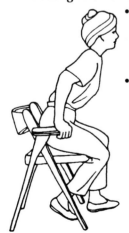

- When raising or lowering yourself into a chair, make a point of positioning one foot in front of the other.
- Keep your back straight and rely on the power of the thigh muscles and arms to push yourself up to a standing position.

Sitting at Your Work Area

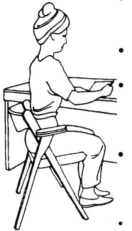

- The work surface (desk, table, etc.) should be the optimal height for the type of work being done.
- The work area should allow for comfortable thigh clearance.
- Work should be kept near the edge of the work surface to eliminate having to reach excessively or lean forward.
- Work should be positioned so that it is at no more than a 90° angle from where you're sitting. Don't reach excessively or lean forward.
- The chair's arm rests (if provided) should be short to enable you to push it close to the work surface.

Driving

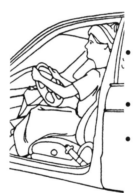

- Keep the car seat close enough to the steering wheel so that your knees are comfortably bent and are higher than your hips.
- Avoid having to stretch your legs to reach the floor pedals since this may strain the lower back.
- Place both hands on the steering wheel.
- If it's comfortable, try placing a small pillow or back rest behind your lower back.

TIPS FOR STANDING

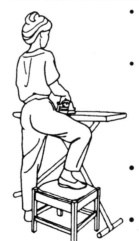

- Prolonged standing at a fixed spot can be hard on the back. Change positions regularly.
- Keep one foot propped up on a stool, book or box to avoid a build-up of back tension. This position is more comfortable because raising the hip slightly eases back strain.
- It's a good idea for women to avoid wearing high heels when standing for any length of time.
- Locking your knees when standing causes the hips to slant forward and produces pressure on the lower back. Your knees should be bent slightly and your feet should face forward.

- Keep your head high and chin comfortably tucked. When you become aware you're starting to lean forward, adjust yourself back to an erect position.

Standing at Your Work Area

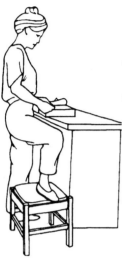

- Your work surface should be at a height that is appropriate for the task. Your feet should face forward.
- The surface you are standing on should be cushioned.
- Use a foot rest to relieve low-back pressure.
- Keep the work in front of you or at no more than a 90° angle to the right or left. Never place the work behind you.
- Keep your work near the ends of the work surface to avoid having to bend or to reach for things.

TIPS FOR SLEEPING

Generally, if you sleep well in a certain position, then that position is not harmful to your back. The following are a few positions we have found to be helpful.

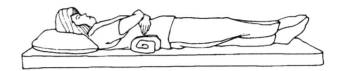

- Back-lying with towel roll under lower back.

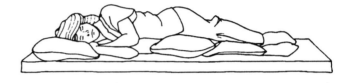

- Side-lying with pillow between legs.

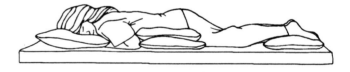

- Lying on stomach with one to two pillows under stomach and ankle.

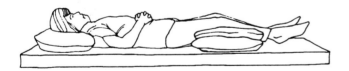

- Back-lying with two pillows under knees.

Lifestyle Counseling Health Check #6
CHOOSING A PRIMARY-CARE PHYSICIAN

RECOMMENDATIONS

1. All adults should establish a working relationship with a primary-care physician which includes a family practice physician, an internist, and for some females, a gynecologist.

2. Record the name of your primary-care physician and the names of any physician specialists in your *Health Questionnaire* located in Appendix A, page 170.

Why Perform

To follow your *Health Check Table* successfully, you must **first** retain the services of a primary-care physician. Finding the right physician may take some research, but the time spent is worth the effort.

The following story is told by one of the authors:

"A few years ago our family relocated to a new city. My periodic physical examination came due, and so I asked the cardiologist working with me for a referral. I acted on his recommendation and scheduled an appointment. I soon learned why this physician was highly recommended.

"Following the routine clinical tests by his nursing staff, I found myself seated next to his desk while he spent quality time talking about my past health history and my current medical status. I was impressed with this physician's interest in my nutritional and exercise habits, how well I was coping with my job and home life, and if I was faithful in wearing my seat belt.

"Following our visit, during which time he made very detailed notes along with an action list, he proceeded to perform a very detailed examination (carefully explaining the procedures and the reason they were being done). I was also impressed during our visit that on several occasions he referred to new studies that he had read about or learned of while attending recent medical conferences."

STEPS TO FOLLOW

The "inside connection" that was used to locate a physician in the above story is not necessary. Use the following tips to assist you in choosing a physician.[269-272]

Primary-Care Physician. The role of the primary-care physician is to assist you in the management of your Health Check Table and to direct you to other medical specialists when necessary. The three major sources of primary-care physicians include:

- **Family Practice Physicians.** These doctors are specialty trained in patient-care and are required to pass a recertification examination every three years (administered by the American Academy of Family Practice) to remain board certified.
- **Internists.** These physicians have specialized in adult internal medicine with specific skills in diagnosing medical problems. Many internists choose to continue their medical education and subspecialize in various medical areas such as cardiology or endocrinology.
- **Gynecologists.** These physicians specialize in female medical care. Some gynecologists choose to emphasize primary-care as part of their medical practice.

Supportive. An important consideration is whether or not the primary-care physician is supportive of the concept of assisting you with your *Health Check Table.*

Ask Friends. Take the time to ask close friends and/or relatives which physician they respect, and what specifically they like about their physicians.

Other Sources. Ask nurses or other allied health personnel that work with the physicians in your community for a physician recommendation. These individuals are often "in the know" when it comes to recommending a quality care physician.

When Relocating. If you move to another city or state, ask your current physician for a physician referral. When settled into your new residence, make it a point to also visit several different neighbors to get their advice on a good physician.

Qualifications. Consider the physician's qualifications. Visit your local library to consult the "Directory of Medical Specialists," or the "American Medical Directory." Among other things, you can learn from these references whether or not physicians are board certified (have successfully passed the examination requirements issued by the respective medical board), or whether they are board-eligible (have completed the necessary residency training but not practiced for a period of at least two years or have not passed the examination of the respective board).

Attending Privileges. Does the physician have attending privileges at a hospital? Most hospitals have a thorough review procedure used to screen physicians applying for privileges.

Keeping Current. Is the physician remaining as current as possible with the rapidly changing medical world? Many physicians have board specialty requirements to complete post-graduate medical education classes each year. For example, the American Board of Family Physicians requires all family practice doctors to recertify every three years in order to maintain their board eligibility.

Practice Type. The type of practice (solo, partnership, or group) that the primary-care physician participates in may be important. The benefits and disadvantages associated with the type of physician practice are discussed in *Lifestyle Counseling Health Check #7, Choosing A Health Care Plan and Medical Care Facility*, page 144.

Professionalism. Are your primary-care physician and staff both capable and courteous? Do they promote an atmosphere of friendliness and give you the opportunity to be part of the decision-making process in following your Health Check Table? Does your physician have a flexible attitude and allow you to disagree if you feel a particular matter needs further clarification or discussion? If you feel intimidated and you're afraid to ask questions regarding your personal health concerns, then participating in your own health care is hindered.

Follow-Up. Does your physician and staff have adequate follow-up procedures? Although the maintenance manual encourages you to keep your own medical records, your primary-care physician should keep accurate and organized records of your health-care procedures.

Doctor's Age and Gender. Finally, you may want to consider the age and gender of your primary-care physician. Some individuals feel more comfortable with a physician of their same sex and age, while others prefer a physician either younger or older than their age and the sex is of no consequence.

Remember, a critical component of following your maintenance manual is to establish a positive relationship with a primary-care physician. If you are without a primary-care doctor, turn to the *Yearly or Periodic Health Check #1, Physical Examination and Health History*, page 76, and schedule an appointment today.

Lifestyle Counseling Health Check #7

CHOOSING A HEALTH CARE PLAN
AND MEDICAL CARE FACILITY

RECOMMENDATIONS

1. **Never** be without medical insurance coverage. If you do not now have medical insurance coverage, follow the recommendations in this section and then take the steps necessary to secure medical insurance.

2. Record the name(s) and policy number(s) of your health insurance carriers in your *Health Questionnaire* located in Appendix A, page 170.

Why Perform

Few professions have changed as drastically in the past decade as has the health insurance field. Health insurance companies now publish thick books to explain various insurance coverage options. No longer do we simply sign a one-page policy that is the same for all employees.

Time and effort are required to choose a health care policy that is best for the needs of you or your family. Take an active role in reviewing available health care plans (costs and benefits) offered by your employer or other health care facilities. Be aware also that some medical/health care plans are now paying for periodic physical examinations and healthy lifestyle counseling.

Finally, just as it is illegal to own and operate an automobile without car insurance — so should you consider it illegal to be without health care coverage. You cannot afford to take such a financial risk.

TYPES OF HEALTH CARE PLANS & POLICIES[269-272]

Keep two tips in mind as you consider the major types of health care policies.

- **Cost** – How do the premium payments compare? Is there a deductible cost (how much) before the insurance provider will pay? Are there co-payments (how much)?
- **Freedom of choice** – How restricted are you in choosing a physician and medical care? Are there options to match your individual health needs?

Fee-for-Service. This is the most widely used type of medical insurance coverage. The patient (and/or employer) simply pays a monthly premium to an insurance company and when the physician is seen, the doctor's office bills the insurance carrier. The largest user of the fee-for-service plan is Medicare and Medicaid.

A major advantage of the fee-for-service coverage is the user's freedom. You are generally not restricted in your selection of a primary-care physician or other medical specialists. However, these types of policies are quite narrow in their approach to covering preventive medicine claims, and unless you have a symptom-of-illness the insurance carrier will not cover the medical costs.

Health Maintenance Organization (HMO). This health insurance plan is increasing in popularity because of the potential to reduce health care costs. You and your employer pay a *fixed* monthly or annual amount and then all health care needs are covered. A positive aspect of many HMOs is that they cover the cost of preventive care services. This means that most (if not all) of the clinical health checks are paid by the HMO — including, in some instances, educational classes.

Although the cost to the person enrolling with an HMO is generally less, there may be less opportunity to choose your physician. Some primary-care physicians feel the HMO interferes with their freedom of practice because of pre-established utilization guidelines.

Preferred Provider Organization (PPO). Also increasing in popularity, the PPO is an attempt to curb medical costs. The PPO consists of physicians (primary-care and other specialists) who independently contract with an insurance company or a large company to provide medical services at a cost lower than the going rate.

The PPO plan may have a broad spectrum of options to choose from, but your options for choosing a doctor may be limited. All medical services you require must be coordinated through your primary-care physician (this is generally a positive point).

TYPES OF PHYSICIAN PRACTICES

Listed below are the types of physician practices to help you further in choosing a health care plan and primary-care physician.[269-272]

Solo Practice. Although the solo practice physician is a traditional part of America, fewer doctors are choosing to "go it alone." If you live in a remote area, your primary-care physician's only choice may be to practice solo. Disadvantages of having a solo practice physician are:

- Your doctor may be limited in seeking advice from colleagues;
- Getting medical help when your doctor is out of town. (This is not always the case — some solo practice doctors will arrange with other primary-care physicians to cover their office practice when necessary and to trade evening and emergency calls.)

Partnership Practice. This practice consists of two or more physicians who share clinical and financial responsibilities. Partnership doctors can reduce expenses and can assist one another in their practices. If your primary-care doctor is part of a partnership practice, your health care needs will generally be covered day and night and follow-up will be consistent.

A possible disadvantage of partnership practice is you may not always see your doctor of choice, but his or her partner. Advance planning may be necessary to make certain you see the physician of preference.

Group Practice. If you live in a city of moderate or larger population, there is likely to be one or more group medical practices. The group practice consists of a number of physicians with varying types of specialties and subspecialties working together in what is often called a clinic. Among the first physicians to introduce the concept of group medical practice were the Mayo brothers of Rochester, Minnesota. From an initial group of three doctors, the Mayo Clinic has grown to almost 1,000 physicians.

The advantages to choosing a primary-care physician who practices in a group setting are:

- A built-in privilege for your doctor to consul colleagues for advice;
- Additional clinical tests can generally be performed in the clinic;
- If necessary, you can be seen by additional specialist doctors in the clinic;
- Doctors in the clinic generally carefully screen new doctors joining their staff;
- An effort is often made to provide patient education services.

Hospital-Based Out-Patient Clinic. A majority of hospitals have out-patient clinics to provide primary-care service for patients. In some instances, the doctor you see will be a physician in training (a resident or intern). Because many of these clinics are established in part to educate young physicians, the cost for services may be significantly lower than that found elsewhere in the community.

One negative factor of a hospital-based out-patient clinic is that you may see a different physician every time you go to the clinic. This does not imply that your medical care will be substandard (often the training physician is very thorough) but establishing a positive relationship with the primary-care physician of your choice is difficult.

Freestanding Primary-Care Centers. These centers have continued to spring up in many cities to provide "around-the-clock" service, and to treat minor emergencies and illnesses such as common respiratory infections.

These facilities are usually operated by hospitals that have contracted with physicians to work back-to-back shifts. Many free-standing centers are now getting involved with primary-care services.

The cost of seeing a physician at a free-standing center is generally much less than the expenses of an emergency room visit. Like the hospital out-patient clinic, these free-standing centers may limit your ability to establish a long-lasting relationship with a primary-care physician.

Lifestyle Counseling Health Check #8

DETERMINING YOUR GENETIC
AND ENVIRONMENTAL RISK

Why Perform

We occasionally learn of individuals who have smoked for 50 years and appear quite healthy, or who have broken the rules of good nutrition and at age 80 their only exercise is acting as pallbearer for friends' funerals.

These incidents seem to suggest that diseases occur in a random or an unpredictable fashion. In actuality, the role of chance in the disease process diminishes rapidly as additional information is discovered about the mechanisms of the disease.

The attitude that "you can't change your genes, so why worry about it" is far from correct. Literally thousands of lives have been favorably impacted because of personal attention to genetic and environmental risk factors. Consider the following evidence:

- A detailed family history can help identify those individuals with a strong tendency to certain major illnesses such as colon cancer and diabetes. These individuals can then focus their preventive measure efforts.[273]
- An understanding of the environmental factors promoting disease development will facilitate effective prevention strategies, delaying the disease process in susceptible individuals.[273]
- Dr. Roger Williams, University of Utah Medical Center, has identified four large families that carry a gene for developing very high blood cholesterol. Although the male population of these families born **since** the turn of the century have died of

coronary heart disease on the average *at age 45*, the male family members born *before 1880* (also carrying the high cholesterol gene) lived from *62 to 81* years of age. The research suggests the pre-1880-born individuals lived longer because of a healthier lifestyle.[273, 274]

- Past studies have shown that the rate of early coronary heart disease is less than one-fourth among men of the Japanese male population when compared to the young men of the United States. However, when Japanese men move to Hawaii or California, their blood cholesterol levels and early coronary heart disease rates rise to match the American male's. Environmental influences may have a great impact on this disease process among individuals who have similar genetic backgrounds.[275]

HOW TO DETERMINE YOUR GENETIC AND ENVIRONMENTAL RISK

To assess your genetic and environmental risk status, you should complete the *Genetic/Environmental Risk* portion of your *Health Questionnaire*, located in Appendix A, page 182. Refer to your questionnaire at this time. Note that this section of your health questionnaire emphasizes the following questions:[273]

- Do you have any medical problems that tend to run in the family?
- Have you any close relatives (parents, grandparents, siblings, aunts, uncles or offspring) who have had premature or early (before the age of 55) heart attack or heart surgery, cancer, diabetes mellitus, high blood pressure, stroke, emotional illness, serious problems with allergies?
- What was the age of onset and treatment of any of your relatives for the reported disease? An early age onset of disease occurring among several relatives would suggest a strong family history.
- What are the vital statistics of your family such as current age or age at death and what was the cause of death (if deceased)?

To complete your personal questionnaire, you may need to contact family members for additional information. For example, if a strong family history for a given disease is indicated, efforts to obtain additional health history information from family relatives is a good idea. A family member who had heart surgery for rheumatic heart disease may be confused with coronary artery disease, or a benign (non-cancerous) growth may be confused with a

certain type of cancer. Remember, if you approach relatives for this information, we suggest that you do so with the understanding that all medical information will be kept confidential — and then keep it that way.[273]

Health Risk Appraisal. Together with completing your *Health Questionnaire* and participating in lifestyle counseling, a Health Risk Appraisal (HRA) can help you identify your risk of disease or disability. HRAs have been developed to tie disease prevention with computer science. Most HRAs include questions about your age and gender, as well as lifestyle habits such as smoking, exercise, and diet. You'll also be questioned about your cholesterol and blood pressure. Your answers to these and other questions are then compared to large population databases and a profile of your risk for certain diseases or health conditions is then developed.

The HRA is often used in community and worksite health promotion programs to identify areas of individual health concern. It's also a good way to motivate participants to take preventive action to reduce their risk for potential health problems.

WHAT'S NEXT?

Review Health Questionnaire. Review your genetic/environmental information with your primary-care doctor and together determine if your *Health Questionnaire* identifies a tendency for a certain disease.

Make Adjustments. Based upon the review of your questionnaire, discuss with your physician whether your *Health Check Table* should be adjusted so certain health checks are performed on a more frequent schedule or whether additional *high-risk* health checks should be part of your health maintenance program.

For example, a family history of early colon cancer might suggest you and your doctor consider a *high-risk* health check referred to as a **colonoscopy** exam. In addition, your doctor may recommend you have colon cancer screening earlier than the standard recommended age.

Keep record. Be certain to keep record of the recommended changes to your *Health Check Table*.

Health Risk Appraisal (HRA). Consider completing an HRA. If you are unaware of a health promotion program in your area that provides an HRA, contact the *Society of Prospective Medicine* (1-317-923-3600) or your state Health Department (Office of Disease Prevention and Health Promotion) for more information about how to obtain an HRA questionnaire.

Lifestyle Counseling Health Check #9
and
Daily Health Check #9

GUIDELINES FOR BETTER SLEEP

RECOMMENDATIONS

1. We recommend that individuals sleep seven to eight hours each night. We also recommend that people review with their doctor the quality of their sleep, and in addition, learn techniques to improve sleep.

2. Although napping is generally discouraged for proper sleep hygiene, a **short duration** nap may have health benefits for certain individuals, providing the practice of napping does not interfere with evening sleep patterns.

Why Perform

We all understand the value of "a good night's sleep." Sleep, like eating, is vitally important for maintaining good health. Our belief, however, is that few people recognize just how important a role sleep plays in how we feel about our personal health — emotionally and physically.

SLEEP: AN ACTIVE PROCESS

Most people view sleep as a time when the body "shuts down." Interestingly, the opposite is true — sleep is an active, complex process in which two types of sleep alternate through the night in roughly 90-minute cycles. These two types of sleep and a simplified listing of what takes place during these types of sleep patterns is outlined below:[276]

Quiet Sleep — Non-Rapid Eye Movement (Non-REM)

- 75 percent of our total sleep time;
- No rapid eye movements;
- Decreased brain metabolism;
- Low, steady metabolic rate;
- Slower frequency and higher amplitude EEG (brain waves).

Active or Paradoxical Sleep –
Rapid Eye Movement (REM)

- 25 percent of total sleep time;
- Rapid eye movements;
- Increased brain metabolism;
- Muscle paralysis;
- Intense dreaming;
- Erratic breathing pattern.

HOW MUCH SLEEP IS REQUIRED?

With age the amount of time spent in deep sleep generally decreases and the fragmentation of our sleep increases. Although the amount of sleep required for each individual varies, most adults require **seven to eight** hours of sleep each night. Most sleep experts agree that less than six and a-half hours of sleep is **too little** for good health.

We encourage patients who almost brag that they function on very little sleep to experiment with increasing their amount of sleep and to monitor their day's production. Often the productivity of the person is not hampered by getting more sleep.

ELEVEN RULES FOR BETTER SLEEP HYGIENE[277]

Consider the following for improving the quality of your sleep:

1. Sleep as much as necessary to feel refreshed and healthy during the day, but not more. Curtailing the time in bed seems to solidify sleep; excessively long times in bed seem related to fragmented and shallow sleep.

2. A regular time of awakening each morning strengthens the daily sleep period and leads to regular times of sleep onset at night. Try to go to sleep about the same time every night. (However, if you don't feel sleepy, don't get into bed.) Follow the same routine every night before going to bed.

3. A steady daily amount of exercise is associated with faster sleep onset, fewer awakenings from sleep, and deeper sleep. However, avoid vigorous exercise just prior to sleep since it tends to disrupt sleep.

4. Occasional loud noises (for example, aircraft fly-overs) disturb sleep even in people who are not awakened by noises and cannot remember them in the morning. Soundproofed bedrooms may help those close to noise.

5. An excessively warm or cold room disturbs sleep.

6. Hunger may disturb sleep; a light snack may help sleep. Warm milk just before bed has been shown to help sleep.

7. Caffeine in the evening disturbs sleep, even in those who feel that it does not. It is best to avoid drinks such as coffee, tea, colas, and soft drinks that contain caffeine after noon. Decaffeinated coffee, decaffeinated or herbal teas, and caffeine-free soft drinks are all good substitute beverages during the afternoon and evening.

8. Alcohol may help tense people fall asleep more easily, but the sleep is often disturbed.

9. People who feel angry and frustrated because they cannot sleep should not try harder and harder to sleep but should turn on the light and do something different.

10. The chronic use of tobacco disturbs sleep.

11. An occasional sleeping pill may be of some benefit, but chronic use is ineffective in most insomniacs and can lead to further disruptions of the sleep period.

(These sleep hygiene rules are printed by permission of Upjohn Pharmaceutical. The rules are taken from "The Sleep Disorders," by Dr. Peter Hauri.)

SLEEP TREATMENT

We spend one-third of our life sleeping, or for some people, trying to sleep. Sleep disorders are becoming more widely recognized as clinicians and patients learn more about the various kinds of sleep disorders (including the typical symptoms). Many major hospitals now have "Sleep Disorder Clinics," to diagnose and treat sleep problems effectively.

You should discuss with your doctor the following questions:

- "What is the quality of your sleep?"
- "Does your night's sleep afford you optimal daytime function with minimal drowsiness?"

In addition to these questions, if you notice any of the symptoms for sleep disorders described on the next page, be certain to bring the matter to the attention of your physician.[276]

DISORDER	SYMPTOMS
Sleep Apnea	1. Excessive daytime sleepiness
	2. Snoring
	3. Nightly apnea (absence of breathing)
	4. Non-refreshing sleep
	5. Morning headache
	6. Repeated nightly arousals without memory
Narcolepsy	1. Excessive daytime sleepiness
	2. Sudden weak knees or jaw when excited
	3. Naps are refreshing
	4. Sleepy when excited
	5. Sleep paralysis
	6. Vivid dreaming at sleep onset
Restless Legs and Nocturnal Myoclonus	1. Excessive daytime sleepiness
	2. Non-refreshing sleep
	3. Restless sensation in legs
	4. Nightly leg jerks
Insomnia	1. Daytime fatigue
	2. Restlessness
	3. Difficulty initiating or maintaining sleep
	4. Remembers repeated nightly arousals
	5. Sleeps less than six hours

A WORD ABOUT NAPPING

Most sleep disorder experts are opposed to the idea of recommending napping because of the increased likelihood of developing sleep disorders or worsening already existing sleep problems. Dr. David Dinges has conducted research on napping and has recently published a medical text on the health benefits of napping.

One of the authors of this book feels that a short nap, such as 10 to 15 minutes, can be very refreshing. Many countries take advantage of a midday "break" (or siesta), so the concept is not new.

Individuals should avoid following the recommendation of taking a nap if the practice interferes with their ability to get to sleep at night. Also, an **extended** nap should be avoided.

High-Risk Health Check #1

FASTING PLASMA GLUCOSE [278]
(SCREENING FOR ABNORMAL BLOOD SUGAR)

RECOMMENDATIONS

1. The following individuals who are high-risk for diabetes mellitus should consider having a periodic fasting blood glucose (blood sugar) test:[278, 386]
   - Persons who are markedly obese;
   - Individuals who have a family history of diabetes;
   - Women with a history of gestational diabetes.

2. Pregnant women should have a 50-gram oral glucose tolerance test for gestational diabetes between 24 and 28 weeks of gestation. If the results of the one-hour blood glucose level is 140 mg/dl or greater, then it is recommended that a three-hour 100-gram oral glucose test be performed to confirm the previous results.[278]

Why Perform

Diabetes mellitus is the seventh major cause of death in the United States.[278, 365, 366] Estimates suggest that 11 million Americans have diabetes mellitus (five million of whom are unaware that they have the disease).[278,279] Type II, or non-insulin-dependent diabetes mellitus (NIDDM), (often referred to as "adult-onset diabetes") accounts for 90 percent of the diabetes cases.[279] Type I diabetes, or insulin-dependent diabetes mellitus (IDDM), generally occurs in the earlier years of life (childhood or adolescent).[278] There is also a condition of glucose intolerance that develops in approximately three percent of non-diabetic women who become pregnant.[278]

Diabetes is a major risk factor for:

- Coronary artery disease and stroke;
- Circulation problems (diabetes accounts for approximately 50,000 amputations each year); [278, 280]
- Neuropathy (a very painful disease of the nerve endings);[279]
- Blindness (diabetes is the leading cause of blindness in the adult population);[278-282]
- Kidney failure;
- Other metabolic complications.[278]

Early detection of diabetes mellitus in individuals without symptoms can help "prevent or delay" the potential complications of this disease.[278] Many of the medical problems associated with diabetes are "directly related to the duration and severity" of high blood sugar.[278, 283-286]

The *greatest* prevention for adult-onset diabetes (NIDDM) is regular exercise (such as a walking program), weight loss, and proper nutrition (see *Daily Health Checks*).[278] There are many adults who have literally removed the threat of potential diabetes complications by pursuing these lifestyle habits.

How Performed

The principal screening test for diabetes mellitus is the fasting blood glucose (blood sugar) test obtained from a simple blood draw. If the results of this test are abnormally high, your physician will help you decide if you should have a more specific test (glucose-tolerance test) to confirm a glucose problem.

High-Risk Health Check #2

BACTERIURIA, HEMATURIA, AND PROTEINURIA [287]
(SCREENING FOR INDIVIDUALS WITHOUT SYMPTOMS FOR BACTERIURIA, HEMATURIA, AND PROTEINURIA)

RECOMMENDATIONS

1. The following persons should be routinely screened for bacteriuria, hematuria, and proteinuria (bacteria, blood or protein in the urine):
   - Individuals with diabetes mellitus;
   - Pregnant women;
   - Persons aged 60 and older and **preschool children.**[287]

Why Perform

Because **hematuria and proteinuria** frequently are the result of kidney or bladder cancer or kidney disease, early detection before other symptoms emerge is important.[287,288] The earlier the detection of bladder cancer, the greater the likelihood of survival.[287,66] Early detection of **bacteriuria** in individuals (especially the elderly) who are without symptoms may result in the prevention of the disorder progressing to the stage of producing symptoms and further clinical problems.[287,289,290]

In addition to recommended screening, it is very important that individuals reduce their risk for bladder and kidney cancer by *not smoking* — cigarette smoking has been linked to 48 percent of the deaths from kidney cancer and 47 percent of the deaths from bladder cancer.[287]

How Performed

The screening test generally used to detect these disorders is a dipstick urinalysis.[291] A paper stick with chemically prepared pads is dipped into the urine sample, and if bacteria, blood or protein is present, the small pad will react by turning a specific color.

High-Risk Health Check #3

HEARING SCREENING

RECOMMENDATIONS

1. Individuals who are exposed to hazardous noise levels should consider a periodic hearing screen. For further explanation regarding the hearing screening test, refer to *Yearly or Periodic Health Check #15, Hearing Test*, page 115.

High-Risk Health Check #4

COLONOSCOPY [58]

RECOMMENDATIONS

1. The following individuals should undergo a colonoscopy, or an air-contrast barium enema, examination. Persons who have:
    *   A family history of polyposis coli (a high number of polyps in the colon, large intestine);
    *   A strong family history of colon cancer.

2. These tests examine the entire colon (or the entire large intestine). For further explanation regarding these risk factors and the subsequent screening test, refer to *Yearly or Periodic Health Check #10, Lower Colon Exam*, page 87.

High-Risk Health Check #5 and #6

RESTING ELECTROCARDIOGRAM
EXERCISE ELECTROCARDIOGRAM STRESS TEST

RESTING ELECTROCARDIOGRAM

To learn more about the recommendations for this screening procedure and how the test is performed, refer to *Yearly or Periodic Health Check #2, Cardiovascular Screening,* page 79.

EXERCISE ELECTROCARDIOGRAM STRESS TEST

To learn more about the recommendations for this screening procedure and how the test is performed, refer to *Yearly or Periodic Health Check #2, Cardiovascular Screening,* page 79.

High-Risk Health Check #7

MAMMOGRAM[292]

RECOMMENDATIONS

1. Women who have a family history of **pre-menopausal detected breast cancer in first-degree relatives** (mother or sisters) should have a mammogram at an age *earlier* than the recommended age of 40. Whether or not mammography should be performed earlier than age 40 because of other risk factors should be discussed with your doctor. For more information regarding mammography and risk factors for developing breast cancer, refer to *Yearly or Periodic Health Check #13 and #14,* page 111.

High-Risk Health Check #8

SCREENING FOR TUBERCULOSIS [293]

RECOMMENDATIONS[293]

1. The following high-risk individuals should be screened for tuberculosis:
   - Household members who live with a person who has tuberculosis;
   - Individuals who are at risk for close contact with this disease such as staff members of tuberculosis clinics, homeless shelters, nursing homes, substance abuse treatment facilities, dialysis units, and correctional institutions;
   - Recent immigrants or refugees from countries in which tuberculosis is common such as Asia, Africa, Central and South American, the Pacific Islands and Caribbean;
   - Residents of nursing homes, correctional institutions, or homeless shelters;
   - Persons with underlying medical disorders such as HIV infection (AIDS virus infection).

Why Perform

Early detection and subsequent treatment of individuals found to have a positive tuberculosis screening test can have beneficial effects for the individual by preventing further progression of the tuberculosis.[293, 294] The process of early detection and treatment can also be beneficial in preventing the spread of tuberculosis to those individuals who may be in close contact with the carrier.[293, 295, 296]

How Performed

For the doctor to determine if you are infected with the bacteria that can cause tuberculosis, a small amount of protein is taken from dead TB bacteria and then injected into your skin. If you have been infected with TB or if you have had a vaccination against TB, then your skin will swell where the dead TB was injected.[297]

If your tuberculin skin test is positive, you should consult with your physician to weigh carefully the risks and benefits of receiving treatment (there are risks involved in receiving the current treatment for positive tuberculin screens).[293] How frequent high-risk groups should receive a tuberculin screening test should also be discussed with your physician.

High-Risk Health Check #9, #10, and #11

DISCUSSION OF OSTEOPOROSIS RISK,
BONE MINERAL SCREENING,
AND HORMONE REPLACEMENT THERAPY

RECOMMENDATIONS[298, 299, 392]

1. Bone mineral screening for osteoporosis is **not** recommended for:
   - Women without symptoms of low-bone mineral content and women at low risk for osteoporosis;
   - Women who are experiencing fractures suggestive of significant bone loss.

2. It may be prudent and desirable to perform bone mineral screening in women who are:
   - At high-risk for osteoporosis and who would not otherwise receive long-term hormone replacement therapy;
   - Receiving long-term steroid therapy for diseases such as rheumatoid arthritis, asthma, lupus, and inflammatory bowel disease;[300]
   - Receiving long-term thyroid replacement therapy for thyroid disorders.

3. Women should be made aware of risk factors for osteoporosis and in addition, receive counseling about the preventive value of weight-bearing exercise (*Daily Health Check #1, Physical Activity Programs*, page 40), and the appropriate use of calcium supplementation (*Daily Health Check #4, Proper Nutrition program*, page 58). Elderly persons should also be made aware of the importance of taking measures to prevent falls (*Lifestyle Counseling Health Check #2, Injury Prevention*, page 127).

4. Hormone replacement therapy should be considered for women who are at risk for osteoporosis and who understand the potential benefits and risks of receiving hormone supplements. [299, 301]

5. Risk factors for osteoporosis include: [298-302]
   - Female, Caucasian or Oriental;
   - Small-framed, petite, thin, fair-complected;
   - Family history of osteoporosis;
   - Early menopause (natural or from surgical removal of ovaries);
   - Amenorrheic (low estrogen levels);
   - Cigarette smoking, drink alcohol in excess;
   - Low calcium diet;
   - High caffeine intake;
   - Physically inactive;
   - Diabetes mellitus;
   - Gastrointestinal problems which decreases calcium absorption;
   - Long-term use of steroid-based medication for medical problems such as asthma, arthritis and lupus;
   - Long-term use of thyroid medication.

   Recognize that certain risk factors (such as amenorrhia) pose a greater risk than others (such as excessive caffeine intake). For this reason, you and your physician should discuss the risk factors you may have for osteoporosis, paying special attention to the degree of risk for each factor.

Why Perform

Osteoporosis (generally occurring in older adults) is a disease that results in a gradual loss of bone substance. For postmenopausal women, osteoporosis causes:

- One to two million fractures each year in the United States (with hip fractures occurring in one-third of the women who live to age 90).[299, 303-306]
- Seventy percent of all fractures in women over age 45 (50 percent of postmenopausal women will at sometime develop a spontaneous fracture).[299, 304, 307]
- Yearly medical costs greater than $7 billion.[299, 308]

How Performed

SCREENING FOR LOW BONE MINERAL CONTENT

Because low bone mineral content (BMC) is a major risk factor for osteoporosis, medical screening tests to effectively detect low BMC have been developed.[299, 309-314] They include:

- The CT scan;
- The dual-photon absorptiometry (DPA);
- The dual-energy X-ray absorptiometry (DEXA).

Because of the expense and the radiation exposure the CT scan is used the least for routine screening.[299] Of the remaining methods (DPA and DEXA), research suggests that DEXA may be the more effective screening tool for BMC.[299, 315, 316]

For women at risk for low BMC or osteoporosis, bone mineral screening can be used for treatment decisions such as whether or not to initiate estrogen replacement therapy. In addition, identifying low BMC can help motivate patients to make lifestyle changes that will reduce the risk of osteoporosis such as quitting smoking, beginning a physical activity program, or reducing the intake of alcohol.[299]

HORMONE REPLACEMENT THERAPY

Hormone replacement therapy can have the following benefits for women:

- Slow bone mineral loss following menopause;[299, 308, 309, 317, 318]
- Reduce bone fractures and vaginal atrophy;
- Decrease deaths from coronary heart disease.[301, 319-325]

Although maintaining adequate calcium intake and physical activity are important for bone loss prevention, they may not be enough. Women should recognize that hormone replacement may also be required for osteoporosis prevention.

Women should be aware also that there are potential risks associated with estrogen replacement therapy such as endometrial cancer.[301, 326-330] Because of the potential risks, all women should carefully discuss with their physician whether or not they should participate in hormone replacement therapy.

Finally, if a woman is using estrogen replacement therapy for *short-term* relief of menopausal symptoms, rather than *long-term* use for bone loss prevention, she should have a bone screening to help her decide on which plan to follow.

CALCIUM REQUIREMENTS

A lifelong reduced intake of calcium may contribute to bone mineral loss and to further development of osteoporosis.[331, 332-336] Whether or not increases in calcium intake slows bone mineral loss or osteoporosis is uncertain.[333,334] Because the potential benefits derived from calcium supplementation far outweigh the minimal risks of moderately increasing calcium intake, women at risk for osteoporosis and bone mineral loss are recommended to increase calcium intake.[331]

Calcium intake recommendations from the National Institutes of Health, The National Research Council, and the University of Connecticut Osteoporosis Center include:

Adult Men	800 – 1,000 mg/day
Adult Women	800 – 1,000 mg/day

Pregnant or Breast Feeding
- Over age 19   1,200 mg/day
- Under age 19   1,600 mg/day

After-Menopause
- Not on Estrogen   1,500 mg/day
- On Estrogen   1,000 mg/day

MEDICINE AND OSTEOPOROSIS – NEW PROMISE

Recent research has shown the medicine *etidronate*, a diphosphonate drug, increases bone density and decreases the rate of bone fractures. This medicine and others may lead to improved care for those who suffer from osteoporosis.

PREVENTING OSTEOPOROSIS THROUGH PHYSICAL ACTIVITY

Physical activity has a favorable impact upon osteoporosis prevention.[337,338] Dr. Gail Dalsky, a research specialist in osteoporosis, has suggested that individuals who have:

- had fractures;
- experienced significant bone mineral loss;
- a high-risk profile for osteoporosis;

should participate in physical activities that will improve balance and strength, thereby reducing the risk of having a fall.

Dr. Dalsky cautions that the physical activities should not place too great a stress on the bones and that the women should progress slowly from non-weight bearing physical activities to gradually including weight-bearing activities.[338] She also advises that some women may **not** be able to engage in physical activities that produce a weight-bearing effect.[338]

Finally, individuals who are at normal risk for osteoporosis should follow standard physical activity guidelines. These guidelines are outlined in *Daily Health Check #1, Physical Activity Programs,* on page 40.

High-Risk Health Check #12

DISCUSSION OF ASPIRIN THERAPY

RECOMMENDATIONS

1. Men who are aged 40 and older and are at significantly increased risk for heart attack should consider low-dose aspirin therapy (325 mg. every other day).

2. Prior to beginning aspirin therapy individuals should discuss with their physician potential benefits and risks and whether aspirin therapy is appropriately indicated.[339]

Why Perform

Several research studies have shown that daily aspirin therapy reduces the risk of death from strokes and heart attack in individuals who:

- Are at increased risk for coronary artery disease;
- Have had a heart attack or bypass heart surgery;
- Have had transient ischemic attacks or thrombolysis.

Two studies evaluating the risks and benefits of aspirin therapy in healthy men have been conducted.[339] The first was carried out by Harvard University and involved 22,000 American physicians. One group of physicians took 325 mg. of aspirin every other day and the other group took a placebo.[339, 340] After four-and-a-half years, the aspirin group had a 47 percent lower rate of fatal and non-fatal heart attacks and a higher number of the type of strokes that are caused by bleeding into the brain (hemorrhagic stroke). The difference in hemorrhaging strokes between the two groups was not statistically different, however.

The second study involved 5,000 male physicians in England who took 500 mg. of aspirin daily (no placebo was given).[339, 341] The study did not show aspirin therapy to reduce heart attack. This study also had an increase in hemorrhagic stroke among physicians taking aspirin, but this was not significant.

How Performed

The general consensus among physicians is that aspirin therapy should be considered as a preventive measure for men over age 40 who have risk factors for heart attacks. Before considering aspirin therapy, review the information below, compiled by The American Heart Association:[342]

1. You should not decide to begin taking aspirin every other day until you've consulted with your personal physician. Aspirin shouldn't be used by everyone. For example, people with a history of certain medical problems, such as liver or kidney disease, peptic ulcer, gastrointestinal bleeding or other bleeding problems, may not be able to take it or may need to adjust how they take it.

2. If you decide, with your doctor's approval, to begin taking aspirin regularly, be sure you know aspirin's possible side effects. Your doctor can tell you what they are. Be sure to report any side effects to your doctor without delay.

3. The use of aspirin should be regulated if you're scheduled for surgery (even relatively minor surgery). Aspirin affects the blood clotting process, prolonging bleeding time. This effect can persist for several days after stopping the drug. Be sure your doctor advises you about taking aspirin in these circumstances.

4. All the CHD risk factors that you may have should be determined and a concerted effort made to reduce them (see *Yearly or Periodic Health Check #2, Cardiac Risk Factor Screening*, page 80, for a listing of CHD risk factors). Aspirin doesn't reverse the blood vessel disorder (atherosclerosis) that underlies heart attack. Instead, aspirin affects the clotting process that occurs where atherosclerosis has narrowed a blood vessel. Controlling the risk factors that contribute to atherosclerosis is still vitally important.

Reproduced with Permission. ©Aspirin and Your Heart *Copyright American Heart Association*

High-Risk Health Check #13

DISCUSSION OF HEMOGLOBIN TESTING

RECOMMENDATIONS

1. Hemoglobin analysis is recommended for the following individuals:[343]
   - Adolescents and young adults who are at risk for hemoglobin disorders such as sickle cell disease;
   - Pregnant black women;
   - Newborns who are at risk for hemoglobin disorders should undergo hemoglobin analysis.

2. Individuals who are at increased risk for hemoglobin disorders include people of Caribbean, Latin American, Asian, Mediterranean, and African descent.

3. Women who are pregnant should be screened for anemia by assessing the hematocrit and hemoglobin level. This screening procedure is discussed in *Yearly or Periodic Health Check #18*, page 119.

Why Perform

Hemoglobin is a protein found within the red blood cell. Hemoglobin assists in the transporting of oxygen to living tissues. Hemoglobin disorders such as sickle cell diseases and thalassemia maladies affect several thousands of infants, adolescents and adults. Sickle cell disease is especially prevalent among the black population. Early detection of hemoglobin disorders can lead to effective antibiotic treatment and can help to identify carriers with the disease trait.

How Performed

The principal test to detect hemoglobin abnormalities is a blood test called hemoglobin electrophoreses. This blood test separates and measures different types of hemoglobin that may be found in the blood.

High-Risk Health Check #14

PREVENTION OF INJURIES IN THE ELDERLY

RECOMMENDATIONS

1. Older adults and those who have older adults living in their home should review *Lifestyle Counseling Health Check #2, Injury Prevention*, page 127, to reduce injuries among the elderly.

High-Risk Health Check #15

PREVENTION OF CHILDHOOD INJURIES

RECOMMENDATIONS

1. To reduce injuries in children, individuals who care for children (in the home and in the automobile) should review *Lifestyle Counseling Health Check #2, Injury Prevention*, page 127.

High-Risk Health Check #16

HEPATITIS B VACCINE

Why Perform

Estimates suggest that one-half to one million people carry the hepatitis B virus (HBV) in the U.S.,[344, 345] more than 300,000 people become infected with HBV yearly,[344, 346] and 5,000 people die from the effects of the virus (4,000 from cirrhosis of the liver and 1,000 from liver cancer).[344, 345]

Tragically, thousands of infants are born each year with HBV because their mothers are carriers; many of these children later develop fatal liver cancer or liver disease.[346-350]

The major benefit derived from early detection of HBV infection is the prevention of *transmission* of the virus to other individuals. In addition, when HBV virus is detected in a woman who is pregnant, research suggests that treatment can help prevent infection in the newborn.[344]

How Performed

A blood sample is required to test for the presence of the HBV virus. This test is called an immunoassay.

High-Risk Health Check #17

MEASLES – MUMPS – RUBELLA VACCINE [351]

RECOMMENDATIONS

1. Individuals who lack immunity to measles and mumps should have a measles-mumps-rubella vaccine. (The vaccination should not be administered during pregnancy.)

Why Perform

A measles-mumps-rubella (MMR) vaccine is performed to produce a long-term (lifetime) immunity against these three diseases.

How Performed

The MMR vaccine is administered by injecting a small amount of the vaccine serum into the arm through a small gauge needle.

High-Risk Health Check #18

SCREENING FOR RUBELLA ANTIBODIES [352]

RECOMMENDATIONS

1. Blood testing for rubella antibodies should be performed on women who are pregnant and who have no evidence of immunity for rubella (do not have proof of rubella vaccination after the first birthday or laboratory evidence of immunity).

2. Pregnant women who meet the criteria above should be counseled regarding the potential risks to the fetus if they should contract rubella and should be vaccinated following delivery and before discharge from the hospital.

3. Non-pregnant woman of childbearing age without immunity for rubella, and who will agree not to become pregnant within the following three months, should be immunized against rubella.

Why Perform

Although a rather minor illness, rubella can cause serious problems for the fetus should a woman become infected with rubella during pregnancy.[352] The incidence of rubella in the U.S. has dropped by 99 percent since the introduction of the rubella vaccine in 1969,[353-355] but 10 to 20 percent of the population older than 15 years lack rubella antibodies.[352] Screening and vaccination of women without the rubella antibodies may eventually lead to the elimination of the rubella problem.

How Performed

A blood sample is required to test for rubella antibodies. A positive test suggests that a person's immune system has responded to the presence of rubella by producing antibodies.

High-Risk Health Check #19 and #20

PNEUMOCOCCAL VACCINE
INFLUENZA VACCINE

RECOMMENDATIONS

1. For recommendations regarding pneumococcal vaccine, refer to *Yearly or Periodic Health Checks #20, #21, and #22, Vaccinations*, page 121.

2. For recommendations regarding influenza vaccine, refer to *Yearly or Periodic Health Checks #20, #21, and #22, Vaccinations*, page 121.

High-Risk Health Check #21

AUSCULTATION FOR CAROTID BRUITS [356]

RECOMMENDATIONS

1. Individuals who have risk factors for cardiovascular disease or cerebrovascular disease should be screened for carotid bruits.

2. Individuals who are at risk for carotid bruits are those with:
   - increased age;
   - high blood pressure;
   - smoking history;
   - coronary heart disease;
   - atrial fibrillation;
   - diabetes;
   - transient ischemic attacks (mini-strokes);
   - previous history of strokes.

Why Perform

The development of atherosclerosis (plaque build up in the arteries of the body) can occur in the major arteries that transport blood to the brain, the carotid arteries. If significant obstruction occurs (i.e., plaque build up) within the carotid arteries, a noise is created as turbulent blood flows across the obstruction. This noise is called a bruit.

A bruit can further lead to a total blockage of blood to the brain or the plaque build up can increase the likelihood of a stroke.[357-359]

How Performed

Individuals who have risk factors (see list in *Recommendations* box) should have their doctor or nurse listen for carotid bruits. A physician or nurse can detect these bruits by listening over the carotid arteries with a stethoscope.

High-Risk Health Check #22
CHLAMYDIAL TESTING [360]

_____

RECOMMENDATIONS

1. The following individuals should undergo testing for chlamydial infection. Those persons who:

   - Attend clinics established for the treatment of sexually transmitted diseases (STD);
   - Attend other health care facilities for high-risk STD groups such as adolescent and family planning clinics;
   - Have other risk factors for chlamydial infection such as:
     - Multiple sexual partners;
     - Sexual partners with multiple sexual contacts;
     - A sexual partner with a chlamydial infection;[361]
   - Are unmarried, under age 20 and who are sexually active;
   - Pregnant women who are unmarried, younger than age 20, have multiple sexual partners or a history of another sexually transmitted disease.[361]

2. The frequency of testing is uncertain and should be determined by the doctor.

Why Perform

Each detection of chlamydial infection in people who are without symptoms can lead to antibiotic treatment and prevention of further complications.[360] For additional information, refer to _Lifestyle Counseling Health Check #4, Preventing Sexually Transmitted Diseases_, page 135.

How Performed

A blood sample taken from a vein or a culture taken from areas of the body that may be producing abnormal secretions such as the penis, the vagina, or the eye are used to test for the presence of chlamydial infection.

High-Risk Health Check #23

GONORRHEA CULTURE [362]

RECOMMENDATIONS

1. The following should be tested for gonorrhea:
    *   Persons with multiple sexual partners or whose sexual partners have multiple sexual contacts;
    *   Prostitutes;
    *   Persons whose sexual contacts have cultural proven gonorrhea;
    *   Persons with a history of repeated episodes of gonorrhea;
    *   Pregnant women at high risk for contacting gonorrhea.

2. The frequency of testing for gonorrhea should be determined by the doctor.

Why Perform

Each detection of gonorrhea can lead to effective treatment and prevention of further complication, and further counseling regarding the consequences of sexually transmitted diseases.[362] For additional information, refer to *Lifestyle Counseling Health Check #4, Preventing Sexually Transmitted Diseases*, page 135.

How Performed

The test is performed by examining the possible discharge from areas such as the penis or the vagina. This test is referred to as a Gram Stain.

High-Risk Health Check #24

VDRL: SCREENING FOR SYPHILIS [363]

RECOMMENDATIONS

1. Screening for syphilis in individuals who are without symptoms is recommended for pregnant women and the following high-risk groups:
    *   Persons who engage in sex with multiple partners in areas where syphilis is prevalent;
    *   Persons who have had sexual contacts with individuals with active syphilis;
    *   Prostitutes.

2. The frequency of testing for syphilis in the high-risk groups should be determined by the individual's doctor.

3. The recommended frequency of testing for pregnant women is during their first prenatal visit and at delivery; and an additional test at 28 weeks into the pregnancy for women who are at increased risk for contacting syphilis during pregnancy.[363]

Why Perform

When syphilis is detected in individuals who are without symptoms, antibiotic treatment can prevent further untoward complications from the infection and prevent further spread of syphilis. For additional information, refer to *Lifestyle Counseling Health Check #4, Preventing Sexually Transmitted Diseases*, page 135.

How Performed

The main screening tests for syphilis are the VDRL (Venereal Disease Research Laboratory) and RPR (rapid plasma reagin) blood tests.[363]

High-Risk Health Check #25

COUNSELING AND TESTING FOR
HUMAN IMMUNODEFICIENCY VIRUS
(HIV – AIDS) [364]

RECOMMENDATIONS

1. Periodic screening for the AIDS virus should be performed on individuals who are:
   - Seeking treatment for sexually transmitted diseases (STD);
   - Homosexual and bisexual men;
   - Past or present intravenous (IV) drug users;
   - With a history of prostitution *or* multiple sexual partners;
   - Women whose past or present sexual partners were infected with HIV (AIDS virus), bisexual or IV drug users;
   - Residents who have lived for a long time in an area with a high prevalence of HIV infection;
   - Recipients of a blood transfusion between 1978 and 1985;
   - Pregnant or considering pregnancy and who are within the high risk categories listed above.

(Individuals listed above should also seek counseling regarding the consequences of contracting the AIDS virus.)

Why Perform

Although it is not currently known whether or not early detection of HIV will lead to improved health outcome for the individual, early discovery of HIV can:
- Help the person alter his/her sexual practices (if applicable) to prevent infection with other sexually transmitted diseases;
- Help prevent the further spread of the AIDS virus;
- Assist the doctor in decisions regarding course and action of treatment for other potential or present medical problems;
- Identify individuals who may qualify for current and/or future treatment methods for the AIDS virus;
- Assist women identified as seropositive (confirmed HIV positive) in their decision regarding avoiding pregnancy;
- Assist women who are already pregnant and seropositive (confirmed HIV positive) with their care for their newborn such as avoiding breast feeding and determining if the child is HIV positive;
- Provide opportunities for further counseling and appropriate support for those individuals who are positive for the AIDS virus (HIV).[364]

For additional information, refer to *Lifestyle Counseling Health Check #4, Preventing Sexually Transmitted Diseases,* page 135.

How Performed

Appropriately established confidentiality procedures should be part of the HIV screening process. Proper counseling by trained medical/health personnel before and following screening also is of vital importance. The test requires that a sample of blood be taken from a vein.

High-Risk Health Check #26

TONOMETRY
(GLAUCOMA CHECK)

> To learn more about the recommendations for this screening procedure and how the test is performed, refer to *Yearly or Periodic Health Check #16, Visual Acuity and Tonometry (Glaucoma Check)*, page 117.

High-Risk Health Check #27

PROSTATE SPECIFIC ANTIGEN (PSA) TEST
(SCREENING FOR PROSTATE CANCER)

RECOMMENDATIONS

1. The following men over age 50 should consult with their physician to determine whether or not they should have a prostate specific antigen (PSA) test.[374, 375] Men who:
   - Have a strong family history of prostate cancer;
   - Have symptoms, or physical exam results suggestive of prostate cancer;
   - Are scheduled to have a prostate resection (TURP);
   - Are undergoing treatment for prostate cancer (surgery, radiation or hormone therapy).

Why Perform

The prostate specific antigen test (PSA test) can be used to assist in determining whether or not a man has prostate cancer. The test results can also be used to help follow the course of prostate cancer. The Early Detection Branch of the National Cancer Institute is now beginning a several year study to investigate whether or not the PSA test should be used as a periodic screening test in conjunction with a digital rectal examination.[374] The National Cancer Institute now recommends that the PSA test be used only for men who meet the criteria listed in the recommendations.

How Performed

Only a sample of venous blood is required to perform the test. The test does not require fasting.

APPENDIX

APPENDIX A

MEDICAL HEALTH QUESTIONNAIRE

The following detailed medical questionnaire is included to assist you and your doctor with your medical history record. It may seem lengthy, but once the questionnaire is completed it will serve as a basis for your maintenance manual for the remainder of your life.

Health Assessment and Medical History Questionnaire

1. GENERAL INFORMATION

A. PERSONAL

Name: _____
(Last)   (First)   (Middle)

Date of Birth: _____
(Month)   (Day)   (Year)

Address: _____

Phone: _____
(Home)   (Work)

Marital Status:

☐ Single ☐ Married ☐ Divorced ☐ Widowed ☐ Separated

Total Number of Children: (including adopted) _____

Race:

☐ Caucasian ☐ Black ☐ Asian ☐ Hispanic ☐ Other

Education: (Check highest level attained)

☐ Grade School ☐ Jr. High ☐ High School ☐ College ☐ Graduate School

Occupation: _____

Blood Type: _____

Sex: _____

Age: _____

What is your Rh Type: _____

B. MEDICAL COVERAGE

Carrier(s) or Provider(s) including Medicare:

_____

_____

Policy or Identification Number(s):

_____

_____

Name of Policy Holder:

_____

_____

Employer and Address:

_____

_____

_____

(Note: When visiting your doctor, please take insurance/Medicare forms with you.)

C. DOCTORS

Primary Care: _____ Eye: _____

Address: _____ Phone: _____ Address: _____ Phone: _____

Specialist: _____ Dentist: _____

Address: _____ Phone: _____ Address: _____ Phone: _____

Specialist: _____ Dentist: _____

Address: _____ Phone: _____ Address: _____ Phone: _____

(The material contained within this questionnaire has been used by permission of the Cardiovascular Genetics Research Clinic, University of Utah School of Medicine, and the Fitness Institute at LDS Hospital. Questions on physical activity are adapted in part from the "Harvard Alumni Health Questionnaire," used by permission of Dr. Ralph Paffenbarger. The psychological information is from "Mending the Body, Minding the Mind" and is used by permission of Dr. Joan Borysenko, Ph.D.)

2. MEDICAL HISTORY

A. MEDICAL ILLNESS

Have you ever been told BY A DOCTOR that you suffer from any of the following health problems?

Medical Illness	Yes	No	AGE AT 1st DIAGNOSIS. Age	Have you taken prescription medication for this health problem? Yes	No	Have you ever been hospitalized for this health problem? Yes	No	Have you ever had any special tests performed for this health problem? Yes	No
1. Heart Attack (Myocardial Infarction [MI], Coronary Thrombosis)	☐	☐	_____	☐	☐	☐	☐	☐	☐
2. Angina Pectoris	☐	☐	_____	☐	☐	☐	☐	☐	☐
3. Rheumatic or other Heart Disease Please list: _____	☐	☐	_____	☐	☐	☐	☐	☐	☐
4. Stroke	☐	☐	_____	☐	☐	☐	☐	☐	☐
5. High Blood Pressure	☐	☐	_____	☐	☐	☐	☐	☐	☐
6. High Blood Pressure during Pregnancy only	☐	☐	_____	☐	☐	☐	☐	☐	☐
7. High Blood Cholesterol or Triglycerides, and/or Low HDL	☐	☐	_____	☐	☐	☐	☐	☐	☐
8. Diabetes	☐	☐	_____	☐	☐	☐	☐	☐	☐
9. Cancer	☐	☐	_____	☐	☐	☐	☐	☐	☐

Do you currently have or have you ever had any of the following: (please indicate the year)

10. _____ anemia	15. _____ malaria	20. _____ mumps	25. _____ varicose veins or phlebitis
11. _____ asthma	16. _____ jaundice or hepatitis	21. _____ polio	26. _____ venereal disease
12. _____ chickenpox	17. _____ measles	22. _____ scarlet fever	27. Other: _____
13. _____ hemorrhoids	18. _____ liver disease	23. _____ thyroid disease	
14. _____ hives	19. _____ mononucleosis	24. _____ typhoid	

HEART DISEASE

28. If you answered "Yes" to Number 1 (**Heart Attack**), circle any of the following that apply:

   a. Hospitalized for _____ days.
   b. Was placed in a Coronary or Intensive Care Unit.
   c. Experienced chest pain for one hour or more.

   Please circle any of the following terms used by your doctor to describe your situation:

   1 - Coronary thrombosis
   2 - Myocardial infarction (MI)
   3 - Congestive heart failure
   4 - Unstable angina
   5 - Other: _____

29. If you had **other heart problems,** circle any of the following that apply:

   a. Congestive heart failure
   b. Rheumatic heart disease
   c. Congenital heart disease
   d. Atrial fibrilation
   e. Paroxysmal atrial tachycardia (PAT)
   f. Premature ventricular contractions (PVC)
   g. Other heart rhythm problems
   h. Cardiomyopathy (diseased heart muscle)
   i. Pulmonary heart disease
   j. Any heart murmurs
   k. Any heart valve problems (stenosis, regurgitation, etc.)
   l. Other: _____

STROKE

30. If you answered "Yes" to Number 4 (**Stroke**), circle any of the following that apply:

   a. My muscles suddenly became weak or paralyzed on one side of my body.
   b. I suddenly had difficulty talking.
   c. I suddenly had partial or complete loss of vision in one eye.
   d. I fainted or passed out (usually not due to a stroke).
   e. I was hospitalized for _____ days.
   f. Some of the above problems were still present to some degree several months after the stroke.
   g. Other: _____

HIGH BLOOD PRESSURE

31. If you answered "Yes" to Number 5 or 6 (**High Blood Pressure**), circle any of the following that apply:

   a. Currently take prescription medication for high blood pressure.
   b. Previously took prescription medication for high blood pressure, but stopped taking it on my own.
   c. Previously took prescription medication for high blood pressure, but my doctor told me to stop.
   d. Only had high blood pressure when I was pregnant.
   e. Do not take prescription medication, but the doctor follows my high blood pressure (see doctor regularly to check blood pressure).

HIGH BLOOD CHOLESTEROL

32. If you answered "Yes" to Number 7 (**High Blood Cholesterol**, etc.), circle any of the following that apply:

   a. Has your blood cholesterol ever been measured ? Yes ☐ No ☐
   b. My highest blood cholesterol level was: _____ Date: _____
   c. My current cholesterol level is: _____ Date: _____
   d. My highest triglyceride level was: _____ Date: _____
   e. My current triglyceride level is: _____ Date: _____
   f. My lowest HDL level was : _____ Date: _____
   g. My current HDL level is: _____ Date: _____
   h. Medication has been prescribed by my doctor for my high blood lipids.

DIABETES

33. If you answered "Yes" to Number 8 (**Diabetes**), circle any of the following that apply:

   a. Insulin injections have been prescribed by my doctor for control of my blood sugar.
   b. Medication (pills or tablets) have been prescribed for control of my blood sugar.
   c. I monitor my urine and/or blood sugar at home as directed by my doctor.
   d. A special diet for control of my blood sugar has been prescribed by my doctor.

CANCER

34. If you answered "Yes" to Number 9 (**Cancer**), please answer the following questions:

   a. The type of cancer your doctor said you had: _____
   b. Did you undergo any surgical therapy for this cancer? ____ yes ____ no
   c. Did you have chemotherapy? ____ yes ____ no
   d. Did you have radiation therapy? ____ yes ____ no

B. MEDICAL PROCEDURES

Tests
(indicate previous tests and year performed:)

	Tests	Year	Was the test normal ?		Operations and Hospitalizations
			Yes	No	(Please list past hospitalization and operations/major procedures)
☐	upper GI X-ray	_____	☐	☐	_____ Year: ___
☐	lower GI X-ray	_____	☐	☐	_____ Year: ___
☐	gallbladder X-ray	_____	☐	☐	_____ Year: ___
☐	proctoscopic exam	_____	☐	☐	_____ Year: ___
☐	chest X-ray	_____	☐	☐	_____ Year: ___
☐	TB skin test	_____	☐	☐	_____ Year: ___
☐	tetanus shot	_____	☐	☐	_____ Year: ___
☐	allergy tests	_____	☐	☐	_____ Year: ___
☐	complete physical examination	_____	☐	☐	_____ Year: ___
☐	electrocardiogram (resting EKG)	_____	☐	☐	_____ Year: ___
☐	exercise electrocardiogram (stress test)	_____	☐	☐	_____ Year: ___
☐	mammogram	_____	☐	☐	_____ Year: ___
☐	pap smear	_____	☐	☐	
☐	colonoscopy	_____	☐	☐	

☐ Other X-rays

Year	Kind of X-ray
_____	_____
_____	_____

C. MEDICATIONS, DRUG REACTION(S) and ALLERGIES

1. MEDICATIONS

(Please list the medications, vitamins and dietary supplements you take, prescription and non-prescription, even ones taken on an occasional basis.)

Name	When did you start this medication?	How often do you take this medication?	Dose

2. DRUG REACTIONS

(Please list any drug reaction you have had and the year you had this reaction.)

Date

Drug:
Side Effect:

Drug:
Side Effect:

Drug:
Side Effect:

Drug:
Side Effect:

Drug:
Side Effect:

3. ALLERGIES

(Please list the things you are allergic to and any reactions you have had.)

Date

Allergic to:
Side Effect:

Allergic to:
Side Effect:

Allergic to:
Side Effect:

Allergic to:
Side Effect:

Allergic to:
Side Effect:

Allergic to:
Side Effect:

3. REVIEW OF SYSTEMS

A. GENERAL REVIEW

(Check the appropriate boxes:)

- ☐ Do you have an intolerance to heat?
- ☐ Do you have an intolerance to cold?
- ☐ Do you often notice excessive fatigue or exhaustion?
- ☐ Do you have difficulty getting to sleep or staying asleep?
- ☐ Have you noticed any unusual thirst?
- ☐ Are you always hungry?
- ☐ Has your appetite disappeared or decreased?
- ☐ Have you noticed any lymph node swelling?
- ☐ Have you ever been exposed to radiation of head or neck? (other than dental or other diagnostic X-rays)
- ☐ Do you ever feel faint?
- ☐ Do you lose feeling in any part of your body?
- ☐ Have you noticed shaking or trembling?
- ☐ Have you ever had convulsions?
- ☐ Have you had excessive bleeding from a cut?
- ☐ Are you prone to bruise easily?
- ☐ Are you bothered with any skin abnormalities?
- ☐ Do you have any physical handicaps?

B. DIGESTIVE SYSTEM

- ☐ Do you notice any discomfort or pain in your upper abdomen or stomach?
- ☐ Do you have much abdominal gas?
- ☐ If you notice pain or discomfort in your abdomen, is it made worse by eating?
  - Is it made better by eating?   ☐ Yes   ☐ No
  - Is it improved with antacids?   ☐ Yes   ☐ No
- ☐ Are you bothered with heartburn, belching or do you have trouble swallowing? (underline which)
- ☐ Are you constipated more than once weekly?
- ☐ Do you have loose bowels for more than one or two days?
- ☐ Have you had any black or bloody stools in the last five years?
- ☐ Have you had any rectal bleeding in the last five years?
- ☐ Are your bowel movements painful?
- ☐ Do you have rectal pain?
- ☐ Do you have a hernia?
- ☐ Do you have hemorrhoids?
- ☐ Have you been told you have diverticulitis?

C. GENITO-URINARY SYSTEM

- ☐ Do you notice pain or burning when urinating?
- ☐ Do you have trouble starting to urinate?
- ☐ Does your urination seem too slow?
- How many times per night do you generally urinate? _____
- How many times per day do you generally urinate? _____
- ☐ Do you have frequent urinary tract infections?
- ☐ Have you had past kidney trouble?

D. MEN

- ☐ Has the force of urine stream markedly decreased?
- ☐ Do you notice any dribbling after stopping urination?
- ☐ Have you noticed any discharge from the penis?
- ☐ Have you been told you have prostate trouble?
- ☐ Do your testicles become tender and swollen?

E. WOMEN

- ☐ Have you noticed any breast lumps?
- ☐ Have you noticed any discharge from your breasts?
- ☐ Are your periods regular with normal flow?
- ☐ Do you ever bleed between periods?
- ☐ Do you have vaginal itching or discharge?
- ☐ Have you ever taken birth control pills?
- ☐ Have you ever taken any hormone (estrogen or progesterone)replacement therapy?
- ☐ Have you ever been pregnant? If yes, how may pregnancies? _____

F. EYES, EARS, NOSE, THROAT and MOUTH

- ☐ Do you wear corrective lenses?
- ☐ Do you ever notice blurred or double vision?
- ☐ Are you bothered with eye pains or itching?
- ☐ Do you have excessive eye watering?
- ☐ Do you have difficulty hearing?
- ☐ Do you have ringing in your ears?
- ☐ Do you often have headaches?
- ☐ Have you had pain or swelling in your neck?
- ☐ Do you have sore areas on your gums?
- ☐ Is your tongue or the inside of your mouth sore?
- ☐ Do you have frequent stuffiness and drainage from your nose?
- ☐ Do you frequently notice drainage in the back of your throat?
- ☐ Are you bothered with nosebleeds?
- ☐ Is your throat sore or hoarse when you don't have a cold?

G. RESPIRATORY SYSTEM

- ☐ Do you ever have periods of wheezing?
- ☐ Do you have a regular cough?
- ☐ Do you often cough up anything?
- ☐ Have you ever coughed up blood?
- ☐ Do you need more than one pillow to sleep?
- ☐ Do you have or have you had the following?
  - ☐ Bronchitis
  - ☐ Emphysema
  - ☐ Pneumonia

4. LIFESTYLE HISTORY (Personal Habits)

A. CIGARETTE SMOKING

1. Please circle the one that applies:

   a. **Smoker:** Have smoked daily for one year or more.

   b. **Ex-smoker:** Have not smoked for at least one year after having smoked daily for at least one year.

   c. **Non-smoker:** Have never smoked daily for at least one year.

2. If **smoker or ex-smoker**, circle **average** amount and indicate number of years smoked. Choose one only.

   a. Less than one pack a day for _____ years.

   b. About one pack a day for _____ years.

   c. One-two packs a day for _____ years.

   d. Two or more packs a day for _____ years.

3. List the last year in which you smoked _____.

4. Do you smoke cigars? _____ yes _____ no _____ cigars per day? _____

5. Do you smoke a pipe? _____ yes _____ no _____ bowls per day? _____

6. Would you like to quit smoking ? _____ yes _____ no

7. Do you use smokeless tobacco? _____ yes _____ no

8. On the average, how many hours per day are you exposed to other people's cigarette smoke?

   _____ 0 hours   _____ 5-8 hours

   _____ 1-2 hours   _____ more than 8 hours

   _____ 3-4 hours

B. ALCOHOL CONSUMPTION

1. Do you drink alcoholic beverages (beer, wine, or liquors)? Please circle the one that applies:

   a. No.

   b. Less than once a month.

   c. Once a month or more with an average of:

   1. _____ 12-16 oz. cans of beer per week.

   2. _____ 4-6 oz. glasses of wine per week.

   3. _____ shots, jiggers or mixed drinks per week.

C. DIETARY INFORMATION

1. How would you describe your tendency to lose weight? (If in doubt circle #3.)

   1) Lose weight easily by cutting food intake slightly.

   2) Lose weight with difficulty, even if I cut my food intake greatly.

   3) Average - neither tendency above noticed.

2. What is your current weight? _____ lbs. What is the most you have ever weighed (excluding pregnancy)? _____ lbs.

3. If you feel you need to lose weight, how much weight would you like to lose? _____ lbs.

4. How do you feel about your current weight?

   1) very satisfied
   2) satisfied
   3) not concerned
   4) dissatisfied
   5) very dissatisfied

5. Do you follow any special diet most of the time?

   1) No
   2) Yes, low calorie
   3) Yes, low fat or low cholesterol
   4) Yes, diabetic
   5) Yes, low salt
   6) Yes, other

6. In a typical week, how many meals or snacks do you eat away from home?

   1) _____ Breakfast (where) _____
   2) _____ Morning Snack (where) _____
   3) _____ Lunch (where) _____
   4) _____ Afternoon Snack (where) _____
   5) _____ Dinner (where) _____
   6) _____ Evening Snack (where) _____

List of Salty Foods:

Bacon or Ham	Salted Crackers
Hot Dogs	Seasoning Salts
Sausage	(celery, garlic, onion)
Bologna and Luncheon	Pickles
Meats	Sauerkraut
Chipped or Corned Beef	Boullion
Smoked or Salted Meats	Catsup
Herring, Sardines	Canned Soups
Potato Chips	Dried Soups
Pretzels	Chili Sauce
French Fries	Mustard
Salted Snacks	Olives
(popcorn, nuts, etc.)	Relishes
Sauces (soy, steak, etc.)	Meat Tenderizers

7. How often do you salt your food from a shaker at the dinner table or eat salty foods such as potato chips, bacon, or other foods listed above?

   1) 2 or more times a day
   2) Once a day
   3) 2-5 times a week
   4) Once a week
   5) Less than once a week
   6) Almost never (I'm on a special low salt diet)

8. When was the last time you used a salt shaker on your food or ate one of the salty foods listed above?

   1) Within the last three meals
   2) A day ago
   3) 2-5 days ago
   4) A week ago
   5) Over a week ago
   6) Over a year ago

9. Do you place specific emphasis of high fiber in your diet? _____ yes _____ no

10. How many cups of coffee containing caffeine do you drink in an average day? ☐

11. How many cups of tea containing caffeine do you drink in an average day? ☐

List of foods high in Cholesterol or Saturated Fat:

Bacon	Sweet Rolls
Hot Dogs	Butter
Sausage	Shortening
Marbled and Fatty Meats	Coconut Oil
(beef, pork, lamb)	Potato Chips
Spare Ribs	French Fries
Fish fried in shortening	Other Fried Foods
Liver or other organ meats	Lard
Hamburger	Cream and Ice Cream
Luncheon Meats	Cheese
Egg Yolks	Butter Rolls
Cakes and Pies	Donuts
Whole Milk	Egg Noodles

12. If you drink coffee or tea, how do you normally drink it?

   1) black, no cream or sugar
   2) cream, no sugar
   3) cream, one spoon of sugar
   4) cream, two spoons of sugar
   5) cream, three or more spoons of sugar
   6) no cream, one spoon of sugar
   7) no cream, two spoons of sugar
   8) no cream, three or more spoons of sugar

13. During the last week, how many days did you experience difficulty in limiting candy eating?

   1 2 3 4 5 6 7 Zero

14. During the past week, how many days did you experience difficulty in limiting your eating of fatty foods?

   1 2 3 4 5 6 7 Zero

15. During the past week, how many days did you plan what you would eat at the start of the day?

   1 2 3 4 5 6 7 Zero

16. During the past week, how many days did you eat your meals at set times?

   1 2 3 4 5 6 7 Zero

17. During the past week, on how many days did you decide not to eat a snack that you wanted, even though the food was available?

   1 2 3 4 5 6 7 Zero

18. How many carbonated soft drinks do you have in a week? ☐☐

19. How many are diet drinks? ☐☐

20. How many of the drinks you consume contain caffeine? (Drinks like Coca Cola, Pepsi, Dr. Pepper, Mountain Dew, contain caffeine.) ☐☐

21. How many cups of hot chocolate do you drink each day? ☐☐

22. How many cups of water do you drink each day? ☐☐

23. When was the last time you ate eggs, whole milk, meat or other high cholesterol foods from the above list?

   1) Within the last three meals
   2) A day ago
   3) 2-5 days ago
   4) A week ago
   5) Over a week ago
   6) Over a year ago

24. How often do you eat any of the foods listed above?

   1) 2 or more times a day
   2) Once a day
   3) 2-5 times a week
   4) Once a week
   5) Less than once a week
   6) Almost never

25. In an average month, how may times do you skip:

   1) Breakfast?
   2) Lunch?
   3) Dinner?

   ☐☐
   ☐☐☐

D. PHYSICAL ACTIVITY INFORMATION

1. Are you currently participating in a physical activity program? _____ yes _____ no

2. Please list the type, the frequency and the duration with which you participate in physical activity, that either includes brisk walking, jogging, swimming, gardening, aerobics, stationary cycling, country cycling, carpentry, calisthentics, etc. (please include only the time you are physically active).

Type of physical activity	Number of times per week	Time Spent in each activity session hours	minutes	Number of weeks per year (approximately)

3. If you walk briskly on a regular basis, how many miles do you walk each session? _____ How long does it take you to walk one mile? _____ (minutes).

4. On a usual weekday and a weekend day, how much time do you spend on the following activities

	Usual weekday hours/day	Usual weekend day hours/day
a. Vigorous activity (digging in the garden, strenuous sports, jogging, chopping wood, sustained swimming, brisk walking, heavy carpentry, bicycling on hills, etc.)		
b. Moderate activity (housework, light sports, regular walking, golf, yard work, lawn mowing, painting, repairing, light carpentry, dancing, bicycling on level ground, etc.)		
c. Light activity (office work, driving a car, strolling, personal care, standing with little motion, etc.)		
d. Sitting activity (eating, reading, desk work, watching TV, listening to radio, etc.)		
e. Sleeping or reclining		

5. Have you ever had any chest discomfort brought on by exercise? _____ yes _____ no (If yes, please be prepared to discuss it with the doctor.)

Circle the number, from 0 (never) to 4 (frequently), that represents the degree to which the following thoughts, feelings, and behaviors have bothered you during the past month.

THOUGHTS

	Never	Rarely	Sometimes	Often	Frequently
1. Awfulizing (taking things to their worst possible outcome)	0	1	2	3	4
2. Blaming myself	0	1	2	3	4
3. Blaming others	0	1	2	3	4
4. Difficulty concentrating	0	1	2	3	4
5. Holding grudges	0	1	2	3	4
6. Thinking and rethinking the same situation	0	1	2	3	4
7. Wishing I could "turn my mind off"	0	1	2	3	4
8. Constantly criticizing other people or situations	0	1	2	3	4
9. Worrying	0	1	2	3	4
10. Thinking something is wrong with my mind	0	1	2	3	4
11. Needing to be right	0	1	2	3	4
12. Feeling out of control	0	1	2	3	4

EMOTIONS

	Never	Rarely	Sometimes	Often	Frequently
1. Afraid of specific places or circumstances	0	1	2	3	4
2. Feeling like a victim	0	1	2	3	4
3. Anxious	0	1	2	3	4
4. Blue	0	1	2	3	4
5. Lonely	0	1	2	3	4
6. Irritable	0	1	2	3	4
7. Wanting to throw things or hit people	0	1	2	3	4
8. Guilty	0	1	2	3	4
9. Feeling unfriendly	0	1	2	3	4
10. Uptight	0	1	2	3	4
11. Hopeless about the future	0	1	2	3	4
12. Wanting to "pull the covers over my head"	0	1	2	3	4
13. Feeling that other people don't like me	0	1	2	3	4
14. Upset over criticism	0	1	2	3	4

BEHAVIORS

	Never	Rarely	Sometimes	Often	Frequently
1. Nail or cuticle biting	0	1	2	3	4
2. Using tobacco in any form	0	1	2	3	4
3. Taking tranquilizers or "street" drugs to change mood	0	1	2	3	4
4. Drinking alcoholic beverages	0	1	2	3	4
5. Chewing gum or sucking candies	0	1	2	3	4
6. Talking a lot	0	1	2	3	4
7. Crying a lot	0	1	2	3	4
8. Sleeping problems (too much or too little)	0	1	2	3	4
9. Eating problems (too much or too little)	0	1	2	3	4
10. Trouble communicating	0	1	2	3	4
11. Avoiding responsibilities	0	1	2	3	4
12. Too much caffeine	0	1	2	3	4

F. SEAT BELT USAGE

1. Do you wear seat belts when riding in or driving motor vehicles?

   _____ no _____ sometimes _____ usually _____ always

G. SLEEP

1. How many hours of sleep do you usually get a night? _____ hours

2. How would you best describe your night's sleep?

   _____ restful _____ difficult to get to sleep

   _____ wake at night and can't get back to sleep

3. Do you take naps during the day on a regular basis?

   _____ yes _____ no

   If yes, how long is your nap? _____ minutes

MEDICAL HEALTH QUESTIONNAIRE 181

5. GENETIC HISTORY

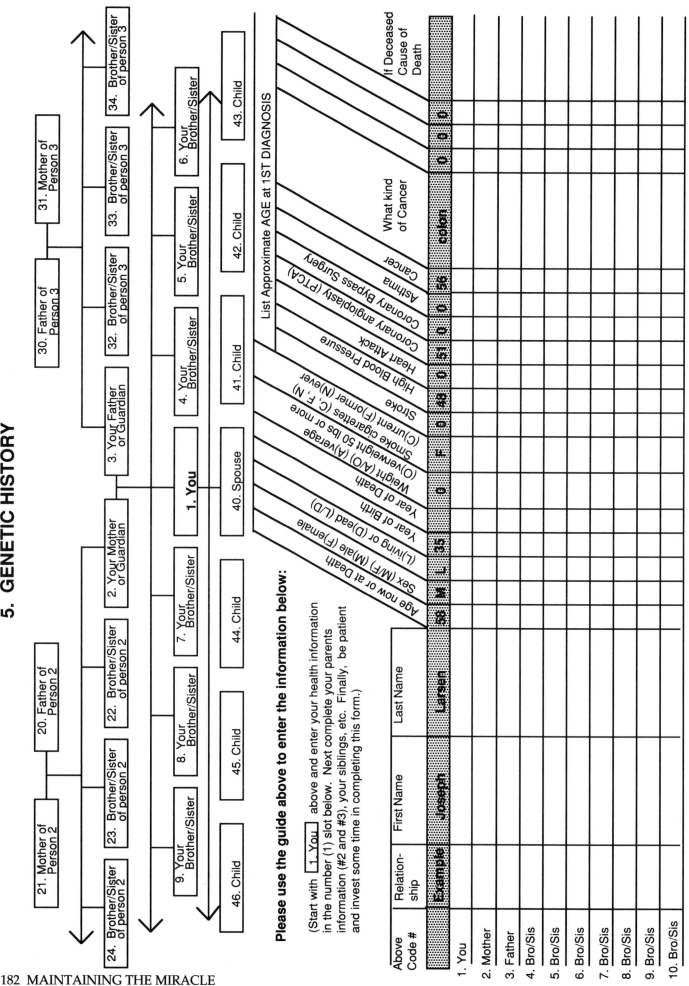

Please use the guide above to enter the information below:

(Start with [1. You] above and enter your health information in the number (1) slot below. Next complete your parents information (#2 and #3), your siblings, etc. Finally, be patient and invest some time in completing this form.)

Above Code #	Relation-ship	First Name	Last Name	Age now or at Death	Sex (M/F) (M)ale (F)emale	(L)iving or (D)ead (L/D)	Year of Birth	Year of Death	Weight (A/O) (A)verage (O)verweight 50 lbs or more	Smoke cigarettes (C, F, N) (C)urrent (F)ormer (N)ever	Stroke	High Blood Pressure	Heart Attack	Coronary angioplasty (PTCA)	Coronary Bypass Surgery	Asthma	Cancer	What kind of Cancer	List Approximate AGE at 1ST DIAGNOSIS	If Deceased Cause of Death
Example		**Joseph**	**Larsen**	**38**	**M**	**L**	**35**		**O**	**F**	**0**	**48**	**0**	**51**	**0**	**56**	**0**	**colon**	**0**	**0 0**
1. You																				
2. Mother																				
3. Father																				
4. Bro/Sis																				
5. Bro/Sis																				
6. Bro/Sis																				
7. Bro/Sis																				
8. Bro/Sis																				
9. Bro/Sis																				
10. Bro/Sis																				

11. Bro/Sis																		
12. Bro/Sis																		
20. Grand-Father																		
21. Grand-Mother																		
22. Ant/Unc																		
23. Ant/Unc																		
24. Ant/Unc																		
25. Ant/Unc																		
26. Ant/Unc																		
27. Ant/Unc																		
28. Ant/Unc																		
30. Grand-Father																		
31. Grand-Mother																		
32. Ant/Unc																		
33. Ant/Unc																		
34. Ant/Unc																		
35. Ant/Unc																		
36. Ant/Unc																		
37. Ant/Unc																		
38. Ant/Unc																		
40. Spouse																		
41. Son/Dau																		
42. Son/Dau																		
43. Son/Dau																		
44. Son/Dau																		
45. Son/Dau																		
46. Son/Dau																		

APPENDIX B

ROCKPORT FITNESS WALKING TEST (RFWT)
AND ROCKPORT WALKING PROGRAM

Drs. James M. Rippe and Ann Ward who direct the University of Massachusetts Medical School, Exercise Physiology and Nutrition Laboratory, recently developed a fitness walking test. Sponsored by The Rockport Walking Institute (a division of the Rockport shoe company), Drs. Rippe and Ward tested 343 men and women over a period of 18 months to formulate a very practical and accurate fitness walking test — and the only requirement is that you walk one mile at a comfortable pace. Instructions for taking the test, how to interpret the results, and how to implement a walking program based upon the results of the test are included in this Appendix.

The information below is reprinted by permission from Dr. Rippe and the Rockport Company. The material is taken from *Dr. James M. Rippe's Complete Book of Fitness Walking*, published by Prentice Hall Press, New York.

"As long as one foot is kept on the ground, the test works for anybody and any kind of walking. (Running is not allowed.) How fit a person is makes no difference. The test works for a swimmer, a tennis player or a sedentary person.

"There are a few limitations to taking this test. A serious orthopedic problem or an injury that makes it difficult for you to walk renders the test impossible. Consult your doctor if you have been inactive and are over 45, or if you have any question as to whether the test is safe for you. *The test is not for people on beta-blocker medication for heart disease or high blood pressure.* (We are hard at work, however, at developing a test that is accurate for such people.)

"To do the Rockport Fitness Walking Test (**RFWT**) all you need to know are your age, sex, the time it takes to walk the mile, and your heart rate immediately after the mile. After that you use the charts developed from the tests we did on our volunteers. The RFWT shows if your fitness level is high, above average, average, below average, or low for age groups 20-29, 30-39, 40-49, 50-59, 60 or higher.

"Before you begin, you need to learn to take your pulse. For that you need a watch with a second hand. And you will need to practice a few times. Here's how.

"While sitting still, place your first and second fingers (not your thumb) gently on your wrist, or on the side of your neck. On your wrist you will feel the pulse in the radial artery, which is just inside the wrist bone on the

thumb side. In your neck the pulse is just below the angle of the jawbone at the level of the Adam's apple. Press gently, otherwise you can get an inaccurate reading.

"Count your pulse for 15 seconds and multiply by four to get your heart rate per minute. That gives you your *resting heart rate*. At the end of the test you are going to take your *exercise heart rate*.

"Once you can take your pulse with confidence, you are ready to take the RFWT. First you need to find a place to take the test. A track is best, since a mile is already measured and you won't be interrupted by car traffic. Health clubs and your local high school normally have quarter-mile tracks you can use. Another alternative is to use your car's odometer to measure out a one-mile course on a flat road with no stop signs or stop lights.

"Wear comfortable loose-fitting clothes and a pair of well-designed walking shoes. As with any exercise, stretch and then walk slowly for two or three minutes to build up your pace, warm up, and accelerate your heart rate before beginning the test.

"Now you are ready. Walk the mile as briskly as possible, trying to maintain as even a pace as you can. When you have finished, note the time in minutes and seconds; then *immediately* take your pulse, since your heart rate slows down rapidly after you stop walking. Count the beats for 15 seconds and multiply by four to get the number of beats per minute. At the end of the test a person's heart rate is typically 25 to 40 beats in 15 seconds. When you multiply that by four you will know your exercise heart rate. Remember your results.

"Here's an example of how it works. On the Rockport Fitness Walking Test a 52-year-old woman walks a mile in 17 minutes and 15 seconds and her heart rate is 132 beats per minute at the end of the mile. On the Relative Fitness Chart for women 50 to 59 years old, she finds 17 minutes and 15 seconds on the horizontal line (the time line) and draws a vertical line to the point where it meets the horizontal line drawn through the 132 on the heart rate line. The point where those two lines intersect on the Relative Fitness Chart is within the average range for 50 to 59 year old women (Figure 1).

"On the Exercise Program Chart for women 50 to 59 years old (Figure 2), again use her heart rate and time results to locate the program designed for her level of fitness, which is called Green. The next day she begins her ideal fitness-walking program (Figure 3). During the first two weeks of the Green program, she follows the routine listed under Week One to Two. She warms up for five to seven minutes and walks one and a half miles at three miles per hour. She should get her heart rate up to 60 to 70 percent of her maximum heart rate, or about 100 beats per minute. After her walk, she cools down and stretches for five to seven minutes. She follows this routine for five days per week. At the end of the second week, she moves into the second phase of the Green program; after the fourth week, the next phase; and so on. When she has finished the 22-week program, she should retest herself with the RFWT to establish her new program.

"To do the same for yourself, take your results from the Rockport Fitness Walking Test. Find your fitness level on the Relative Fitness Chart for your age and sex (Figure 4). Next find your exercise program among the Exercise Program graphs for your age and sex (Figure 4). Follow the color-coded 20-week exercise program that corresponds with the Exercise Program graph (Figure 5).

"This test is your instrument panel as you begin your fitness-walking program. It tells you how far and how fast to go. As you follow the program, it also informs you how far you have come. Watching your progress is good for motivation.

"At the end of each 20-week program, retest yourself with RFWT just as you did at the beginning. From this test, gauge your progress, and on the basis of your second result start another program. Repeat the whole process every 20 weeks until you reach the fitness level you want. Once you have reached the Yellow, Red, or Orange level of fitness and are satisfied with the way you feel, then you can adopt the Yellow or Red or Orange maintenance program for a lifetime of fitness.

"For optimal benefits follow each program carefully and don't skip any of the phases of the program. The major advantage of adhering to this fitness-walking schedule is that it is carefully designed to begin with a degree of difficulty suited for your aerobic capacity and to increase in difficulty as your aerobic capacity improves."

FIGURE 1

Example of Relative Fitness Chart for 50- to 59-Year-Old Woman

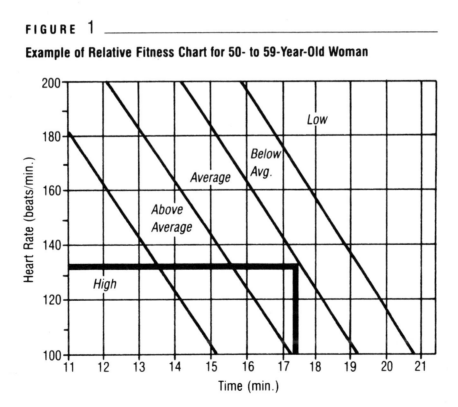

FIGURE 2

Example of Exercise Program Chart for 50- to 59-Year-Old Woman

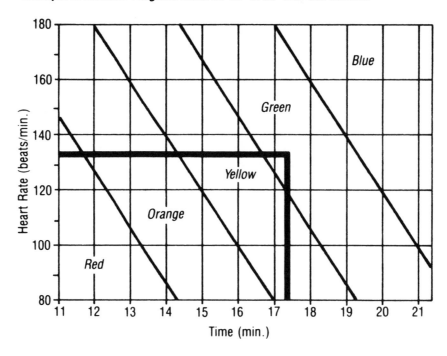

FIGURE 3

GREEN PROGRAM

Week	1–2	3–4	5–6	7	8–9	10–12	13	14	15–16	17–18	19–20
WARM-UP (mins. before walk stretches)	5–7	5–7	5–7	5–7	5–7	5–7	5–7	5–7	5–7	5–7	5–7
MILEAGE	1.5	1.75	2.0	2.0	2.25	2.5	2.75	2.75	3.0	3.25	3.5
PACE (mph)	3.0	3.0	3.0	3.5	3.5	3.5	3.5	4.0	4.0	4.0	4.0
HEART RATE (% of max)	60–70	60–70	60–70	70	70	70	70	70–80	70–80	70–80	70–80
COOL-DOWN (mins. after walk stretches)	5–7	5–7	5–7	5–7	5–7	5–7	5–7	5–7	5–7	5–7	5–7
FREQUENCY (times per week)	5	5	5	5	5	5	5	5	5	5	5

*At the end of the twenty-week fitness-walking protocol, retest yourself to establish your new program.

FIGURE 4

Relative Fitness Levels and Exercise Programs for the Rockport Fitness Walk-ing Test

**20–29-Year-Old Males
Relative Fitness Level**

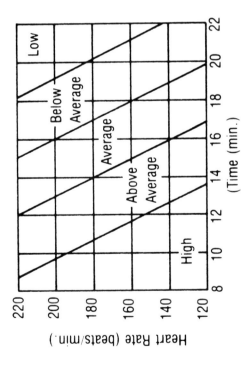

**20–29-Year-Old Females
Relative Fitness Level**

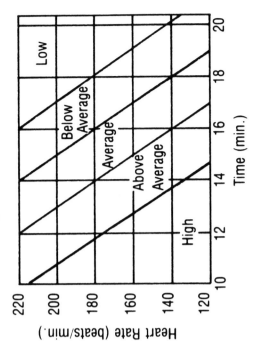

**20–29-Year-Old Males
Exercise Program**

**20–29-Year-Old Females
Exercise Program**

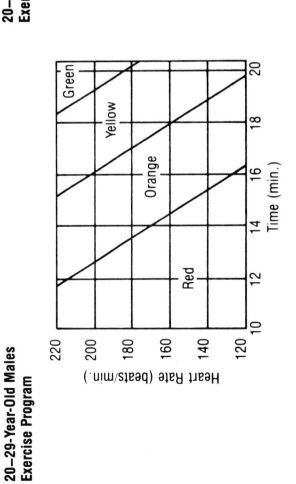

30–39-Year-Old Females
Relative Fitness Level

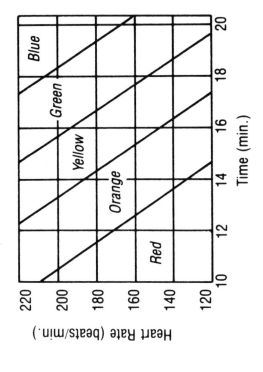

30–39-Year-Old Females
Exercise Program

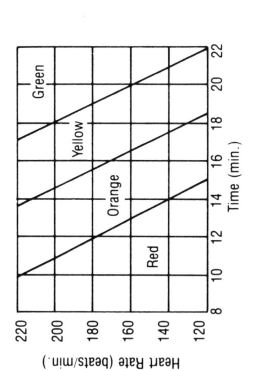

30–39-Year-Old Males
Relative Fitness Level

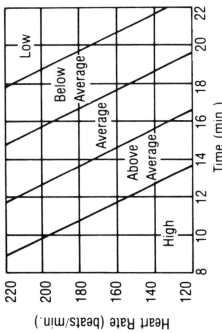

30–39-Year-Old Males
Exercise Program

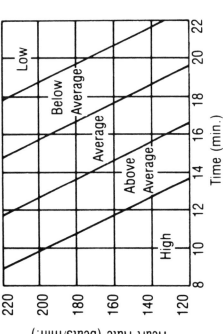

40–49-Year-Old Females
Relative Fitness Level

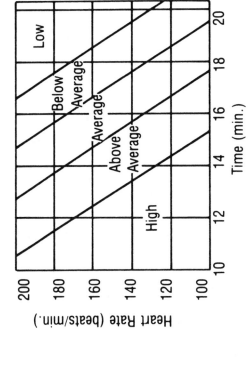

40–49-Year-Old Females
Exercise Program

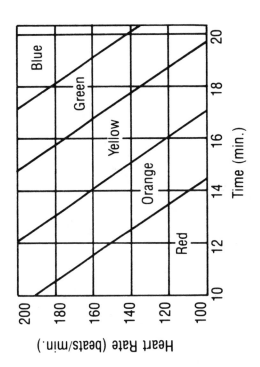

40–49-Year-Old Males
Relative Fitness Level

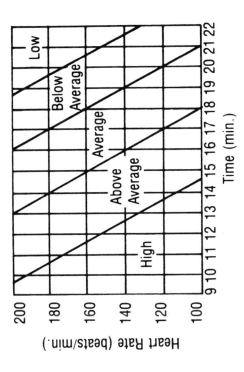

40–49-Year-Old Males
Exercise Program

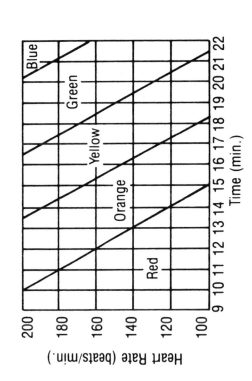

50–59-Year-Old Females
Relative Fitness Level

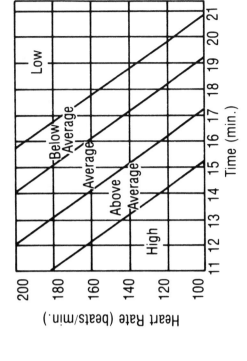

50–59-Year-Old Females
Exercise Program

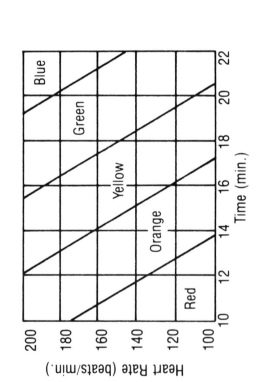

50–59-Year-Old Males
Relative Fitness Level

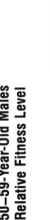

50–59-Year-Old Males
Exercise Program

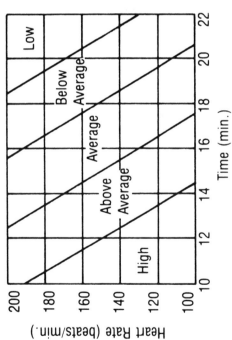

**60 + Year-Old Males
Relative Fitness Level**

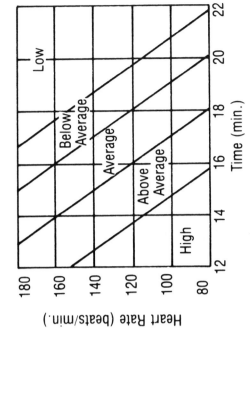

**60 + Year-Old Females
Relative Fitness Level**

**60 + Year-Old Males
Exercise Program**

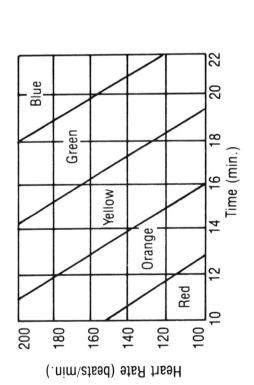

**60 + Year-Old Females
Exercise Program**

FIGURE 5

Fitness Walking Programs

BLUE PROGRAM*

Week	1–2	3–4	5	6	7–8	9	10	11	12–13	14	15–16	17–18	19–20
WARM-UP (mins. before walk stretches)	5–7	5–7	5–7	5–7	5–7	5–7	5–7	5–7	5–7	5–7	5–7	5–7	5–7
MILEAGE	1.0	1.25	1.5	1.5	1.75	2.0	2.0	2.0	2.25	2.5	2.5	2.75	3.0
PACE (mph)	3.0	3.0	3.0	3.5	3.5	3.5	3.75	3.75	3.75	3.75	4.0	4.0	4.0
HEART RATE (% of max)	60	60	60	60–70	60–70	60–70	60–70	70	70	70	70	70–80	70–80
COOL-DOWN (mins. after walk stretches)	5–7	5–7	5–7	5–7	5–7	5–7	5–7	5–7	5–7	5–7	5–7	5–7	5–7
FREQUENCY (times per week)	5	5	5	5	5	5	5	5	5	5	5	5	5

*At the end of the twenty-week fitness-walking protocol, retest yourself to establish your new program.

GREEN PROGRAM*

Week	1–2	3–4	5–6	7	8–9	10–12	13	14	15–16	17–18	19–20
WARM-UP (mins. before walk stretches)	5–7	5–7	5–7	5–7	5–7	5–7	5–7	5–7	5–7	5–7	5–7
MILEAGE	1.5	1.75	2.0	2.0	2.25	2.5	2.75	2.75	3.0	3.25	3.5
PACE (mph)	3.0	3.0	3.0	3.5	3.5	3.5	3.5	4.0	4.0	4.0	4.0
HEART RATE (% of max)	60–70	60–70	60–70	70	70	70	70	70–80	70–80	70–80	70–80
COOL-DOWN (mins. after walk stretches)	5–7	5–7	5–7	5–7	5–7	5–7	5–7	5–7	5–7	5–7	5–7
FREQUENCY (times per week)	5	5	5	5	5	5	5	5	5	5	5

*At the end of the twenty-week fitness-walking protocol, retest yourself to establish your new program.

YELLOW PROGRAM*

Week	1	2	3–4	5	6–8	9–10	11–12	13–14	15	16–17	18–20
WARM-UP (mins. before walk stretches)	5–7	5–7	5–7	5–7	5–7	5–7	5–7	5–7	5–7	5–7	5–7
MILEAGE	2.0	2.25	2.5	2.75	2.75	3.0	3.0	3.25	3.5	3.5	4.0
PACE (mph)	3.0	3.0	3.0	3.0	3.5	3.5	4.0	4.0	4.0	4.5	4.5
HEART RATE (% of max)	70	70	70	70	70	70	70–80	70–80	70–80	70–80	70–80
COOL-DOWN (mins. after walk stretches)	5–7	5–7	5–7	5–7	5–7	5–7	5–7	5–7	5–7	5–7	5–7
FREQUENCY (times per week)	5	5	5	5	5	5	5	5	5	5	5

*At the end of the twenty-week fitness-walking protocol, you may either retest yourself and move to a new fitness-walking category or follow the Yellow Maintenance Program for a lifetime of fitness walking.

ORANGE PROGRAM*

Week	1	2	3–4	5	6	7	8	9–10	11–14	15–20
WARM-UP (mins. before walk stretches)	5–7	5–7	5–7	5–7	5–7	5–7	5–7	5–7	5–7	5–7
MILEAGE	2.5	2.75	3.0	3.25	3.25	3.5	3.75	4.0	4.0	4.0
PACE (mph)	3.5	3.5	3.5	3.5	4.0	4.0	4.0	4.0	4.5	4.5
INCLINE/WEIGHT										+**
HEART RATE (% of max)	70	70	70	70	70–80	70–80	70–80	70–80	70–80	70–80
COOL-DOWN (mins. after walk stretches)	5–7	5–7	5–7	5–7	5–7	5–7	5–7	5–7	5–7	5–7
FREQUENCY (times per week)	5	5	5	5	5	5	5	5	5	3

*At the end of the twenty-week fitness-walking protocol, follow the Orange/Red Maintenance Program for a lifetime of fitness walking.
**During weeks 15–20, arm weights or incline may be added to increase intensity.

RED PROGRAM*

Week	1	2	3	4	5	6	7–20
WARM-UP (mins. before walk stretches)	5–7	5–7	5–7	5–7	5–7	5–7	5–7
MILEAGE	3.0	3.25	3.5	3.5	3.75	4.0	4.0
PACE (mph)	4.0	4.0	4.0	4.5	4.5	4.5	4.5
INCLINE/WEIGHT							+**
HEART RATE (% of max)	70	70	70	70–80	70–80	70–80	70–80
COOL-DOWN (mins. after walk stretches)	5–7	5–7	5–7	5–7	5–7	5–7	5–7
FREQUENCY (times per week)	5	5	5	5	5	5	3

*At the end of the twenty-week fitness-walking protocol, turn to the Orange/Red Maintenance Program for a lifetime of fitness walking.
**During weeks 15–20, arm weights or incline may be added to increase intensity.

YELLOW MAINTENANCE PROGRAM

WARM-UP: 5–7 minutes before walk stretches

AEROBIC WORK OUT: mileage: 4.0; pace: 4.5 mph

HEART RATE: 70–80% of maximum

COOL-DOWN: 5–7 minutes after walk stretches

FREQUENCY: 3–5 times per week

WEEKLY MILEAGE: 12–20 miles

ORANGE/RED MAINTENANCE PROGRAM

WARM-UP: 5–7 minutes before walk stretches

AEROBIC WORK OUT: mileage: 4.0; pace: 4.5 mph
weight/incline: Add weights to upper body or add hill walking as needed to keep heart rate in target zone (70–80% of predicted maximum).

HEART RATE: 70–80% of maximum

COOL-DOWN: 5–7 minutes after walk stretches

FREQUENCY: 3–5 times per week

WEEKLY MILEAGE: 12–20 miles

APPENDIX C

DAILY ACTIVITY LOGS

Included in this appendix is a physical activity log. Use this log to record your daily physical activity (see *Daily Health Check #1, Physical Activity Programs*, page 46, for a description of how to use the physical activity portion of this log). You can also use the log to keep track of your participation in muscle resistance or flexibility activities (see *Daily Health Checks #2 and #3*, pages 47 and 53) or your body weight (see *Daily Health Check #6*, page 69). Finally, use the log to note whether or not you have done "something for yourself" during the day, or whether or not you have participated in meditation/deep relaxation (see *Daily Health Check #5, Stress Management Program*, page 63).

We suggest you make several copies of the log for extended use.

Days	Date	Physical Activity Type	Minutes			Distance (optional)	Activity Heart Rate (10 sec.)	Weight (pounds)	Meditation/ Relaxation (Yes or No)	Did Something For Self (Yes or No)
			Warm-up	Exercise	Cool-Down					

Days	Date	Physical Activity Type	Minutes			Distance (optional)	Activity Heart Rate (10 sec.)	Weight (pounds)	Meditation/ Relaxation (Yes or No)	Did Some-thing For Self (Yes or No)
			Warm-up	Exercise	Cool-Down					

Days	Date	Physical Activity Type	Minutes			Distance (optional)	Activity Heart Rate (10 sec.)	Weight (pounds)	Meditation/ Relaxation (Yes or No)	Did Some-thing For Self (Yes or No)
			Warm-up	Exercise	Cool-Down					

| Days | Date | Physical Activity Type | Minutes | | | Distance (optional) | Activity Heart Rate (10 sec.) | Weight (pounds) | Meditation/ Relaxation (Yes or No) | Did Some-thing For Self (Yes or No) |
			Warm-up	Exercise	Cool-Down					

Days	Date	Physical Activity Type	Minutes			Distance (optional)	Activity Heart Rate (10 sec.)	Weight (pounds)	Meditation/ Relaxation (Yes or No)	Did Some- thing For Self (Yes or No)
			Warm-up	Exercise	Cool-Down					

Days	Date	Physical Activity Type	Minutes			Distance (optional)	Activity Heart Rate (10 sec.)	Weight (pounds)	Meditation/ Relaxation (Yes or No)	Did Some-thing For Self (Yes or No)
			Warm-up	Exercise	Cool-Down					

APPENDIX D

MUSCLE STRENGTH TESTS

Note: **If you have a history of back problems, or if performing these tests bothers your back, we suggest you avoid taking these tests.**

Two tests are included for assessing body strength:
- Abdominal test;
- Upper-body test.

Abdominal. Lie on your back (use a soft surface) with your knees in a bent position (about 45 degrees). Knees should remain bent throughout the entire test sequence. The test includes four sets of slow *curl-ups*, each set becoming more difficult.

Set One: Keeping your hands and arms to your side (see Figure 1), slowly curl-up your upper body; beginning with your head, then your shoulders and following through by raising from your waist until the body is generally flexed (see Figure 2). Concentrate on **not** "jerking" your upper body forward — the curl-up should be slow and deliberate. With your arms in this position, attempt to do five consecutive curl-ups.

Set Two: Arms should be folded across the chest (see Figure 3). Attempt to do five more consecutive curl-ups slowly (see Figure 4).

Set Three: Move the arms to the back of your head (see Figure 5). In this position you will be tempted to jerk forward, using the leverage of your hands secured behind your head (see Figure 6). Make every attempt to perform the curl-ups slowly and smoothly. Attempt five consecutive curl-ups in this position.

Set Four: The arms should be extended above your body and remain behind your head as you perform the curl-up (see Figure 7). Attempt to complete five consecutive curl-ups (see Figure 8). Remember to keep your arms behind your head as you come forward.

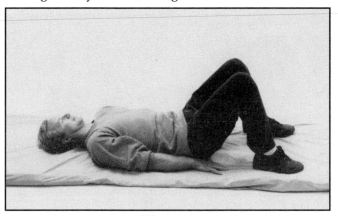

Figure 1

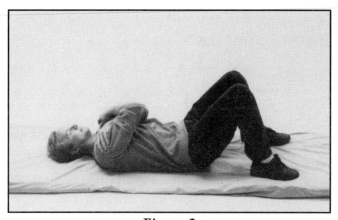

Figure 3

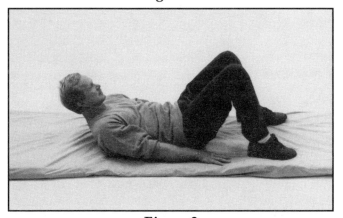

Figure 2

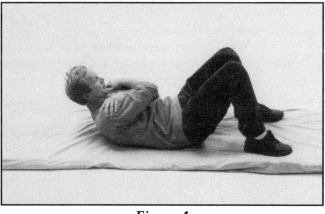

Figure 4

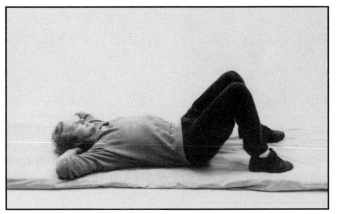

Figure 5

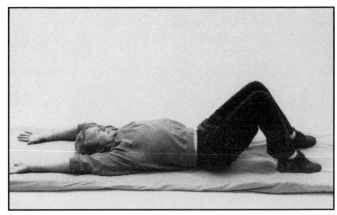

Figure 7

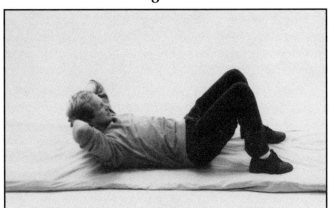

Figure 6

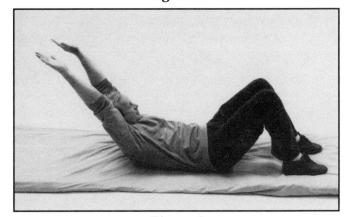

Figure 8

INTERPRETING THE RESULTS

The ratings for this abdominal test are shown below:

Less than five curl-ups completed: Very Poor
Five curl-ups completed (Set One):   Poor
Ten curl-ups completed (Set Two):   Average
Fifteen curl-ups completed (Set Three):   Good
Twenty curl-ups completed (Set Four):   Excellent

Upper-body Test. This test primarily assesses the strength of the arms, chest, shoulder and abdominal muscles and is referred to as the "push-up" test. Those of you who served in the military or were a pledge in a fraternity will be quite familiar with this test.

Women: Refer to Figures 9 and 10. Make certain that you keep the body straight from the knees to the head, and as you lower your body, bend from the knees rather than from the waist. The test is designed to have you do as many push-ups as you can. You should not stop between push-ups for more than three to four seconds.

Men: Refer to Figures 11 and 12. To start the test begin in the up position. The body should be lowered until approximately three to four inches from the floor, keeping the back straight and then once again raising your body to the up position. **Do not** hold your breath during the test. Breath freely during each push-up.

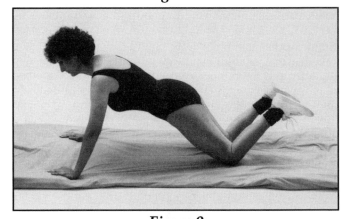

Figure 9

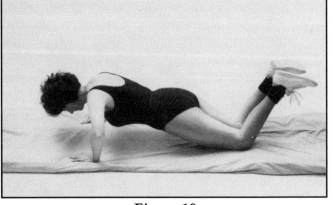

Figure 10

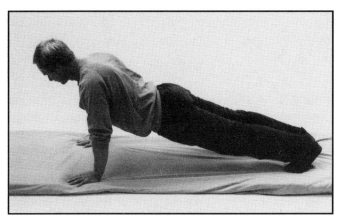

Figure 11

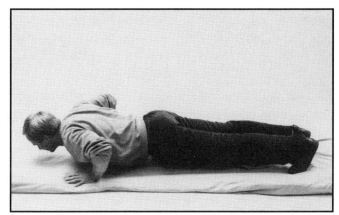

Figure 12

INTERPRETING THE RESULTS

The fitness categories for this test are illustrated in Table 1.

Table 1. Norms and Percentiles by Age Groups and Gender for Push-ups

Norms												
Age (yrs)	15–19		20–29		30–39		40–49		50–59		60–69	
Gender	M	F	M	F	M	F	M	F	M	F	M	F
Excellent	≥39	≥33	≥36	≥30	≥30	≥27	≥22	≥24	≥21	≥21	≥18	≥17
Above average	29–38	25–32	29–35	21–29	22–29	20–26	17–21	15–23	13–20	11–20	11–17	12–16
Average	23–28	18–24	22–28	15–20	17–21	13–19	13–16	11–14	10–12	7–10	8–10	5–11
Below average	18–22	12–17	17–21	10–14	12–16	8–12	10–12	5–10	7–9	2–6	5–7	1–4
Poor	≤17	≤11	≤16	≤9	≤11	≤7	≤9	≤4	≤6	≤1	≤4	≤1

Percentiles												
Age (yrs)	15–19		20–29		30–39		40–49		50–59		60–69	
Gender	M	F	M	F	M	F	M	F	M	F	M	F
95	50	46	48	37	36	36	30	32	28	30	25	30
90	43	38	41	32	32	31	25	28	24	23	24	25
85	39	33	36	30	30	27	22	24	21	21	18	17
80	35	31	34	26	27	24	21	22	17	17	16	15
75	32	28	32	24	25	22	20	20	15	15	13	13
70	31	26	30	22	24	21	19	18	14	13	11	12
65	29	25	29	21	22	20	17	15	13	11	11	12
60	27	23	27	20	21	17	16	14	11	10	10	10
55	26	21	25	18	20	16	15	13	11	10	10	9
50	24	20	24	16	19	14	13	12	10	9	9	6
45	23	18	22	15	17	13	13	11	10	7	8	5
40	22	16	21	14	16	12	12	10	9	5	7	4
35	21	15	20	13	15	11	11	10	8	4	6	3
30	20	14	18	11	14	10	10	7	7	3	6	2
25	18	12	17	10	12	8	10	5	7	2	5	1
20	16	11	16	9	11	7	8	4	5	1	4	—
15	14	9	14	7	10	6	7	3	5	1	3	—
10	11	6	11	5	8	4	5	2	4	—	2	—
5	8	4	9	2	5	1	4	—	2	—	—	—

(Based on data from the Canada Fitness Survey, 1981. Reprinted from **Canadian Standardized Test of Fitness (CSTF) Operations Manual**, 3rd Ed. With the permission of Fitness Canada, Fitness and Amateur Sport Canada, Ottawa, 1986.)

APPENDIX E

BODY FLEXIBILITY TESTS

There is no single *best test* for assessing total flexibility because a person may be flexible in one joint but not in another. It is possible, however, to get a general idea of one's flexibility. Listed below are the following flexibility tests:

- The simple, non-quantifiable assessment;
- The sit-and-reach test.

The Simple, Non-Quantifiable Tests. Try the suggested flexibility moves listed below. (*Note:* **You should not bounce or force yourself when doing these tests**):

1. Can you turn your head to the right or the left without difficulty?
2. Can you touch your chin to your chest without difficulty?
3. Can you reach your arms over your shoulders and touch your back between the shoulder blades?
4. Can you straighten your arms behind you and then grasp your hands together?
5. Can you twist your trunk to the left and to the right so your chest is almost 90 degrees to your legs?
6. Can you bend over without experiencing back pain?
7. Can you touch your toes?
8. Lying on your back, with one leg bent in a 45-degree angle, can you raise the other leg to a 90-degree position, and then reverse leg positions and do this with the other leg?
9. Can you point your toes and feet forward so they are straight with your legs and then point them towards your head to reach a 45-degree angle?

Sit-and-Reach Test.[369] This test is designed to assess the flexion of your lower-back and hips as well as the extensibility of your hamstring muscles (the large muscles in the back of your upper leg). Sit on the floor with your legs extended in front of you and knees and backs of legs pressed flat to the surface of the floor (knees and legs must remain in this position throughout the test).

You will need to attach a ruler or meter stick to a block with the 26 cm. mark secured at the point where your feet contact the block.[369, 370] Place your index fingers of both hands together and then reach forward towards the ruler as far as possible (see Figure 1). The farthest distance you can reach on the measuring stick should be noted (do not bounce during the test). You may want to do a little stretching for a minute prior to the test. Repeat the test three times and then take the greatest measurement.[369]

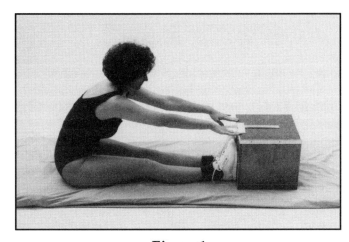

Figure 1

INTERPRETING THE RESULTS

Fitness categories for this test are illustrated in Table 1 (next page).

Table 1. *Norms and Percentiles by Age Groups and Gender for Trunk Forward Flexion (cm)*

Norms

Age (yrs)	15–19		20–29		30–39		40–49		50–59		60–69	
Gender	**M**	**F**	**M**	**F**	**M**	**F**	**M**	**F**	**M**	**F**	**M**	**F**
Excellent	≥ 39	≥ 43	≥ 40	≥ 41	≥ 38	≥ 41	≥ 35	≥ 38	≥ 35	≥ 39	≥ 33	≥ 35
Above average	34–38	38–42	34–39	37–40	33–37	36–40	29–34	34–37	28–34	33–38	25–32	31–34
Average	29–33	34–37	30–33	33–36	28–32	32–35	24–28	30–33	24–27	30–32	20–24	27–30
Below average	24–28	29–33	25–29	28–32	23–27	27–31	18–23	25–29	16–23	25–29	15–19	23–26
Poor	≤ 23	≤ 28	≤ 24	≤ 27	≤ 22	≤ 26	≤ 17	≤ 24	≤ 15	≤ 24	≤ 14	≤ 23

Percentiles

Age (yrs)	15–19		20–29		30–39		40–49		50–59		60–69	
Gender	**M**	**F**	**M**	**F**	**M**	**F**	**M**	**F**	**M**	**F**	**M**	**F**
95	44	47	44	45	43	45	40	43	41	43	44	40
90	42	44	42	43	40	42	37	40	38	40	35	37
85	39	43	40	41	38	41	35	38	35	39	33	35
80	38	42	38	40	37	39	34	37	32	37	30	34
75	36	41	37	39	35	38	32	36	30	36	28	33
70	35	40	36	38	34	37	30	35	29	35	26	31
65	34	38	34	37	33	36	29	34	28	33	25	31
60	33	37	33	36	32	35	28	33	27	32	24	30
55	31	36	32	35	31	34	26	32	26	31	23	28
50	30	35	31	34	29	33	25	31	25	30	22	28
45	29	34	30	33	28	32	24	30	24	30	20	27
40	28	33	29	32	27	31	23	29	22	29	18	26
35	27	32	27	31	26	30	21	28	20	28	17	25
30	26	31	26	29	24	28	20	26	18	26	16	24
25	24	29	25	28	23	27	18	25	16	25	15	23
20	22	27	23	26	21	25	16	24	15	23	14	23
15	19	25	21	25	20	23	14	22	14	22	13	20
10	17	23	18	22	17	21	12	19	12	19	11	18
5	13	18	14	18	13	16	8	14	7	13	8	13

(Based on data from the Canada Fitness Survey, 1981. Reprinted from **Canadian Standardized Test of Fitness (CSTF) Operations Manual**, 3rd Ed. With the permission of Fitness Canada, Fitness and Amateur Sport Canada, Ottawa, 1986.)

APPENDIX F

NUTRITION GOAL SHEETS

Each of the 11 goal sheets contains three columns: "Ready to Work on This;" "Satisfied and Not Ready to Change;" and "Doing This Already." When you move to a new goal sheet, take a minute or two and with a pencil, check the column that appropriately corresponds to your current nutritional status. The goal is to gradually move towards the **"Doing This Already"** column.

If you feel strongly that you are satisfied with your current nutritional habit with regards to one of the goals, and you do not want to change at this time, consider returning to this goal in a six to 12 month period and then re-evaluate your feelings towards this goal.

Take six to eight weeks and work on a specific goal sheet. Give yourself time to determine how the changes are affecting your health. We think you'll be pleasantly surprised.

(*Note:* **Included within some of the goal sheets are additional nutritional tips to assist you in making desired nutritional changes.**)

EATING MORE FISH
Check which category you are now in for each goal.

	DOING THIS ALREADY	SATISFIED AND NOT READY TO CHANGE	READY TO WORK ON THIS
1. Eat three to six ounces of fish or three ounces of shellfish three to four times a week.			
2. Eat fish prepared by grilling, baking, poaching, etc., but not frying or sauteing in lots of oil.			
3. Have a wide variety of fish recipes my family likes.			
4. Use only a small amount of low calorie dressing or "lite" mayonnaise mixed with yogurt in tuna salad or for other seafood salads.			
5. Order fish at least half the time when eating out.			
6. Serve fish dishes to company.			
7. Eat a higher omega-3 fat fish once a week, like salmon, trout, sardines, anchovies or herring.			
8. Avoid taking fish oil supplements unless you have discussed this with an M.D. and read labels carefully for Vitamin A & Vitamin D content (too much of these vitamins can be toxic).			

© Cardiovascular Genetics Clinic of the University of Utah School of Medicine

CHOOSING LOW-FAT CHEESES
Check which category you are now in for each goal.

GOALS

	DOING THIS ALREADY	SATISFIED AND NOT READY TO CHANGE	READY TO WORK ON THIS
1. I always use low-fat cottage cheese in place of regular creamed cottage cheese.			
2. I use lower fat/cholesterol cheeses like part-skim mozzarella, Hickory Farms Lites, Weight Watchers or Lifetime Block Cheese, cottage cheese or Golden Image (a filled cheese) in place of cheddar or other high-fat cheeses in recipes. These products are six grams of fat or less/ounce.			
3. When using grated cheese as a topping, I calculate the number of ounces from the package weight, and use only one ounce per person.			
4. I either do not snack on cheese, or I snack on only very low-fat cheeses like St. Otho, Laughing Cow Reduced Calories Wedges, Lifetime Natural Cheeses, low-fat cottage cheese, processed low-fat cheese slices, or other cheeses that are three grams of fat or less/ounce.			
5. I either do not use sliced cheese, or else I use the low-fat cheese slices, like Weight Watchers or Lite-line.			
6. I use low-fat cottage cheese to make Mock Sour Cream (1 cup low-fat cottage cheese, 2 TB. buttermilk or yogurt and one-half to one tsp. freshly squeezed lemon juice, blend until smooth) for potato topper, dips in place of sour cream, or for toppings or cream cheese.			
7. I use a low-fat cream cheese like Kraft Light Philadelphia in place of regular cream cheese, or else substitute Mock Sour Cream or Part Skim Milk Ricotta Cheese for all or part of the cream cheese in recipes or spreads.			
8. I can find low-fat cheeses in the stores where I shop.			
9. I buy regular high-fat cheeses less than once per month.			

READING LABELS AND GROCERY SHOPPING
Check which category you are now in for each goal.

1. I/my family nearly always buy healthy, low-fat foods when I/we shop for groceries and I/we avoid buying "junk food" or unplanned items.			
2. My/our carts are usually full of fruits, vegetables, grains, cereals, legumes, and low-fat dairy products (along with the non-food items).			
3. I/we can comfortably make dietary changes fit into our food budget.			
4. I/we regularly examine food labels to help make decisions about what to buy.			

© Cardiovascular Genetics Clinic of the University of Utah School of Medicine

	DOING THIS ALREADY	SATISFIED AND NOT READY TO CHANGE	READY TO WORK ON THIS
5. I/we often use the label to calculate the percent of calories from fat. Using this number, I choose the lowest fat brands or, when the percent fat is over 30, I/we "dilute the fat" with other meal items (like breads, potatoes, etc.).			
6. I/we do not buy foods which contain egg yolk, butter, coconut oil, lard, or palm oil, unless I/we decide it is present in small amounts.			
7. Most weeks I/we do not buy chocolate, dried foods, chips, fatty meats, high-fat cheeses, margarine or oils, or other high-fat foods.			
8. I/we have a system for keeping plenty of good food in the house, so I/we can have low-fat meals and snacks prepared easily, without extra trips to the store or stopping for fast foods.			

HOLIDAY EATING

Check which category you are now in for each goal.

1. I plan ahead for holiday meals and parties by making the rest of my diet very low fat.			
2. I prepare holiday foods using low-fat substitutes: replacing whole eggs with egg whites, substituting skim evaporated milk for cream or whole milk, using light mayonnaise and non-fat yogurt for sour cream.			
3. Before social events, I pre-plan the foods that I will and will not eat. I consider portion sizes, seconds, and how much food I will leave on the plate.			
4. I remove the skin from the turkey before I eat it, and I prepare the turkey stuffing with broth or bouillon rather than butter, margarine or gravy.			
5. I prepare the gravy after removing the fat from the drippings.			
6. I fill up on complex carbohydrate foods like bread or rolls, salads, vegetables and rice or potatoes, and eat them with little added fat.			
7. I don't leave holiday munchies out. Instead, I put them away after serving. However, I make sure that vegetable slices, bread sticks, and low-fat crackers such as rye krisp, are available for snacking.			
8. I replace real mayonnaise with non-fat yogurt, light mayonnaise or blended cottage cheese in dips, spreads and other recipes.			

© Cardiovascular Genetics Clinic of the University of Utah School of Medicine

LEGUMES: DRY BEANS, PEAS AND LENTILS

Legumes are low in fat, tasty, high in complex carbohydrate and fiber, and they have zero cholesterol content. To avoid possible bloating and excessive gas from beans, add a small quantity of beans to your diet every day, and within a period of a month you should be able to consume large amounts of legume dishes without the worry of discomfort. A good approach for including legumes into your diet is to start adding a tablespoon of garbanzo beans on a salad or eating a small serving of baked beans or bean soup each day.

Check which category you are now in for each goal.

	GOALS		
	DOING THIS ALREADY	SATISFIED AND NOT READY TO CHANGE	READY TO WORK ON THIS
1. I regularly eat legumes (dried beans and peas) and consume about two cups per week (for women and children) or four cups per week (for men and teenagers).			
2. I keep a variety of canned or dried legumes on hand.			
3. I can prepare legumes easily, either by using them canned, planning ahead to soak and/or pressure cook the dried beans, or by another system that works for me. (DO NOT PRESSURE COOK FOAMY BEANS LIKE SOYBEANS OR LENTILS.)			
4. I have at least seven dishes that I like that include a variety of legumes, which include tofu; pinto, red kidney, lima, black, soy or garbanzo beans; red or brown lentils, or black-eyed, yellow or split peas.			
5. I can eat beans without being miserable with gas or cramping.			
6. I often eat legumes for meatless, cheeseless lunches or dinners.			
7. I eat bean dips for appetizers or snacks. These include refried bean dip, hummous or tofu dips.			
8. When I buy canned bean products (like baked beans or refried beans), I choose brands which are low in fat.			

EATING OUT AND EATING WHILE TRAVELING

Check which category you are now in for each goal.

1. <u>BREAKFAST</u> — I either do not eat out for breakfast, or else I almost always choose a low-fat, low-cholesterol meal.			
2. <u>LUNCH</u> — I either do not eat out for lunch, or else I take my own low-fat, low-cholesterol lunch, or else I almost always choose a low-fat, low-cholesterol meal.			
3. <u>DINNER</u> — I either do not eat out for dinner more than once a month, or else I almost always choose a low-fat, low-cholesterol meal.			
4. For fast inexpensive dining, I go to eating places that have low-fat foods.			
5. For special occasions, I usually go to places at which I can order low-fat foods I enjoy. (About once every six months or so, I splurge on a higher fat favorite.)			

	DOING THIS ALREADY	SATISFIED AND NOT READY TO CHANGE	READY TO WORK ON THIS
6. I usually ask for low-fat substitutes: skim milk instead of whole milk, margarine in place of butter, or low-calorie salad dressing or salad dressing "on the side." I avoid eating butter, fried foods, sour cream, gravy, rich desserts, and other fatty foods.			
7. I fill up on the complex carbohydrate foods: bread and rolls (without spread), salads without regular dressing, potatoes without butter or sour cream, rice and vegetables.			
8. I eat low-fat snacks like bread, crackers, fruit, yogurt, or popcorn before a meal that might be high in fat.			
9. I have found ethnic restaurants that I enjoy that serve Italian, Asian (Chinese, Vietnamese, Thai, Japanese) or Middle Eastern foods which have low-fat choices.			
10. I often choose low-fat fish or seafood dishes that are prepared with little fat.			

SNACKS AND DESSERTS

Check which category you are now in for each goal.

	DOING THIS ALREADY	SATISFIED AND NOT READY TO CHANGE	READY TO WORK ON THIS
1. When I/my children snack between meals, I/they choose foods which are low in fat, like fruit, vegetables, low-fat chips (homemade) and crackers, low-fat yogurt, sherbet, sorbet, popsicles, breads, muffins or bagels, cereals, etc.			
2. I keep a good supply of low-fat snacks on hand, and do not eat the high-fat types like chips, most cookies and candy bars, ice cream, etc.			
3. For treats away from home (either at work or at restaurants, malls or movies), I/my children usually choose lower fat foods instead of the high-fat doughnuts, desserts, ice cream, chips, candy bars, etc.			
4. When I am offered a special high-fat food at work or by friends or family, I can respond gracefully and either avoid eating it at all, or eat only a small amount.			
5. I limit treat splurges (high-fat foods like chips and dip, cheesecake, candy bars, etc.) to not more than once every two months.			
6. When we have dessert, I/my family usually eat low-fat choices like fruits, quick breads, sherbets or sorbet, or low-fat baked items like apple crisp, angel food cake, etc.			
7. When I cook, I always use low-cholesterol, low-saturated fat substitutes (egg whites or egg substitutes instead of whole eggs, low-fat yogurt for sour cream, margarine for butter, evaporated skim milk, etc.).			
8. I eat snacks and desserts only if I am really hungry, and not just out of habit.			

RECIPE SUBSTITUTIONS AND CHANGES

This goal sheet should be correlated with Phase I information, pages 59 to 60.

Check which category you are now in for each goal.

	DOING THIS ALREADY	SATISFIED AND NOT READY TO CHANGE	READY TO WORK ON THIS
1. I always use skim milk for whole milk, and margarine or butter substitute (like Butter Buds) for butter in recipes.			
2. I always use egg whites or egg substitutes in recipes in place of the egg yolks.			
3. I use "light" mayonnaise or "light" Miracle Whip mixed with low-fat yogurt in place of regular mayonnaise in recipes.			
4. I use low-fat yogurt or cottage cheese in place of sour cream or IMO-type products.			
5. I use low-fat cottage cheese, part skim-milk mozzarella, or other low-fat cheeses in recipes in place of regular cheese.			
6. I almost always use less fat than the recipe calls for.			
7. I almost always use less salt or salt substitute in recipes.			
8. I do not prepare any foods by deep-fat frying or pan frying.			
9. I purchase mixes that do not contain egg yolks, such as pancake mix without the eggs included.			
10. I do not use regular whipped cream or Cool Whip-type products for toppings or in recipes.			
11. I substitute cocoa for chocolate.			
12. I keep evaporated skim milk on hand to use in place of cream.			
13. When recipes call for ground beef, I use lean ground turkey or very lean beef, and cut the amount to two to three ounces per person.			
14. I always remove the skin before cooking chicken.			

GOALS

INCLUDING CHILDREN IN HEALTHY EATING

These goals are primarily for families with children who have high cholesterol levels.

Check which category your children are now in.

	DOING THIS ALREADY	SATISFIED AND NOT READY TO CHANGE	READY TO WORK ON THIS
GOALS			
1. My children eat ample amounts of legumes, whole grains, fruits, vegetables and low-fat dairy products at mealtimes.			
2. When my children snack between meals, they choose foods which are low in fat, like fruit, vegetables, low-fat chips (homemade) and crackers, skim milk or low-fat yogurt, sherbet, sorbet, popsicles, breads, muffins or bagels, cereals, etc.			
3. My children eat fish, poultry, meat or cheese only once a day, and have fish two to four times per week.			
4. At home, my children avoid egg yolks, butter, whole or 2% milk, ice cream, chocolate and other high-fat, high-cholesterol foods and ingredients.			
5. My children almost always choose the lowest fat choices at fast food places and other restaurants.			
6. Other caretakers for my children (relatives, baby-sitters, etc.) understand the dietary restrictions and serve low-fat, low-cholesterol foods to the children.			
7. For school children: I have made arrangements so my child can receive a low-fat, low-cholesterol lunch on school days.			

MEATLESS MEALS

Check which category you are now in for each goal.

1. I usually have two meals per day that contain no meat, fish, poultry, or cheese.			
2. I have a wide variety of meatless, egg yolk-less breakfasts that I enjoy.			
3. There are a variety of meatless foods that I enjoy for lunch or supper.			
4. I can pack an enjoyable sack lunch or dinner that does not include a sandwich using meat, poultry, fish, or cheese.			
5. I regularly eat legumes (dried beans and peas) and consume about two cups per week (for women and children) or four cups per week (for men and teenagers).			
6. I eat three to five servings of whole grains or vegetables at each meal with no added fat or only small amounts of margarine, spread, or regular salad dressing.			
7. When I get hungry between meals, I eat low-fat, high-fiber snacks like low-fat crackers, homemade tortilla chips, unbuttered popcorn, pretzels, fresh fruit, etc.			

KEEPING ON TRACK IN THE FUTURE

This sheet is to help you see what changes you have made by following the nutritional goal sheets, and to see what further steps you can take. These goals summarize the low-fat, low-cholesterol diet according to the topics discussed in these goal sheets. Check if you're doing these regularly.

		PERFORM REGULARLY
1.	Almost ALL of my meals and snacks include mostly grains, cereals, legumes, fruits, and vegetables, with small amounts of fish, poultry, lean meat and low-fat cheeses, and no high-fat, high-cholesterol foods like egg yolk, butter, chocolate, regular cheese, or steak.	
2.	I eat a very low-fat diet, using little margarine, oils, salad dressings, mayonnaise, or Miracle Whip, chocolate or other fats, and I cook with only small amounts of vegetable fats.	
3.	I carefully read labels to choose brands low in fat and avoid buying products with egg yolk, coconut oil, palm oil, lard, butter, hydrogenated fats, etc.	
4.	I always use low-fat products like skim milk, non-fat yogurt, egg whites or egg substitutes, and low-fat cheeses.	
5.	I eat three to six ounces of fish or three ounces of shellfish two to four times a week.	
6.	I usually have two meals per day which contain no meat, fish, poultry or regular cheese.	
7.	I/we have a system for keeping plenty of foods in the house, so I can have low-fat meals and snacks prepared easily, without extra trips to the store or stopping for fast foods.	
8.	I regularly eat legumes (dried beans and peas) and consume about two cups per week (for women and children) or four cups per week (for men and teenagers).	
9.	When I snack between meals, I choose low-fat foods like fruits, vegetables, chips (homemade) and crackers, skim milk or low-fat yogurt, sherbet, sorbet, popsicles, breads, muffins, or bagels, etc.	
10.	I can respond to offers of not-allowed foods from friends and relatives, and can gracefully refuse these, or plan ahead to include small amounts of higher fat foods in my diet that day.	
11.	I enjoy a wide variety and large servings of vegetables, grains, cereals and fruits.	
12.	I use lower fat/cholesterol cheeses like part-skim mozzarella, Hickory Farms Lites, Weight Watchers or Lifetime Block Cheeses, cottage cheese or Golden Image (a filled cheese) in place of cheddar or other high-fat cheeses in recipes. These products are six grams of fat or less per ounce.	
13.	I stay on the low-fat diet when I go out to eat.	
14.	I have reduced other heart disease risk factors—I do not smoke; I am at a healthy weight; I get aerobic exercise three to four times a week, and my blood pressure is normal.	

KEEPING ON TRACK IN THE FUTURE (continued on next page)

RATE YOURSELF:

How many questions could you check as DOING REGULARLY?

13-14 CHECKS: **EXCELLENT!** You've worked hard, made many changes, and are eating a very healthy diet. We expect your risk of heart disease to have decreased markedly. Now your job is to continue these excellent habits.

8-12 CHECKS: You are working hard. We encourage you to keep up the good work and continue to make gradual improvements in your eating habits.

4-7 CHECKS: You have probably not made enough changes to drop your cholesterol to the lowest possible level. We encourage you to continue working with the goal sheets and to become very familiar with the nutritional tips in this section.

0-3 CHECKS: Time to recommit to making gradual dietary changes. We suggest you review this section.

APPENDIX G

MEASURING BODY COMPOSITION (% BODY FAT)

This test will help you determine your ideal body weight. The test is designed to determine how much lean body mass (the entire body without any fat) a person has and then calculate the ideal body weight on the basis of that measurement. This test is superior to a height-weight chart because there is wide variation in body type and build. For example, if you have inherited a muscular body, you should weigh more than if you have inherited a slender body because the basic nonfat portion of your body — the lean body mass — will be larger.

The generally accepted **good range** of percent body fat for men and women is:

Men: **15-21% Fat**   Women: **21-27% Fat**

PREDICTING BODY FAT FOR WOMEN

To get a good estimate of the percentage of body fat, you should measure the following areas with a cloth tape measure. Pull the tape lightly but firmly around the areas to be measured and measure over the bare skin if possible. You should be sure to keep the tape level during the measurement and take two or three measurements at each of the following sites to get a good average:

- **HIPS** — measure around the hips at the maximum girth.
- **ABDOMEN** — measure around the waist at the umbilicus (belly button).
- **HEIGHT** — measure the height in inches.

COMPUTATION FORM

Hips Average
Measurement _____ Constant A _____
(from Table 1, pg. 216)

Abdomen Average
Measurement _____ Constant B _____

Add A and B _____

Height
in Inches _____ Constant C _____

(A plus B) minus C = _____ % Body Fat

Put the average of your measurements in the blank space on the computation form. Now look at the "hips" column in Table 1. Note that there is a number to the right side of each hip measurement. This number is a "constant" and is used in the computation of percent body fat from the measurements you have taken. Write down the constant for each measurement you have made on the computation form to the right side of the measurement. Now add constant A to constant B and subtract constant C. The number you have left is percent body fat.

An example may be helpful. If a lady had an average hip circumference of 42 inches and an average abdominal circumference of 28 and was 64 inches tall, we would get the following calculations:

Hips Average
Measurement __42__ Constant A __50.24__

Abdomen Average
Measurement __28__ Constant B __19.91__

Add A and B __70.15__

Height
in Inches __64__ Constant C __39.00__

(A plus B) minus C __70.15 - 39 = 31.15__

% Body Fat: __31.15%__

According to these measurements, she is about 31 percent fat.

Table 1. *Conversion Constants to Predict Percent Body Fat (Women)*

	Hips		Abdomen		Height
In.	*Constant A*	*In.*	*Constant B*	*In.*	*Constant C*
30	33.48	20	14.22	55	33.52
31	34.87	21	14.93	56	34.13
32	36.27	22	15.64	57	34.74
33	37.67	23	16.35	58	35.35
34	39.06	24	17.06	59	35.96
35	40.46	25	17.78	60	36.57
36	41.86	26	18.49	61	37.18
37	43.25	27	19.20	62	37.79
38	44.65	28	19.91	63	38.40
39	46.05	29	20.62	64	39.01
40	47.44	30	21.33	65	39.62
41	48.84	31	22.04	66	40.23
42	50.24	32	22.75	67	40.84
43	51.64	33	23.46	68	41.45
44	53.03	34	24.18	69	42.06
45	54.43	35	24.89	70	42.67
46	55.83	36	25.60	71	43.28
47	57.22	37	26.31	72	43.89
48	58.62	38	27.02	73	44.50
49	60.02	39	27.73	74	45.11
50	61.42	40	28.44	75	45.72
51	62.81	41	29.15	76	46.32
52	64.21	42	29.87	77	46.93
53	65.61	43	30.58	78	47.54
54	67.00	44	31.29	79	48.15
55	68.40	45	32.00	80	48.76
56	69.80	46	32.71	81	49.37
57	71.19	47	33.42	82	49.98
58	72.59	48	34.13	83	50.59
59	73.99	49	34.84	84	51.20
60	75.39	50	35.56	85	51.81

From *The Complete Book of Physical Fitness*, A.G. Fisher and R.K. Conlee, used by permission.

PREDICTING BODY FAT FOR MEN.

Two measurements are needed to calculate the percent body fat of men. First, measure your waist at the umbilicus (belly button) and then have someone measure your wrist circumference just in front of the wrist bones where the wrist bends. Now subtract the wrist measurement from the waist measurement and enter the chart with this number and your weight.

For example, if your waist is 34 inches, and your wrist is seven inches, the difference is 27 (34 - 7 =27). If you weigh 175 pounds, go down the "27" column in Table 2 (page 217) to 175 and read 15 percent fat.

Record your waist measurement_____

Record your wrist measurement_____

Difference_____

Now enter the column in Table 2 with this difference and go down to your weight.

This number is your percent fat_____

Table 2. *Body Fat Percentages From the Penrose-Nelson-Fisher Equations*
Waist Minus Wrist (Inches)

WT (LBS)	29	29.5	30	30.5	31	31.5	32	32.5	33	33.5	34	34.5	35	35.5	36
120	31	33	35	37	39	41	43	45	47	49	50	52	54	56	58
125	30	32	33	35	37	39	41	43	45	46	48	50	52	54	56
130	28	30	32	34	36	37	39	41	43	44	46	48	50	52	53
135	27	29	31	32	34	36	38	39	41	43	44	46	48	50	51
140	26	28	29	31	33	34	36	38	39	41	43	44	46	48	49
145	25	27	28	30	31	33	35	36	38	39	41	43	44	46	47
150	24	26	27	29	30	32	34	35	36	38	40	41	43	44	46
155	23	25	26	28	29	31	33	34	35	37	38	40	41	43	44
160	22	24	25	27	28	30	32	33	34	35	37	38	40	41	43
165	22	23	24	26	27	29	31	31	33	34	36	37	38	40	41
170	21	22	24	25	26	28	30	30	32	33	34	36	37	39	40
175	20	22	23	24	25	27	29	29	31	32	33	35	36	37	39
180	19	21	22	23	24	26	28	28	30	31	32	34	35	37	37
185	19	20	21	22	23	25	27	27	29	30	31	33	34	36	36
190	18	19	20	22	23	24	26	26	28	29	30	32	33	35	35
195	18	19	20	21	22	24	25	26	27	28	30	31	32	34	34
200	17	18	19	20	22	23	24	25	26	28	29	30	31	33	33
205	17	18	19	20	21	23	23	25	26	27	28	29	30	32	32
210	16	17	18	19	21	22	23	24	25	26	27	28	29	31	32
215	16	17	18	19	20	21	22	23	24	26	26	28	29	30	31
220	15	16	17	18	19	21	22	22	23	24	25	27	28	30	30
225	15	16	17	18	19	20	21	22	24	24	26	26	28	29	29
230	14	15	16	17	18	20	21	22	23	23	25	24	27	28	28
235	14	15	16	17	18	19	20	21	23	23	24	26	26	27	28
240	14	14	16	17	18	19	20	20	22	23	24	24	26	27	27
245	13	14	15	16	17	18	20	20	21	22	23	24	25	26	27
250	13	14	15	16	17	19	19	20	21	22	23	24	24	26	26
255	13	14	14	15	16	17	19	19	21	21	22	23	24	25	25
260	12	13	14	15	16	18	18	19	20	21	22	23	23	24	25
265	12	13	14	15	16	17	18	18	20	21	21	22	23	24	24
270	12	13	13	15	16	16	17	18	19	19	20	21	22	23	24
275	11	12	13	14	15	16	17	17	19	19	20	21	22	23	23
280	11	12	13	14	15	16	16	17	18	18	19	20	21	22	22
285	11	11	12	13	14	15	16	16	18	18	19	19	20	22	22
290	10	11	12	13	14	15	15	16	17	17	18	19	20	21	22
295	10	11	12	12	13	14	15	16	16	17	18	19	20	21	21
300	10	11	11	12	13	14	15	16	16	17	18	19	19	20	21

WT (LBS)	22	22.5	23	23.5	24	24.5	25	25.5	26	26.5	27	27.5	28	28.5
120	4	6	8	10	12	14	16	18	20	21	23	25	27	29
125	4	6	7	9	11	13	15	17	19	20	22	24	26	28
130	3	5	7	9	11	12	14	16	18	20	21	23	25	27
135	3	5	7	8	10	12	13	15	17	19	20	22	24	26
140	3	5	6	8	10	11	13	15	16	18	19	21	23	24
145	3	4	6	7	9	11	12	14	15	17	19	20	22	23
150	2	4	5	7	9	10	12	13	15	16	18	19	21	23
155	2	4	5	7	8	10	11	13	14	16	17	19	20	22
160	2	3	5	6	8	9	11	12	14	15	17	18	19	21
165	2	3	5	6	8	9	10	12	13	15	16	17	19	20
170	2	3	4	6	7	9	10	11	13	14	15	17	18	19
175	2	3	4	5	7	8	10	11	12	13	15	16	17	19
180	1	3	4	5	7	8	9	10	12	13	14	16	17	18
185	1	3	4	5	6	8	9	10	11	13	14	15	16	18
190	1	2	4	5	6	7	8	10	11	12	13	14	16	17
195	1	2	3	5	6	7	8	9	11	12	13	14	15	16
200	1	2	3	4	6	7	8	9	10	11	12	14	15	16
205	1	2	3	4	5	6	8	9	10	11	12	13	14	15
210	0	2	3	4	5	6	7	8	9	10	12	13	14	15
215	0	2	3	4	5	6	7	8	9	10	11	12	13	14
220	0	1	3	4	5	6	7	8	9	10	11	12	13	14
225	0	1	2	3	4	6	6	7	8	9	11	12	13	13
230	0	1	2	3	4	5	6	7	8	9	10	11	12	13
235	0	1	2	3	4	5	6	7	8	9	10	11	12	13
240	0	1	2	3	4	5	6	7	8	8	9	11	12	12
245	0	1	2	3	4	5	6	7	7	8	9	10	11	12
250	0	1	2	3	4	5	6	6	7	8	9	10	11	11
255	0	1	2	3	4	5	5	6	7	8	9	10	10	11
260	0	1	2	3	3	4	5	6	7	7	8	9	10	11
265	0	1	2	3	3	4	5	6	6	7	8	9	10	11
270	0	1	1	3	3	4	5	5	6	7	8	8	9	10
275	0	0	1	2	3	4	4	5	6	7	7	8	9	10
280	0	0	1	2	3	4	4	5	6	6	7	8	9	10
285	0	0	1	2	3	4	4	5	6	6	7	8	9	9
290	0	0	1	2	3	4	4	5	5	6	7	8	9	9
295	0	0	1	2	3	4	5	5	6	7	8	9	9	9
300	0	0	1	2	4	4	5	6	6	7	8	9	9	9

Penrose, Nelson and Fisher, "Generalized Body Composition Prediction
Equation for Men Using Simple Measurement Techniques.
Medicine and Science in Sports and Exercise
Vol. 17, No. 2, April, 1985.

Table 2. Body Fat Percentages From the Penrose-Nelson-Fisher Equations
Waist Minus Wrist (Inches)

WT (LBS)	50	49.5	49	48.5	48	47.5	47	46.5	46	45.5	45	44.5	44	43.5
120	99	99	99	99	99	99	99	99	97	95	93	91	89	87
125	99	99	99	99	99	98	96	95	93	91	89	87	85	84
130	99	99	99	98	96	94	93	91	89	87	86	84	82	80
135	99	98	96	94	92	91	89	87	86	84	82	80	79	77
140	96	94	92	91	89	87	86	84	82	81	79	77	76	74
145	92	91	89	87	86	84	83	81	79	78	76	75	73	71
150	89	87	86	84	83	81	80	78	77	75	74	72	70	69
155	86	85	83	82	80	79	77	76	74	73	71	70	68	67
160	83	82	80	79	77	76	75	73	72	70	69	68	66	64
165	81	79	78	76	75	74	72	71	69	68	67	65	64	62
170	78	77	75	74	73	71	70	69	67	66	64	63	62	60
175	76	74	73	72	70	69	68	66	65	64	63	61	60	59
180	74	72	71	70	68	67	66	65	63	62	61	59	58	57
185	71	70	69	68	66	65	64	63	61	60	59	58	56	55
190	69	68	67	66	65	63	62	61	59	58	57	56	55	54
195	68	66	65	64	63	62	60	59	58	57	56	55	53	52
200	66	65	63	62	61	60	59	58	57	55	54	53	52	51
205	64	63	62	61	60	58	57	56	55	54	53	52	51	49
210	62	61	60	59	58	57	56	55	54	53	51	50	49	48
215	61	60	59	58	57	56	54	53	52	51	50	49	48	47
220	59	58	57	56	55	54	53	52	51	50	49	48	47	46
225	58	57	56	55	54	53	52	51	50	49	48	47	46	45
230	57	56	55	54	53	52	51	50	49	48	47	46	45	44
235	55	54	53	52	51	51	50	49	48	47	46	45	44	43
240	54	53	52	51	50	50	48	47	46	46	45	44	42	42
245	53	52	51	50	49	49	47	46	45	45	44	43	41	41
250	52	51	50	49	48	48	46	45	44	44	43	42	41	40
255	51	50	49	48	47	47	45	44	44	43	42	41	40	39
260	50	49	48	47	46	46	44	43	43	42	41	40	39	38
265	49	48	47	46	45	45	43	43	42	41	40	39	38	37
270	48	47	46	45	44	44	43	42	41	40	39	38	37	37
275	47	46	45	44	43	43	42	41	40	39	38	37	36	36
280	46	45	44	43	43	42	41	40	39	38	38	37	36	35
285	45	44	43	43	42	41	40	39	39	38	37	36	35	34
290	44	43	43	42	41	40	39	39	38	37	36	35	35	34
295	43	43	42	41	41	39	39	38	37	36	36	35	34	33
300	43	42	41	40	39	39	38	37	36	36	35	34	33	33

WT (LBS)	43	42.5	42	41.5	41	40.5	40	39.5	39	38.5	38	37.5	37	36.5
120	85	83	81	79	77	76	74	72	70	68	66	64	62	60
125	82	80	78	76	74	72	71	69	67	65	63	61	59	58
130	78	77	75	73	71	69	68	66	64	62	61	59	57	55
135	75	74	72	70	68	67	65	63	62	60	58	56	55	53
140	72	71	69	68	66	64	63	61	59	58	56	54	53	51
145	70	68	67	65	63	62	60	59	57	55	54	52	51	49
150	67	66	64	63	61	60	58	57	55	53	52	50	49	47
155	65	64	62	61	59	58	56	55	53	52	50	49	47	46
160	63	61	60	59	57	56	54	53	51	50	48	47	46	44
165	61	60	58	57	55	54	52	51	50	48	47	45	44	43
170	59	58	56	55	54	52	51	49	48	47	45	44	43	41
175	57	56	55	53	52	51	49	48	47	45	44	43	41	40
180	56	54	53	52	50	49	48	47	45	44	43	41	40	39
185	54	53	51	50	49	48	46	45	44	43	41	40	39	38
190	52	51	50	49	48	46	45	44	43	41	40	39	38	37
195	51	50	49	47	46	45	44	43	41	40	39	38	37	35
200	50	48	47	46	45	44	43	41	40	39	38	37	36	35
205	48	47	46	45	44	43	41	40	39	38	37	36	35	34
210	47	46	45	44	43	42	40	39	38	37	36	35	34	33
215	46	45	44	43	42	41	39	38	37	36	35	34	33	32
220	45	44	43	42	41	40	38	37	36	35	34	33	32	31
225	44	43	42	41	40	39	37	36	35	34	33	32	31	30
230	43	42	41	40	39	38	36	35	34	34	33	32	31	30
235	42	41	40	39	38	38	35	34	33	33	32	31	30	29
240	41	40	39	38	37	37	34	33	32	32	31	30	29	28
245	40	39	38	37	36	36	34	33	31	31	30	30	28	28
250	39	38	37	36	35	35	33	32	31	31	29	29	28	27
255	38	37	36	35	34	34	32	31	30	30	28	28	27	26
260	37	36	35	35	34	33	31	30	30	29	28	27	27	26
265	36	36	35	34	33	32	31	30	29	29	28	27	26	25
270	36	35	34	33	32	31	30	29	28	28	27	26	25	25
275	35	34	33	32	31	30	29	28	28	27	27	26	25	24
280	34	33	33	32	30	30	28	27	27	27	26	25	24	23
285	34	33	32	31	30	29	28	27	27	26	26	25	24	23
290	33	32	31	31	29	28	28	26	26	26	25	24	23	22
295	32	32	31	30	29	28	28	26	26	25	25	24	23	22
300	32	31	30	29	29	28	27	26	26	25	24	23	22	22

COMPUTING LEAN BODY MASS

Although it is interesting to see how much of the body is fat, you need to compute lean body mass (LBM) to compute a realistic body weight.

To compute lean body mass:

1. Multiply the body weight in pounds by the percent fat. This will give pounds of fat on the body. For example, the lady in our example was 31 percent fat. If she weighed 160 pounds, she would have about 49.6 pounds of fat.

    Total Weight x % Fat = lbs. of fat
    160 x .31 (31%) = 49.6 lbs. of fat

2. To determine the LBM, simply subtract pounds of fat from total body weight.

    Total Weight - Pounds of Fat = LBM
    160 lbs. total weight - 49.6 lbs. fat = 110.4 lbs. LBM

Anything not fat is lean, so the fat and lean components must add up to the total body weight.

This LBM is the "real" person without any fat. Obviously, you can't weigh less than your LBM, nor can you get along without any fat. All of us need at least some fat to support the internal organs and to give shape to our frame. The very leanest men sometimes get as low as two to three percent fat while the leanest women are from 9 to eleven percent fat.

COMPUTING A REALISTIC WEIGHT GOAL

To compute a realistic weight, you must decide what percent fat you are willing to have. A realistic beginning goal for the woman in our example may be 25 percent. Enter Table 3 with the LBM and go across to the percent fat goal to get a realistic weight goal. For our example lady, whose LBM is 110 pounds, the realistic weight would be about 146 pounds.

This may be a higher weight than our example lady would care to achieve, but it is realistic, and she would be about 25 percent fat if she achieved that weight.

Another factor needs to be considered. Sometimes the LBM goes up or down during the weight loss process. An extremely heavy person may have a larger LBM than usual because the muscle mass hypertrophied (got larger) from carrying all the weight around. When this person loses fat, he may also lose LBM because the load on the muscles is decreased.

On the other hand, an inactive person may have a decreased LBM because he is so inactive. When this person begins an exercise program, he may experience a gain in LBM back to some normal level. This gain in lean tissue can be discouraging because it may counteract the loss of fat, and the total body weight may stay about the same or even increase, even though the person is losing fat nicely.

You should check your hip and waist measurements each month to determine what is happening to LBM and percent fat. If the LBM changes, you can compute a new realistic weight goal based on this change. The measurements will also permit seeing the circumference changes as they occur.

Table 3. *Total Body Weight at Various Fat Percentages Based on Lean Body Mass*

% Fat Goal

LBM	10	13	16	19	22	25
90	100	103	107	111	115	120
95	105	109	113	117	121	126
100	111	114	119	123	128	133
105	116	120	125	129	134	140
110	122	126	130	135	141	146
115	127	132	136	141	147	153
120	133	137	142	148	153	160
125	138	143	148	154	160	166
130	144	149	154	160	166	173
135	150	155	160	166	173	180
140	155	160	166	172	179	186
145	161	166	172	179	185	193
150	166	172	178	185	192	200
155	172	178	184	191	198	206
160	177	183	190	197	205	213
165	183	189	196	203	211	220
170	188	195	202	209	217	226
175	194	201	208	216	224	233
180	200	206	214	222	230	240
185	205	212	220	228	237	246

LBM in pounds

APPENDIX H

UNDERSTANDING YOUR URINE AND BLOOD TESTS

The following information has been condensed from material listed in an excellent book, *The People's Book of Medical Tests*[141] by Drs. Sobel and Ferguson (published by Summit Books, a division of Simon and Schuester, New York). We appreciate their permission to use this information. Please note that the "normal" lab values listed in this section may vary from laboratory to laboratory. For this reason, we suggest you discuss with your doctor any blood or urine results that are outside of the "normal" range listed in this material.

URINALYSIS

1. *Color*
   Parameter: Urine can vary a great deal based upon a person's state of hydration and also based upon foods that are eaten or medications that are taken.
   Why Tested: For routine screening and to identify any abnormal symptoms.
   Normal Values: Colorless to dark yellow or amber (this varies based upon the concentration of the urine; the darker the urine the more concentrated).
   Possible Concern if Value is Abnormal: An unusual color of the urine may be the result of medicine or food. The color can also vary as the result of infection or blood constituents.

2. *Specific Gravity (SG)*
   Why Tested: Determine the density of the urine compared to water.
   Normal Values: 1.003 to 1.035
   Possible Concern if Value is Abnormal: An increased value may be the result of dehydration or excessive sugar or protein in the urine. A decreased value may suggest a high body fluid volume. The cause may be due to an excess of fluid intake, diuretic medicines, or kidney problems.

3. *pH*
   Why Tested: To determine the acidity of the urine.
   Normal Values: 4.6 to 8.0
   Possible Concern if Value is Abnormal: An increased pH (less acidic) may indicate a diet high in vegetables or citrus fruit. Antacid type medications may also cause a high pH. A decreased pH (less than 6.0, more acidic) is more common when the urine is captured in the morning. Low values measured during the day can be caused by high doses of Vitamin C, lung disease, diabetes (uncontrolled), and other factors that cause dehydration as well as some medications.

4. *Glucose (sugar)*
   Why Tested: To check for glucose abnormalities in the body.
   Normal Values: No glucose present.
   Possible Concerns if Value is Abnormal: An abnormal test (glucose in the urine) may need to be followed with a blood-sugar test to screen for diabetes. Small amounts of glucose in the urine may not be abnormal. To be certain discuss this with your doctor.

5. *Ketones*
   Why Tested: To determine if excess fat is being burned by the body as fuel (ketones are by-products of fat metabolism).
   Normal Values: No ketones present.
   Possible Concerns if Value is Abnormal: If large amounts of ketones are present in the urine, this may be suggestive of diabetes. Ketones can also be present when a person does not have enough carbohydrate in his diet, sometimes the result of a very low carbohydrate weight loss program or severe vomiting.

6. *Protein*
   Why Tested: One of the functions of the kidney is to filter the smaller sized protein from the blood and then eventually return the protein into the blood. Normally, no protein should be present in the urine.
   Normal Values: No protein present.
   Possible Concern if Value is Abnormal: May suggest kidney infection or kidney problems. There are several other possible causes for protein in the urine such as fever, excessive exercise and pregnancy. In addition, some individuals get small amounts of protein in their urine when they stand up to give the urine sample.

7. Red Blood Cells and Hemoglobin
Why Tested: In normal conditions, red blood cells (RBC) and hemoglobin are not found in the urine.
Normal Values: No RBC or hemoglobin present.
Possible Concern if Value is Abnormal: This may suggest problems with the urinary tract (kidney, ureter, bladder or urethra). Hemoglobin in the urine can also be the result of strenuous exercise when red blood cells have been excessively damaged, or certain drugs may also break down a large number of RBC resulting in the appearance of hemoglobin in the urine.

8. Bilirubin
Why Tested: Bilirubin is a waste product from the breakdown of hemoglobin and is not usually found in the urine.
Normal Values: No bilirubin present.
Possible Concern if Value is Abnormal: May suggest a problem with the liver or it may suggest a blocked bile duct.

9. Urobilinogen
Why Tested: Urobilinogen is a by-product of the breakdown of bilirubin (see bilirubin above). Urobilinogen is a yellow colored substance and small amounts of it are found in the urine.
Normal Values: Only small amounts of urobilinogen should be present (0.1 – 1.1 for women; 0.3 – 2.1 for men; measured in Ehrlich units).
Possible Concern if Value is Abnormal: May suggest liver problem or an excessive breakdown of RBC (red blood cells). May suggest a bile blockage or any other problem that prevents the normal release of bilirubin into the intestines.

10. White Blood Cells (WBC)
Why Tested: White blood cells (WBC) are defense cells of the body designed to fight infection.
Normal Values: Generally no WBC in the urine. Please note, however, that it is not uncommon for a few (0-5) cells to contaminate the urine sample during the time of collection. These WBC may come from the hands or the skin areas over which the urine stream passes.
Possible Concern if Value is Abnormal: May suggest urinary tract infection. A few WBC (0-5) are generally of no concern.

BLOOD TESTS

A. COMPLETE BLOOD COUNT (CBC) TEST

1. White Blood Cell Count (WBC)
Parameter: The defense cells of the body, WBC fight infection and foreign organisms.
Why Tested: To check for infection. To monitor leukemia.
Normal Values: 4,500 to 11,000/mm^3
Possible Concern if Value is Abnormal: An elevated WBC count may indicate an infection. Very high values of WBC may suggest leukemia. A decreased WBC count may suggest a problem in WBC production, viral infection, or the responses of certain drugs.

2. Hematocrit (Hct)
Parameter: The red blood cells (RBC) of the body carry oxygen from the lungs to the body and carbon dioxide from the body to the lungs. The percent of the blood that is red blood cells is called the "hematocrit."
Why Tested: To check for anemia. Also to check for too many RBC, a condition called polycythemia.
Normal Values: Men: 40% - 54%; Women: 37% to 47%
Possible Concern if Value is Abnormal: A decreased value may suggest anemia. Anemia can occur from menstrual bleeding or from ulcers or other intestinal problems. An increased value may indicate polycythemia, the result of a number of disorders such as not enough oxygen or not enough blood volume.

3. Hemoglobin
Parameter: Within the mature red blood cell is a protein called hemoglobin. Hemoglobin carries oxygen to the body and carbon dioxide away from the body.
Why Tested: Same as for hematocrit above.
Normal Values: Men: 14 - 18 g/dl; Women: 12-16 g/dl
Possible Concern if Value is Abnormal: Same as for hematocrit, above.

4. Red Blood Cell Indices
Parameter: To help determine the size of RBC and the concentration of hemoglobin, the following indices are measured:
MCV (mean corpuscular volume) – this determines whether RBC are normal in size.
MCH (mean corpuscular hemoglobin) – this indicates the weight of the hemoglobin within an RBC.
MCHC (mean corpuscular hemoglobin concentration) – this indicates the amount of hemoglobin in the average RBC.

Why Tested: To further determine the cause for anemia.

Normal Values: MCV – 80 - 96 cubic microns; **MCH** – 27 - 31 picograms (pg); **MCHC** – 32% - 36%

Possible Concern if Value is Abnormal: An increased MCV may suggest anemia resulting from insufficient folic acid or vitamin B12, or alcoholism. A decreased MCV and MCHC may be due to anemia resulting from a lack of iron.

5. *Platelet Count*

Parameter: Platelets are important for the process of blood clotting. They are manufactured by the bone marrow of the body.

Why Tested: To further examine bleeding problems or excessive bruising.

Normal Values: 150,000 - 400,000 per cubic millimeter (mm³).

Possible Concern if Value is Abnormal: An increased platelet value is referred to as thrombocytosis and may be the result of certain cancers, inflammatory diseases, leukemia, and a variety of other potential medical problems. Pregnancy and excessive exercise can also cause the platelet count to rise. A decreased platelet value, thrombocytopenia, may suggest problems with the destruction of platelets or a problem with the manufacture of platelets such as bone marrow disease or various kinds of anemia. Certain drugs can also cause a drop in platelets.

B. SMAC-20

1. *Alkaline Phosphatase*

Why Tested: One of the important enzymes located within the bones and the liver is alkaline phosphatase. The presence of alkaline phosphatase in the blood can be the result of the breakdown of liver cells (due to possible damage) or the growth of bone (which may be normal or abnormal bone growth).

Normal Values: 20-90 International units per liter (IU/l)

Possible Concern if Value is Abnormal: An increased value may suggest possible liver problems such as hepatitis or cirrhosis. Elevated values may also indicate various bone growth abnormalities. In addition, there are a number of drugs that can affect the level of alkaline phosphatase. Please note that for pregnant women and for children whose bones are still growing, the values of alkaline phosphatase may be greater than normal.

2. *Bilirubin (Total and Direct)*

Why Tested: Within the red blood cell is a protein called hemoglobin. When the red blood cell and hemoglobin are broken down, one of the by-products of the hemoglobin is bilirubin. One of the functions of the liver is to further break down bilirubin, where it is ultimately emptied into the intestines. Bilirubin is brownish-yellow in color and it is this by-product that gives color to the stool. Before bilirubin is processed in the liver, it is referred to as *indirect* bilirubin. After the liver has further processed bilirubin, it is called *direct* bilirubin. Both total and direct bilirubin values can be used to aid in interpretation of possible health problems such as liver disorders.

Normal Values: Direct – less than 0.3 milligrams per deciliter (mg/dl); Total – 0.1-1.2 milligrams per deciliter (mg/dl)

Possible Concern if Value is Abnormal: An increased value may suggest a greater than normal breakdown of red blood cells — conditions in which the liver is not removing the normal amount of bilirubin from the blood. Increased blood bilirubin values might also suggest a possible blockage of the gallbladder or the bile ducts.

3. *BUN (Blood Urea Nitrogen)*

Why Tested: To test kidney function. When protein is broken down in the liver, a by-product is urea nitrogen (BUN). The kidney clears the BUN by excreting it through the urine.

Normal Values: 8-23 milligrams per deciliter (mg/dl)

Possible Concern if Value is Abnormal: An increased value may suggest kidney disease. In addition, the problem could be due to dehydration or medical problems that result in significant protein breakdown. A decreased value may suggest liver problems or extreme fluid consumption. Malnutrition has also been shown to decrease BUN values.

4. *Calcium (Ca⁺⁺)*

Why Tested: Calcium has several important functions in the body, including the building of bone and teeth, and aiding in the function of the heart. Calcium is measured to make certain the value is normal because of its varied function within the body.

Normal Values: 9.2-11.0 milligrams per deciliter (mg/dl)

Possible Concerns if Value is Abnormal: An increased value may suggest a significant dietary intake of foods high in calcium such as milk, extended bed rest, bone-related cancers, or kidney problems. A decreased value may suggest a reduced amount of albumin protein, a reduced dietary intake of foods containing calcium, pregnancy, or problems with the kidney or the parathyroid gland (the gland that regulates the release of calcium from the bones.

5. CO_2 Content

Why Tested: As part of the body's metabolism process, carbon dioxide (CO_2) is produced. This CO_2 is carried by the blood to the lungs to be exhaled. This test checks the ability of the gas (CO_2) to be exchanged in the lungs.

Normal Values: 22–38 millimoles/liter (mM/L)

Possible Concern if Value is Abnormal: An increased value may suggest a problem that is affecting the lung's ability to clear out carbon dioxide. Certain hormone related diseases, excessive vomiting, and certain drugs can cause CO_2 to be elevated in the blood. A decreased value may be the result of diabetes, kidney problems, aspirin overdose, or an overdose of ammonium chloride.

6. Chloride (Cl^-)

Why Tested: To determine if the level of this mineral is normal in the body. Chloride is an electrolyte that helps balance water inside and outside our cells.

Normal Values: 95–103 milliequivalents per liter (mEq/L)

Possible Concern if Value is Abnormal: An increased value may suggest lung disease like emphysema or pneumonia or hormone problems. Other factors like starvation or gastrointestinal disorders can cause increased CO_2 values. A decreased value may suggest kidney failure, hyperventilation, excessive diarrhea or an overdose of drugs like aspirin.

7. Cholesterol

(Please see the *Yearly or Periodic Health Check #9*, page 105).

8. Creatinine

Why Tested: When muscle tissue is broken down (metabolized) one of the waste products is creatinine. The creatinine is then filtered by the kidney. To help determine if the kidneys are functioning properly in filtering the blood of waste products, creatinine levels can be measured in the blood and the urine.

Normal Values: 0.6-1.2 milligrams/deciliter (mg/dl)

Possible Concern if Value is Abnormal: An increased value may suggest kidney disease. A decreased value may be the result of kidney damage or the result of kidney problems.

9. GGTP (Gamma Glutamyl Transpeptidase)

Why Tested: This enzyme is found in the liver; when liver cells are damaged, this enzyme is released into the blood. The test is used to look for liver damage or liver disease.

Normal Values: 0-60 units per liter (U/l)

Possible Concern if Value is Abnormal: An increased value may suggest liver damage from diseases such as alcoholism.

10. Glucose

Why Tested: Glucose (sometimes referred to as blood sugar) is a major source of energy for the body. This test is a screening test for diabetes, low blood sugar, or certain hormone problems.

Normal Values: 70-110 milligrams/deciliter (mg/dl)

Possible Concern if Value is Abnormal: An increased value may suggest diabetes or hormone problems. The elevated glucose can also occur with pregnancy. A decreased value may suggest low blood sugar problems (hypoglycemia) or certain hormone problems.

11. LDH (Lactic Dehydrogenase)

Why Tested: LDH is an enzyme found in several organ tissues of the body, such as the liver and the heart. The routine LDH can be used to look at liver problems, anemia, certain kinds of cancer, and other medical concerns.

Normal Values: 80 - 120 International units per liter (IU/l)

Possible Concern if Value is Abnormal: An increased value may suggest liver disease or certain kinds of cancer.

12. Phosphorus

Why Tested: Phosphorus is an important mineral used by the body for bone production and to aid in the body's metabolism.

Normal Values: 2.3-4.7 milligrams/deciliter (mg/dl)

Possible Concern if Value is Abnormal: An increased value may suggest a disease of the bones, kidney disease, a significant increase of Vitamin D, or under production of the parathyroid. A decreased value may be the result of alcoholism, excessive production of the parathyroid, kidney problems or too little Vitamin D.

13. Potassium (K^+)

Why Tested: Like chloride, potassium helps balance the water inside and outside of our cells. Potassium can affect the contraction of the heart muscle. Potassium levels can also be used to look at kidney function.

Normal Values: 3.8 to 5.0 milliequivalents per liter (mEq/L)

Possible Concern if Value is Abnormal: An increased value (hyperkalemia) may suggest failure of the kidneys, liver disease, or diabetes. A decreased value (hypokalemia) may be the result of certain hormone disorders, or the result of fluid loss (this can occur from diuretic drugs). Anything that excessively reduces body fluids like diarrhea, vomiting, or laxatives can also cause decreased potassium.

14. *Serum Protein (Total blood protein, serum albumin, serum globulin)*

Why Tested: This test is primarily used to test liver function. The blood has a significant amount of protein (the major proteins are globulin and albumin). While albumin protein helps keep blood fluid balance in the body, the globulin protein mainly helps in the defense system of the body.

Normal Values: Total Protein – 6-7.8 grams per deciliter (g/dl); Albumin – 3.2-4.5 grams per deciliter (g/dl); Globulin – 2.3-3.5 grams per deciliter (g/dl)

Possible Concerns if Value is Abnormal: An increased value may suggest kidney problems or conditions that can lead to dehydration such as diarrhea or excessive vomiting. Some infections and arthritis may also cause increased protein values. A decreased value may suggest conditions associated with malnutrition, kidney problems, or blood loss. Other medical problems such as diabetes and toxemia may also cause a protein decrease.

15. *SGOT (Serum Glutamic Oxaloacetic Transaminase)*

Why Tested: SGOT is an enzyme that is located primarily in the liver and the heart. The test primarily looks at liver status.

Normal Values: 10–40 International units per liter (IU/l)

Possible Concerns if Value is Abnormal: An increased value may suggest liver disease, blood clots in the lung, some infections such as mononucleosis, and muscular dystrophy.

16. *SGPT (Serum Glutamic Pyruvic Transaminase)*

Why Tested: One of the enzymes found within the liver is SGPT. When the liver is damaged, this enzyme is released into the blood.

Normal Values: 10-30 units per milliliter (U/ml)

Possible Concern if Value is Abnormal: An increased value may suggest liver problems that damage the liver cells such as hepatitis and alcoholism.

There are also many drugs that may cause liver cell damage and thereby increase the levels of SGPT.

17. *Sodium (Na⁺)*

Why Tested: Sodium is a very important electrolyte in the body, helping to balance water inside and outside of the cell. Sodium is measured to make sure there are no kidney or adrenal gland problems and to verify that this electrolyte value is normal.

Normal Values: 136–142 milliequivalents per liter (mEq/L)

Possible Concern if Value is Abnormal: An increased value may suggest hormonal problems, kidney disease, dehydration or too much salt in one's diet. A decreased value may suggest excessive sodium loss from disorders such as diarrhea, kidney problems, excessive sweating. It may also suggest hormonal problems related to the adrenal gland, inadequate salt in the diet, or heart failure.

18. *Uric Acid*

Why Tested: When the body breaks down cells, uric acid is one of the constituents. Certain medical problems such as gout or kidney disease can result in increased uric acid values. Increased uric acid can eventually lead to kidney stones.

Normal Values: Men – 4.0 - 8.5 milligrams per deciliter (mg/dl); Women – 2.7 - 7.3 milligrams per deciliter (mg/dl)

Possible Concern if Value is Abnormal: An increased value may suggest gout tendencies or medical problems that relate to excessive breakdown of body cells such as certain kinds of cancer. Certain medications may cause an increase in uric acid as well as certain types of kidney problems. A decreased value may suggest a kidney problem. If patients are being treated for gout with a medicine, the uric acid may be lowered.

APPENDIX I

ADDITIONAL SAFETY TIPS
FOR PARTICIPATING IN PHYSICAL ACTIVITY

(This information is reproduced with permission © Exercise Standards, 1990. Copyright American Heart Association. Source: Fletcher GF, Froelicher VF, Hartley H, Haskell WL, Pollock ML. Circulation 1990; Volume 82(6): pages 2286-2322.)

1. **Exercise only when feeling well.**
   Wait until symptoms and signs of a cold or the flu (including fever) have been absent two days or more before resuming activity.

2. **Do no exercise vigorously soon after eating.**
   Wait at least two hours. Eating increases the blood flow requirements of the intestinal tract. During vigorous exercise, the muscle's demand for blood may exceed the ability of the circulation to supply both the bowel and the muscles, depriving organs of blood, resulting in cramps, nausea, or faintness.

3. **Adjust exercise to the weather.**
   Exercise should be adjusted to environmental conditions. Special precautions are necessary when exercising in hot weather, and signs of overheating may not be recognized. It is difficult to define when it is too hot to exercise since air temperature is greatly influenced by humidity and wind, which are not easy to measure. The following guidelines are recommended for a noncompetitive workout: If air temperature is more than 70° F, slow the pace, be alert for signs of heat injury, and drink adequate fluids to maintain hydration. A good rule to follow is to exercise at the usual workout pace (rating of perceived exertion three to five), which will be a slower pace or lower work intensity. Adaptation to moderate levels of heat is gradual, requiring 12 to 14 days. Accommodation to extreme heat never occurs.
   Signs of heat injury may be varied at the onset; hence, any symptom should be regarded as evidence of heat overload. The following indications of heat stress are particularly likely to occur: headache, dizziness, faintness, nausea, coolness, cramps, and palpitations. If any of these indicates are present, stop exercising immediately and go to a cool environment. If the air temperature is over 80° F, exercise in the early morning or late afternoon in shaded areas to avoid the heat.

Air-conditioned shopping malls are popular. Exercise is better tolerated if humidity is low and there is a breeze. Exercise in the heat causes excessive fluid loss, so adequate fluid intake is important before, during, and after each session.

4. **Slow down for hills.**
   Watch for hills. When ascending hills in the exercise course, decrease speed to avoid overexertion. Again, a useful guide is to maintain the same rating of perceived exertion as in a usual workout.

5. **Wear proper clothing and shoes.**
   Dress in loose-fitting comfortable clothes made of porous material appropriate for the weather. Use sweat suits only for warmth. Never use exercise clothing made of rubberized nonporous material. In direct sunlight, wear light-colored clothing and a cap. Wear shoes designed for exercise (walking, jogging, etc.).

6. **Understand personal limitations.**
   Everyone should undergo periodic medical examinations. When under a physician's care, ask if there are limitations that might interfere with the program.

7. **Select appropriate exercises.**
   Cardiovascular (aerobic) exercises should be a major component of activities. However, flexibility and strengthening exercises should also be considered for a well-rounded program.

8. **Be alert for symptoms.**
   If the following symptoms occur, contact a physician before continuing exercise. Although any symptom should be clarified, the following are particularly important:
   a. Discomfort in the upper body, including the chest, arm, neck, or jaw, during exercise. The discomfort may be of any intensity and may be present as an aching, burning, tightness, or sensation of fullness.

b. Faintness accompanying the exercise. Sometimes brief light-headedness may follow unusually vigorous exercise or too short a cool-down at the end of the session. If a "fainting spell" or feeling of faintness occurs during exercise, discontinue the activity until after a checkup by a physician.

c. Shortness of breath during exercise. During exercise, rate and depth of breathing should not be so difficult that talking is an effort, wheezing develops, or more than five minutes are required for recovery.

d. Discomfort in bones and joints either during or after exercise. There may be slight muscle soreness when beginning exercise, but if back or joint pain develops, discontinue exercise until after a checkup by a physician.

9. **Watch for the following signs of over-exercising.**

   a. Inability to finish. Training sessions should be completed with reserve.

   b. Inability to converse during the activity. Breathing normally increases during exercise but should not be uncomfortable. When a conversation cannot be conducted during exercise because of trouble breathing, the conditioning activity may be too intense.

c. Faintness or nausea after exercise. A feeling of faintness after exercise may occur if the activity is too intense or has been stopped too abruptly. In any event, decrease the intensity of the workout and prolong the cool-down period.

d. Chronic fatigue. During the remainder of the day or evening after exercise, an individual should feel stimulated, not tired. If too fatigued during the day, intensity and/or duration of the workout should be decreased.

e. Sleeplessness. If unable to sleep well despite feelings of fatigue, the amount of activity should be decreased until symptoms subside. Insomnia is particularly likely during distance training. A proper training program should make it easier, not more difficult, to have a good night's rest.

f. Aches and pains in the joints. Although there may be some muscle discomfort, joints should not hurt or feel stiff. Check exercise procedures, particularly stretching and warm-up exercises, to ensure that you are using the correct technique. Muscle cramping and back discomfort may also indicate poor technique. If symptoms persist, check with a physician before continuing.

10. **Start slowly and progress gradually. Allow time to adapt.**

REFERENCES

1. Fries JF. Aging, natural death, and the compression of morbidity. N Engl J Med 1980; 303(3):130-135.
2. National Center for Health Statistics. Health in the United States, 1978. Hyattsville, Md.: National Center for Health Statistics, 1978. (DHEW publication no. (PHS)78-1232).
3. Fries JF, Ehrlich GE, eds. Prognosis: contemporary outcomes of disease. Bowie, Md.: Charles Press, 1980.
4. Ekelund LG, Haskell WL, Johnson JL, et al. Physical fitness as a predictor of cardiovascular mortality in asymptomatic North American men: The lipid research clinics mortality follow-up study. N Engl J Med 1988; 319:1379-1384.
5. Leon AS, Connell J, Jacobs DR, Rauramaa R. Leisure-time physical activity levels and risk of coronary heart disease and death. JAMA 1987; 258:2388-2395.
6. Centers for Disease Control. Protective effect of physical activity on coronary heart disease: Progress in chronic disease prevention. MMWP 1987; 36(26):426-430.
7. Blair SN, Kohl HW, Paffenbarger RS, et al. Physical fitness and all-cause mortality: A prospective study of healthy men and women. JAMA 1989; 262:2395-2401.
8. Paffenbarger RS, Hyde RT, Wing AL, et al. Physical activity, all-cause mortality, and longevity of college alumni. N Engl J Med 1986; 314:605-613.
9. Report of the U.S. Preventive Services Task Force. Exercise counseling. In: Guide to Clinical Preventive Services. Health and Human Services, Prepublication copy 1989, pp. 198-202.
10. Harris SS, Casperson CJ, DeFriese GH, et al. Physical activity counseling for healthy adults as a primary preventive intervention in the clinical setting: Report of the U.S. Preventive Services Task Force. JAMA 1989; 261:3590-3598.
11. Astrand P-O. Exercise physiology and its role in disease prevention and in rehabilitation. Arch Phys Med Rehabil 1987; 68:305-309.
12. Tipton CM, Vailas AC, Matthes RD. Experimental studies on the influences of physical activity on ligaments, tendons and joints: A brief review. In: Astrand P-O, Grimby G (eds). Physical Activity in Health and Disease. Acta Med Scand Symposium Series no 2. Stockholm, Almqvist & Wiksell International, 1986. pp. 157-168.
13. Atha J. Strengthening muscle. Exerc Sport Sci Rev 1981; 9:1-73.
14. Astrand P-O, Rodahl K. Textbook of Work Physiology (Ed 3). New York: McGraw-Hill, 1986.
15. Caspersen CJ. Physical activity epidemiology: Concepts, methods, and applications to exercise science. In: Pandolf KB, ed. Exercise and Sciences Reviews: Volume 17 Baltimore: Williams and Wilkins, 1989, pp. 423-474.
16. American College of Sports Medicine Position Stand. The recommended quantity and quality of exercise for developing and maintaining cardiorespiratory and muscular fitness in healthy adults. Med Sci Sports Exer 1990; 22(2):265-274.
17. Pollock ML, Wilmore JH. Exercise in Health and Disease: Evaluation and Prescription for Prevention and Rehabilitation. Philadelphia: W.B. Saunders Company, 1990, pp. 202-236.
18. Committee on Diet and Health, Food and Nutrition Board, Commission on Life Sciences, National Research Council. Diet and Health: Implications for Reducing Chronic Disease Risk. National Academy Press, Washington, D.C., 1989.
19. U.S. Department of Health and Human Services. The Surgeon General's Report on Nutrition and Health 1988; Public Health Service. U.S. Government Printing Office, Washington, D.C.,(GPO Stock no. 017-001-00465-1).
20. Report of the U.S. Preventive Services Task Force. Nutritional counseling. In: Guide to Clinical Preventive Services. Health and Human Services, Prepublication copy, 1989, pp. 203-209.
21. Turnbridge WMG, Evered DC, Hall R, et al. The spectrum of thyroid disease in a community: The Whickham survey. Clin Endocrinol 1977; 7:481-493.
22. National Heart, Lung, and Blood Institute. Eating to Lower Your High Blood Cholesterol. GPO: S/N 017-043-00118-4, 1987.
23. Report of the U.S. Preventive Services Task Force. Screening for depression. In: Guide to Clinical Preventive Services. Health and Human Services, Prepublication copy, 1989, pp. 173-175.
24. Katon W. The epidemiology of depression in medical care. Int'l J Psychiatry Med 1987; 17:93-112.
25. Prestidge BR, Lake CR. Prevalence and recognition of depression among primary care outpatients. J Fam Pract 1987; 25:67-72.
26. Rosenthal MP, Goldfarb NI, Carlson BL, et al. Assessment of depression in a family practice center. J Fam Pract 1987; 25:143-149.
27. Kamerow DB. Controversies in family practice: Is screening for mental health problems worthwhile? J Fam Pract 1987; 25:181-184.
28. Johnstone A, Goldberg D. Psychiatric screening in general practice: A controlled trial. Lancet 1976; 1:605-608.
29. Rucker L, Frye EB, Cygan RW. Feasibility and usefulness of depression screening in medical outpatients. Arch Intern Med 1986; 146:729-731.
30. Kessler LG, Cleary PD, Burke JD. Psychiatric disorders in primary care. Arch Gen Psychiatry 1985; 42:583-587.
31. Report of the U.S. Preventive Services Task Force. Screening for suicidal intent. In: Guide to Clinical Preventive Services. Health and Human Services, Prepublication copy, 1989, pp. 176-178.
32. National Institute of Mental Health. Depression: What we know. Washington, D.C.: Department of Health and Human Services, 1985. (Publication no. DHHS (ADM) 85-1318.)
33. Blumenthal SJ. Suicide: A guide to risk factors, assessment, and treatment of suicidal patients. Med Clin North Am 1988; 72:937-971.

34. Blumenthal SJ, Kupfer DJ. Generalizable treatment strategies for suicidal behavior. Ann NY Acad Sci 1986; 487:327-339.

35. Martin RL, Cloninger R, Guze SB, et al. Mortality in a follow-up of 500 psychiatric outpatients. Arch Gen Psychiatry 1985; 42:58-66.

36. Jamison KR. Suicide and bipolar disorders. Ann NY Acad Sci 1986; 487:301-315.

37. Monk M. Epidemiology of suicide. Epidemiol Rev 1987; 9:51-69.

38. Report of the U.S. Preventive Services Task Force. Screening for abnormal bereavement. In: Guide to Clinical Preventive Services. Health and Human Services, Prepublication copy, 1989, pp. 170-172.

39. Bornstein PE, Clayton PJ, Halikas JA, et al. The depression of widowhood after 13 months. Br J Psychiatry 1973; 122:561-566.

40. Osterweis M, Solomon F, Green M, eds. Bereavement: Reactions, consequences and care. A report of the Institute of Medicine. Washington, D.C.: National Academy Press, 1984.

41. Benson, H. The Relaxation Response. New York: Avon Books, 1975.

42. Report of the U.S. Preventive Services Task Force. Screening for obesity. In: Guide to Clinical Preventive Services. Health and Human Services, Prepublication copy, 1989, pp. 76-78.

43. Foster WR, Burton BT, eds. National Institutes of Health consensus conference: Health implications of obesity. Ann Intern Med 1985; 103:977-1077.

44. Blackburn GL, Kanders BS. Medical evaluation and treatment of the obese patient with cardiovascular disease. Am J Cardiol 1987; 60:55G-55G.

45. Remington D, Fisher G, Parent E. How To Lower Your Fat Thermostat. Provo, UT: Vitality House International, Inc., 1983.

46. Holbrook JH. Periodic health examination for adults In: BM Stults and WH Dere, eds. Practical Care of the Ambulatory Patient. Philadelphia: W.B. Saunders Co., 1989, pp 415-435.

47. Report of the U.S. Preventive Services Task Force. Screening for asymptomatic coronary artery disease. In: Guide to Clinical Preventive Services. Health and Human Services, Prepublication Copy, 1989, pp. 3-7.

48. Grundy SM, Greenland P, Herd A, et al.. Cardiovascular and risk factor evaluation of healthy American adults. Circulation 1987; 75(6):1340A-1360A.

49. Amsterdam EA, Laslett L, Holly R. Exercise and sudden death. Cardiol Clin 1987; 5:337-343.

50. Guidelines for exercise testing: A report of the American College of Cardiology/American Heart Association Task Force on assessment of cardiovascular procedures. JACC 1986; 8(3):725-738.

51. National Center for Health Statistics. Advance report of final mortality statistics, 1986. Monthly Vital Statistics Report [Suppl], vol. 37, no. 6. Hyattsville, Md.: Public Health Service, 1988. (Publication no. DHSS (PHS) 88-1120.)

52. American Heart Association. 1989 heart facts. Dallas, Texas: American Heart Association, 1988.

53. American College of Sports Medicine. Health appraisal, risk assessment, and safety of exercise: a committee report. Chaired by S Blair, 1989 (in press).

54. U.S. Department of Health and Human Services. The 1988 report of the Joint National Committee on detection, evaluation, and treatment of high blood pressure. Arch Int Med 1988; 148(5):10223-1038.

55. Mayo Clinic Health Letter. White coat hypertension. 1989; 7(5):5.

56. DeCosse JJ. Cancer of the colon and rectum. In: Holleb AI, ed. The American Cancer Society Cancer Book: Prevention, Detection, Diagnosis, Treatment, Rehabilitation, Cure. New York: Doubleday and Company, Inc., 1986, pp. 341-61.

57. National Cancer Institute. Colorectal cancer - rationale for early detection guidelines. In: Working Guidelines for Early Cancer Detection: Rationale and Supporting Evidence to Decrease Mortality. Early Detection Branch, Division of Cancer Prevention and Control, National Cancer Institute, 1987, pp. 17-22.

58. Report of the U.S. Preventive Services Task Force. Screening for colorectal cancer. In: Guide to Clinical Preventive Services. Health and Human Services, Prepublication copy, 1989, pp. 32-37.

59. Morganthau T. "The president has cancer" (Ronald Reagan). Newsweek, 1985; July 29: pp.16-18.

60. National Cancer Institute Annual Review, 1987. Unpublished Data.

61. Morson BC. Genesis of colorectal cancer. In: Sherlock P, Zamcheck N, eds. Clinics in Gastroenterology. Philadelphia: W.B. Saunders Co. 1976; pp. 505-525.

62. Winawer SJ, Sherlock P. Surveillance for colorectal cancer in average risk patients, familial high-risk groups, and patients with adenomas, CA 1982; 50:2609.

63. Crespi M, Weissman GS, Gilbertsen VA, et al. The role of proctosigmoidoscopy in screening for colorectal neoplasia. CA 1984; 34(3):158-166.

64. Winawer SJ, Sherlock P, Schottenfeld D, et al. Screening for colon cancer. Gastroenterology 1976; 70:783-789.

65. Report of the U.S. Preventive Services Task Force. Screening for prostate cancer. In: Guide to Clinical Preventive Services. Health and Human Services, Prepublication copy, 1989, pp. 42-44.

66. American Cancer Society. Cancer statistics, 1989. CA 1989; 39:3-20.

67. National Cancer Institute. Prostate cancer - rationale for early detection guidelines. In: Working Guidelines for Early Cancer Detection: Rationale and Supporting Evidence to Decrease Mortality. Early Detection Branch, Division of Cancer Prevention and Control, National Cancer Institute, 1987, pp. 26-31.

68. Murphy GP, Cummings KM, Mettlin CJ. Cancer of the male reproductive system. In: Holleb AI, ed. The American Cancer Society Cancer Book: Prevention, Detection, Diagnosis, Treatment, Rehabilitation, Cure. New York: Doubleday and Company, Inc., 1986, pp. 509-531.

69. Dere WH, Burt RW, Stults BM. Cancer prevention in primary care. In: BM Stults, WH Dere, eds. Practical Care of the Ambulatory Patient. Philadelphia: W.B. Saunders Co., 1989, pp 436-445.

70. Sobel DS, Ferguson T. Sigmoidoscopy. In: The People's Book of Medical Tests. New York: Summit Books, 1985, p. 337.

71. Hertz RE, Dedish MR, Day E. Value of periodic examinations in detecting cancer of the rectum and colon. Postgrad Med 1960; 27:290-294.

72. Dales LG, Friedman GD, Collen MF. Evaluating periodic multiphasic health checkups: A controlled trial. J Chronic Dis 1979; 32:385-404.

73. Dales LG, Friedman GD, Ramcharan S, et al. Multiphasic checkup evaluation study. Outpatient clinic utilization, hospitalization, and mortality experience after seven years. Prev Med. 1973; 2:221-235.

74. Gilbertsen VA. Proctosigmoidoscopy and polypectomy in reducing the incidence of rectal cancer. CA 1974; 34:936-939.

75. Gilbertsen VA, Nelms JM. The prevention of invasive cancer of the rectum. CA 1978; 41:1137-1139.

76. Nivatvongs S, Fryd DS. How far does the proctosigmoidoscope reach? A prospective study of 1,000 patients. N Engl J Med 1980; 303:380-382.

77. Winnan G, Berci G, Panish J, et al. Superiority of the flexible to the rigid sigmoidoscope in routine proctosigmoidoscopy. N Engl J Med 1980; 302:1011-1012.

78. Marks G, Boggs W, Castro AF, et al. Sigmoidoscopic examinations with rigid and flexible fiberoptic sigmoidoscopes in the surgeon's office: A comparative prospective study of effectiveness in 1,012 cases. Dis Colon Rectum 1979; 22:162-168.

79. Weissman GS, Winawer SJ, Sergi M, et al. Preliminary results of a multicenter evaluation of a 30 cm flexible sigmoidoscope by nonendoscopists. Gastrointest Endosc 1982; 28:150.

80. Sobel DS, Ferguson T. Sigmoidoscopy. In: The People's Book of Medical Tests. New York: Summit Books, 1985, pp. 436-445.

81. Report of the U.S. Preventive Services Task Force. Screening for skin cancer. In: Guide to Clinical Preventive Services. Health and Human Services, Prepublication copy, 1989, pp. 48-51.

82. Friedman RJ, Rigel DS, Kopf AW. Early detection of malignant melanoma: The role of physician examination and self-examination of the skin. CA 1985; 35:130-151.

83. Fitzpatrick TB, Rhodes AR, Sober AJ. Prevention of malignant melanoma by recognition of its precursors. N Engl J Med 1985; 312:115-116.

84. Fitzpatrick TB. Skin cancer. In: Holleb AI, ed. The American Cancer Society Cancer Book: Prevention, Detection, Diagnosis, Treatment, Rehabilitation, Cure. New York: Doubleday and Company, Inc., 1986, pp. 532-547.

85. National Cancer Institute. Melanoma–rationale for early detection guidelines. In: Working Guidelines For Early Cancer Detection: Rationale and Supporting Evidence to Decrease Mortality. Early Detection Branch, Division of Cancer Prevention and Control, National Cancer Institute. 1987, pp. 5-8.

86. American Cancer Society. Cancer facts and figures–1987. New York: American Cancer Society, 1987.

87. Friedman RJ, Rigel DS, Kopf AW. Early detection of malignant melanoma: The role of physician examination and self-examination of the skin. CA 1985; 35(3):130-151.

88. Hartley JW, Fletcher WS. Improved survival of patients with Stage II melanoma of the extremity using hyperthermic isolation perfusion with 1-phenylalanine mustard. J Surg Oncol 1987; 36:170-174.

89. Cassileth BR, Lusk EJ, Guerry D, et al. "Catalyst" symptoms in malignant melanoma. J Gen Intern Med 1987; 2:1-4.

90. Report of the U.S. Preventive Services Task Force. Screening for testicular cancer. In: Guide to Clinical Preventive Services. Health and Human Services, Prepublication copy, 1989, pp. 52-54.

91. National Cancer Institute. Testicular cancer: rationale for early detection guidelines. In: Working Guidelines for Early Cancer Detection: Rationale and Supporting Evidence to Decrease Mortality. Early Detection Branch, Division of Cancer Prevention and Control, National Cancer Institute, 1987, pp. 23-25.

92. Sobel DS and Ferguson T. Testicular self-examination. In: The People's Book of Medical Tests. New York: Summit Books, 1985, pp.218-219.

93. Murphy GP, Cummings KM, Mettlin CJ. Cancer of the male reproductive system. In: Holleb AI, ed. The American Cancer Society Cancer Book: Prevention, Detection Diagnosis, Treatment, Rehabilitation, Cure. New York: Doubleday and Company, Inc., 1986, pp. 521-528.

94. Report of the U.S. Preventive Services Task Force. Screening for thyroid disease. In: Guide to Clinical Preventive Services. Health and Human Services, Prepublication copy, 1989, pp. 71-75.

95. Stockwell RM, Barry M, Davidoff F. Managing thyroid abnormalities in adults exposed to upper body irradiation in childhood: a decision analysis. Should patients without palpable nodules be scanned and those with scan defects be subjected to subtotal thyroidectomy? J Clin Endocrinol Metab. 1984; 58:804-812.

96. Krenning EP, Ausema L, Bruining HA, et al. Clinical and radiodiagnostic aspects in the evaluation of thyroid nodules with respect to thyroid cancer. Eur J Cancer Clin Oncol 1988; 24:299-304.

97. Sobel DS and Ferguson T. Thyroid function tests. In: The People's Book of Medical Tests. New York: Summit Books, 1985, pp. 108.

98. National Cancer Institute. Oral cancer - rationale for early detection guidelines. In: Working Guidelines for Early Cancer Detection: Rationale and Supporting Evidence to Decrease Mortality. Early Detection Branch, Division of Cancer Prevention and Control, National Cancer Institute, 1987, pp. 32-34.

99. Report of the U.S. Preventive Services Task Force. Screening for oral cancer. In: Guide to Clinical Preventive Services. Health and Human Services, Prepublication copy, 1989, pp. 61-63.

100. Baker HW. Cancers of the mouth, pharynx, and larynx. In: Holleb AI, ed. The American Cancer Society Cancer Book: Prevention, Detection, Diagnosis, Treatment, Rehabilitation, Cure. New York: Doubleday and Company, Inc., 1986, pp. 444-459.

101. Department of Health and Human Services. Reducing the health consequences of smoking: 25 years of progress. A report of the Surgeon General. Rockville, Md.: Department of Health and Human Services, 1989. (Publication no. DHHS (PHS) 89-8411.)

102. National Cholesterol Education Program. Report of the expert panel on detection, evaluation, and treatment of high blood cholesterol in adults. U.S. Department of Health and Human Services, Public Health Service. 1988; NIH Publication No. 88-2925.

103. Report of the U.S. Preventive Services Task Force. Screening for high blood cholesterol. In: Guide to Clinical Preventive Services. Health and Human Services, Prepublication copy, 1989, pp. 8-15.

104. National Center for Health Statistics. Advance report of final mortality statistics, 1985. Monthly Vital Statistics Report [Suppl], vol. 37, no. 6. Hyattsville, Md.: Public Health Service, 1988. (Publication No. DHHS [PHS] 88-1120.)

105. Lipid Research Clinics Program. The Lipid Research Clinics Coronary Primary Prevention Trial Results: II. The relationship of reduction in incidence of coronary heart disease to cholesterol lowering. JAMA 1984; 251:365-74.

106. The Expert Panel. Report of the national cholesterol education program expert panel on detection, evaluation, and treatment in high blood cholesterol in adults. Arch Intern Med 1988; 148:36-69.

107. Blankenhorn DM, Nessim SA, Johnson RL, et al. Beneficial effects of combined colestipol-niacin therapy on coronary atherosclerosis and coronary venous bypass grafts. JAMA 1987; 257:3233-3240.

108. Martin MJ, Hulley SB, Browner WS, et al. The plasma lipoproteins as risk factors: Comparison of electrophoretic and ultracentrifugation results. Metabolism 1982; 31:773-777.

109. Gusberg SB. Cancer of the female reproductive tract. In: Holleb AI, ed. *The American Cancer Society Cancer Book: Prevention, Detection, Diagnosis, Treatment, Rehabilitation, Cure.* New York: Doubleday and Company, Inc., 1986, pp. 487-500.

110. National Cancer Institute. Cancer of the cervix - rationale for early detection guidelines. In: *Working Guidelines for Early Cancer Detection: Rationale and Supporting Evidence to Decrease Mortality.* Early Detection Branch, Division of Cancer Prevention and Control, National Cancer Institute, 1987, pp. 14-16.

111. Report of the U.S. Preventive Services Task Force. Screening for cervical cancer. In: *Guide to Clinical Preventive Services.* Health and Human Services, Prepublication copy, 1989, pp. 38-41.

112. Day NE. Effect of cervical cancer screening in Scandinavia. Obst & Gynec 1984; 63:714-718.

113. Sobel DS and Ferguson T. Pap smear. In: *The People's Book of Medical Tests.* New York: Summit Books, 1985, pp. 179-182.

114. National Cancer Institute. Breast cancer: rationale for early detection guidelines. In: *Working Guidelines for Early Cancer Detection: Rationale and Supporting Evidence to Decrease Mortality.* Early Detection Branch, Division of Cancer Prevention and Control, National Cancer Institute, 1987, pp. 9-13.

115. Habbema JD. van Oortmarssen GJ, van Putten DJ, et al. Age-specific reduction in breast cancer mortality by screening: An analysis of the results of the Health Insurance Plan of Greater New York study. JNCI 1986; 77:317-320.

116. Scanlon EF, Strax P. Breast cancer. In: Holleb AI, ed. *The American Cancer Society Cancer Book: Prevention, Detection, Diagnosis, Treatment, Rehabilitation, Cure.* New York: Doubleday and Company, Inc., 1986, pp. 341-361.

117. Report of the U.S. Preventive Services Task Force. Screening for hearing impairment. In: *Guide to Clinical Preventive Services.* Health and Human Services, Prepublication copy, 1989, pp. 129-134.

118. National Center for Health Statistics. Prevalence of selected chronic conditions, United States, 1979-81. Vital and Health Statistics, series 10, no. 155. Washington, D.C.: Government Printing Office, 1986. (Publication no. DHSS [PHS] 86-1583.)

119. Department of Labor, Occupational Safety and Health Administration. Occupational noise exposure: hearing conservation amendment. Fed Reg. 1981; 46:4078-4180.

120. Cross AW. Health screening in schools. Part I. J Pediatr 1985; 107:487-494.

121. Herbst KRG. Psychosocial consequences of disorders of hearing in the elderly. In: Hinchcliffe R, ed. *Hearing and Balance in the Elderly.* Edinburgh: Churchhill Livingstone, 1983.

122. Bess FH, Lichtenstein MJ, Logan SA, et al. Hearing impairment as a determinant of function in the elderly. J Am Geriatr Soc (in press).

123. Stults BM. Preventive health care for the elderly. West J Med 1984; 141:832-845.

124. Lichtenstein MJ, Bess FH, Logan SA. Validation of screening tools for identifying hearing-impaired elderly in primary care. JAMA 1988; 259:2875-2878.

125. Strome M. Hearing loss and hearing aids. Harvard Medical School Health Letter. 1989; 14(6):5-8.

126. National Society to Prevent Blindness. Vision problems in the U.S.: Facts and figures. National Society to Prevent Blindness. New York, NY.

127. National Society to Prevent Blindness. Your eyes - for a lifetime of sight. National Society to Prevent Blindness. New York, NY.

128. Report of the U.S. Preventive Services Task Force. Screening for glaucoma. In: *Guide to Clinical Preventive Services.* Health and Human Services, Prepublication copy, 1989, pp. 124-128.

129. Podgor MJ, Leske MC, Ederer F. Incidence estimates for lens changes, macular changes, open-angle glaucoma, and diabetic retinopathy. Am J Epidemiol 1983; 118:206-212.

130. Report of the U.S. Preventive Services Task Force. Screening for diminished visual acuity. In: *Guide to Clinical Preventive Services.* Health and Human Services, Prepublication copy, 1989, pp. 120-123.

131. National Center for Health Statistics. Prevalence of selected chronic conditions, United States, 1979-81. Vital and Health Statistics, series 10, no. 155. Washington, D.C.: Government Printing Office, 1986. (Publication no. DHHS [PHS] 86-583.)

132. Phelps CD. Glaucoma. Primary Care 1982; 9:729-741.

133. National Society to Prevent Blindness. Glaucoma – sneak thief of sight. National Society to Prevent Blindness, Schaumburg, Il.

134. Johnson, C. and A. Mushlin. Routine Laboratory Testing. In: Stults BM, WH Dere, eds. *General Medical Practice, in Practical Care of the Ambulatory Patient.* Philadelphia: W.B. Saunders Company, 1989, pp. 446-455.

135. Fraser CG, Smith BC, and Peake MJ. Effectiveness of an outpatient urine screening program. Clin Chem 1977; 23:2216-2218.

136. Kiel DP, Moskowitz MA. The urinalysis: a critical appraisal. Med Clin North Am 1987; 71:607-624.

137. Elwood PC, Waters WE, Benjamin IT, et al. Mortality and anemia in women. Lancet 1974; 1:891-894.

138. Elwood PC, Waters WE, Green WJ, et al. Evaluation of a screening survey for anemia in adult non-pregnant women. Br Med J 1967; 4:714-717.

139. Rich EC, Crowson TW, and Connelly DP. Effectiveness of differential leukocyte count in case findings in the ambulatory care setting. JAMA 1983; 249:633-636.

140. Cebul RD, Beck JR. Biochemical profiles. Applications in ambulatory screening and preadmission testing of adults. Ann Intern Med 1987; 106:403-413.

141. Sobel DS, Ferguson T. *The People's Book of Medical Tests*. New York: Summit Books, 1985, pp. 42-146.

142. Report of the U.S. Preventive Services Task Force. Adult immunizations. In: *Guide to Clinical Preventive Services*. Health and Human Services, Prepublication copy, 1989, pp. 246-250.

143. Williams WW, Hickson MA, Kane MA, et al. Immunization policies and vaccine coverage among adults: the risk for missed opportunities. Ann Intern Med 1988; 108:616-625.

144. Shapiro ED, Clemens JD. A controlled evaluation of the protective efficacy of pneumococcal vaccine for patients at high risk of serious pneumococcal infections. Ann Intern Med 1984; 101:325-330.

145. Shapiro ED, Austrian R, Adair RK, et al. The protective efficacy of pneumococcal vaccine. Clin Res 1988; 36:470A. Abstract.

146. Bolan G, Broome CV, Facklam RR, et al. Pneumococcal vaccine efficacy in selected populations in the United States. Ann Intern Med 1986; 104:1-6.

147. Sims RV, Steinmann WC, McConvile JH, et al. The clinical effectiveness of pneumococcal vaccine in the elderly. Ann Intern Med 1988; 108:653-657.

148. Meiklejohn G. Effectiveness of monovalent influenza A-prime vaccine during the 1957 influenza A-prime epidemic. Am J Hyg 1958; 67:237-249.

149. Frame PS. A critical review of adult health maintenance: Part II Prevention of infectious diseases. J Fam Prac 1986; 22(5):417-422

150. Centers for Disease Control. Tetanus–United States, 1985-1986. MMWR. 1987; 36:477-481.

151. Brand DA, Acampora D, Gottlieb LD, et al. Adequacy of antitetanus prophylaxis in six hospital emergency rooms. N Engl J Med 1983; 309:636-640.

152. Fatal Diphtheria – Wisconsin. MMWR. 1982; 31:553-555.

153. Immunization Practices Advisory Committee. Prevention and control of influenza. MMWR. 1988; 37:361-364.

154. LaForce FM. Immunizations, immunoprophylaxis, and chemoprophylaxis to prevent selected infections. JAMA 1987; 257(18):2464-2470.

155. Sisk JE, Riegelman RK. Cost effectiveness of vaccination against pneumonia: an update. Ann Intern Med 1986; 104:79-86.

156. Immunizations Practices Advisory Committee. Pneumococcal polysaccharide vaccine. MMWR. 1989; 38:64-68,73-75.

157. Semel JD, Seskind C. Severe febrile reaction to pneumococcal vaccine. JAMA 1979; 241:1792.

158. Report of the U.S. Preventive Services Task Force. Screening for alcohol and other drug abuse. In: *Guide to Clinical Preventive Services*. Health and Human Services, Prepublication copy, 1989, pp. 182-89.

159. Kamerow DB, Pincus HA, Macdonald DI. Alcohol abuse, other drug abuse, and mental disorders in medical practice. JAMA 1986; 255:2054-2057.

160. Clark WB, Midanik L. Alcohol use and alcohol problems among U.S. adults: Results of the 1979 national survey. In: National Institute on Alcohol Abuse and Alcoholism. Alcohol consumption and related problems. Alcohol and Health Monograph 1. Rockville, Md.: National Institute on Alcohol Abuse and Alcoholism, 1982. (Publication no. DHHS [ADM] 82-1190.)

161. Berkelman RL, Ralston M, Herndon J, et al. Patterns of alcohol consumption and alcohol-related morbidity and mortality. MMWR CDC Surveill Summ 1986; 35:1SS-5SS.

162. Stoudemire A, Wallack L, Hedemark N. Alcohol dependence and abuse. In: Amler RW, HB Dull, eds. *Closing the Gap: The Burden of Unnecessary Illness*. New York: Oxford University Press, 1987, pp. 9-18.

163. West LJ, Maxwell DS, Noble EP, et al. Alcoholism. Ann Intern Med 1984; 100:405-416.

164. National Center for Health Statistics. Advance report of final mortality statistics, 1986. Monthly Vital Statistics Report (Suppl), vol. 37, no. 6. Hyattsville, Md.: Public Health Service, 1988. (Publication no. DHSS [PHS] 88-1120.)

165. Report of the U.S. Preventive Services Task Force. Counseling to prevent tobacco use. In: *Guide to Clinical Preventive Services*. Health and Human Services, Prepublication copy, 1989, pp. 193-197.

166. Centers for Disease Control. Smoking-attributable mortality and years of potential life lost – United States, 1984. MMWR 1987; 36:693-697.

167. Department of Health and Human Services. The health consequences of smoking: a report of the Surgeon General. Rockville, Md.: Department of Health and Human Services, 1982. (Publication no. DHSS (PHS) 82-50179.)

168. National Academy of Sciences. Environmental tobacco smoke: Measuring exposures and assessing health effects (Appendix D). Washington, D.C.: National Academy Press, 1986.

169. Fiorem MC, Novotny TE, Pierce JP, et al. Trends in cigarette smoking in the United States: The changing influence of gender and race. JAMA 1989; 261:49-55.

170. Doll R, Peto R. Mortality in relation to smoking: 20 years' observations on male British doctors. Br Med J 1976; 2:1525-36.

171. Rogot E, Murray JL. Smoking and causes of death among U.S. veterans: 16 years of observation. Public Health Rep 1980; 95:213-22.

172. Eraker SA, Marshall HB, Kirscht JP. Smoking cessation: A five-stage plan. In: *Practical Care of the Ambulatory Patient*. Stults BM, Dere WH, eds. Philadelphia: W.B. Saunders Company, 1989, pp.430-435.

173. Tarr JE, Macklin M. Cocaine. Pediatr Clin North Am 1987; 34:319-331.

174. Greenstein RA, Resnick RB, Resnick E. Methadone and naltrexone in the treatment of heroin dependence. Psychiatr Clin North Am 1984; 7:671-679.

175. Jones RT. Marijuana: Health and treatment issues. Psychiatr Clin North Am 1984; 7:703-712.

176. Gold MS, Washton AM, Dackis CA. Cocaine abuse: Neurochemistry, phenomenology, and treatment. Natl Inst Drug Abuse Res Monogr Ser 1985; 61:130-150.

177. Wheeler K, Malmquist J. Treatment approaches in adolescent chemical dependency. Pediatr Clin North Am 1987; 34:437-447.

178. Booth W. AIDS and drug abuse: No quick fix. Science 1988; 239:717-719.

179. Hutchings DE. Methadone and heroin during pregnancy: A review of behavioral effects in human and animal offspring. Neurobehav Toxicol Teratol 1982; 4:429-434.

180. Bennett WI, Goldfinger SE, Johnson GT. *Your Good Health.* Cambridge: Harvard University Press, 1987, pp. 458.

181. Report of the U.S. Preventive Services Task Force. Counseling to prevent motor vehicle injuries. In: *Guide to Clinical Preventive Services.* Health and Human Services, Prepublication copy, 1989, pp. 210-14.

182. Report of the U.S. Preventive Services Task Force. Counseling to prevent household and environmental injuries. In: *Guide to Clinical Preventive Services.* Health and Human Services, Prepublication copy, 1989, pp. 215-21.

183. Smith GS, Falk H. Unintentional injuries. In: Amler RW, HB Dull, eds. *Closing the Gap: The Burden of Unnecessary Illness.* New York: Oxford University Press, 1987, pp. 143-63.

184. Report of the U.S. Preventive Services Task Force. Screening for Violent Injuries. In: *Guide to Clinical Preventive Services.* Health and Human Services, Prepublication copy, 1989, pp. 179-181.

185. National Center for Health Statistics. Current estimates from the National Health Interview Survey, United States, 1982. Vital and Health Statistics, series 10, no. 150. Washington, D.C.: Government Printing Office, 1985. (Publication no. DHSS [PHS] 85-1578.)

186. National Center for Health Statistics. Advance report of final mortality statistics. Monthly Vital Statistics Report (Suppl), vol. 37, no. 6. Hyattsville, Md.: Public Health Service, 1988. (publication no. DHSS [PHS] 88-1120.)

187. Centers for Disease Control. Deaths from motor vehicle-related injuries, 1978-1984. MMWR CDC Surv Summ 1988; 37:5-12.

188. Baker SP, O'Neill B, Karpf R. *The Injury Fact Book.* Lexington, Mass.: DC Heath, 1984.

189. Centers for Disease Control. Premature mortality due to alcohol-related motor vehicle traffic fatalities – United States, 1987. MMWR 1988; 37:753-755.

190. Department of Transportation. Final regulatory impact assessment on amendments to Federal Motor Vehicle Safety Standard 208, Front Seat Occupant Protection. Washington, D.C.: Department of Transportation, 1984. (Publication no. DOT HS 806-572.)

191. Decker MD, Dewey MJ, Hutcheson RH, et al. The use and efficacy of child restraint devices: The Tennessee experience, 1982 and 1983. JAMA 1984; 252:2571-2575.

192. Scherz R. Fatal motor vehicle accidents of child passengers from birth through 4 years of age in Washington State. Pediatrics 1981; 68:572-575.

193. National Highway Traffic Safety Administration. A report to the congress on the effect of motorcycle helmet use repeal – a case report for helmet use. Washington, D.C.: Department of Transportation, 1980. (Publication no. DOT HS 805-312.)

194. Centers for Disease Control. Public health surveillance of 1990 injury control objectives for the nation. MMWR CDC Surveillance Summary, vol. 37, no. SS-1, 1988.

195. US Fire Administration. An evaluation of residential smoke detector performance under actual field conditions: Final report. Emmitsburg, Maryland: Federal Emergency Management Agency, 1980.

196. Jensen GF, Christiansen C, Boesen J, et al. Epidemiology of post-menopausal spinal and long bone fractures: A unifying approach to postmenopausal osteoporosis. Clin Orthoped 1982; 166:75-81.

197. Rubenstein LZ, Robbins AS. Evaluation of falls in elderly persons. In: Stults BM, Dere WH, eds. *Practical Care of the Ambulatory Patient.* W.B. Saunders Company, Philadelphia, 1989, pp. 263-269.

198. Wintemute GJ, Kraus JF, Teret SP, et al. The epidemiology of drowning in adulthood: Implications for prevention. Am J Prev Med 1988; 4:343-348.

199. Dietz PE, Baker SP. Drowning: Epidemiology and prevention. Am J Public Health 1974; 64:303-312.

200. Budnick EK. Estimating effectiveness of state-of-the-art detectors and automatic sprinklers on life safety in residential occupancies. Washington, D.C.: Department of Commerce, National Bureau of Standards, National Engineering Laboratory, Center for Fire Research, 1984. (Publication no. NBSIR 84-2819.)

201. Hall JR Jr. A decade of detectors: Measuring the effect. Fire 1985; 79:37-43.

202. Federal Bureau of Investigation. Uniform crime reports for the United States, 1986. Washington, D.C.: Government Printing Office, 1987.

203. Rosenberg ML, Gelles RJ, Holinger PC, et al. Violence: Homicide, assault, and suicide. In: Amler RW, Dull HB, eds. *Closing the Gap: The Burden of Unnecessary Illness.* New York: Oxford University Press, 1987; 164-178.

204. National Institute of Mental Health. The evaluation and management of rape and sexual abuse: A physician's guide. National Center for Prevention and Control of Rape. Rockville, Md.: National Institute of Mental Health, 1985. (Publication no. DHSS [ADM] 85-1409.)

205. Department of Health and Human Services. Report of the Secretary's Task Force on Black and Minority Health. Volume V: Homicide, suicide, and unintentional injuries. Washington, D.C.: Government Printing Office, 1986.

206. Silverman MM, Lalley TL, Rosenberg ML, et al. Control of stress and violent behavior: Mid-course review of the 1990 health objectives. Public Health Report 1988; 103:38-49.

207. Stark E, Flitcraft A, Zuckerman D, et al. Wife abuse in the medical setting: An introduction for health personnel. Monograph Series No. 7. Rockville, Md.: National Clearinghouse on Domestic Violence, 1981.

208. McLeer SV, Anwar R. A study of battered women presenting in an emergency department. Am J Public Health 1989; 79:65-66.

209. Cupoli JM. Is it child abuse? Patient Care 1988; April:28-51.

210. American Medical Association. AMA diagnostic and treatment guidelines concerning child abuse and neglect. Chicago, Ill: American Medical Association, 1985.

211. Mehta P, Dandrea LA. The battered woman. Am Fam Physician 1988; 37:193-199.

212. Report of the U.S. Preventive Services Task Force. Counseling to prevent dental disease. In: *Guide to Clinical Preventive Services.* Health and Human Services, Prepublication copy, 1989, pp. 236-239.

213. American Dental Association. Periodontal Disease: Don't Wait Till It Hurts. Produced in cooperation of the American Academy of Periodontology, Copyright of the American Dental Association, 1988.

214. American Dental Association. Gum Disease: The Warning Signs, Basic Flossing, Basic Brushing. Copyright, American Dental Association, 211 East Chicago Avenue, Chicago, Ill. 1984.

215. Suomi JD, Greene JC, Vermillion JR, et al. The effect of controlled oral hygiene procedures on the progression of periodontal disease in adults: Results after third and final year. J Periodontal 1971; 42:152-160.

216. Horowitz AM, Suomi JD, Peterson JK, et al. Effects of supervised daily dental plaque removal by children after 3 years. Community Dent Oral Epidemiol 1980; 8:171-176.

217. Lang NP, Cumming BR, Loe H. Toothbrush frequency as it is related to plaque development and gingival health. J Periodontal 1973; 44:398-405.

218. Ripa LW. Professionally (operator) applied topical fluoride therapy: A critique. Clin Prev Dent 1982; 4:3-10.

219. Idem. The current status of pit and fissure sealants: A review. Can Dent Assoc J 1985; 5:367-380.

220. Mertz-Fairhurst EJ, Fairhurst CW, Williams JE, et al. A comparative clinical study of two pit and fissure sealants: 7-year results in Augusta, Georgia. J Am Dent Assoc 1984; 109:252-255.

221. Report of the U.S. Preventive Services Task Force. Counseling to prevent human immunodeficiency virus infection and other sexually transmitted diseases. In: Guide to Clinical Preventive Services. Health and Human Services, Prepublication copy, 1989, pp. 222-228.

222. Centers for Disease Control. Human immunodeficiency virus infection in the United States: a review of current knowledge. MMWR (Suppl 6) 1987; 36:1-20.

223. Idem. Quarterly report to the Domestic Policy Council on the prevalence and rate of spread of HIV and AIDS, United States. MMWR 1988; 37:551-559.

224. Centers for Disease Control. Chlamydia trachomatis infections: Policy guidelines for prevention and control. MMWR (Suppl 3) 1985; 34:53S-74S.

225. Nahmias AJ, Keyserling HL, Kerrick GM. Herpes sim-plex. In: Remington JS, Klein JO, eds. Infectious Disease of the Fetus and Newborn Infant. Philadelphia: W.B. Saunders, 1983:636-678.

226. Hellinger FJ. Forecasting the personal medical care costs of AIDS from 1988 through 1991. Public Health Rep 1988; 103:309-319.

227. Report of the U.S. Preventive Services Task Force. Screening for syphilis. In: Guide to Clinical Preventive Services. Health and Human Services, Prepublication copy, 1989, pp. 89-92.

228. Stramm WE, Handsfield HH, Rompalo Am, et al. The association between genital ulcer disease and acquisition of HIV infection in homosexual men, JAMA 1988; 260:1429-1433.

229. Holmberg SD, Stewart JA, Gerber AR, et al. Prior herpes simplex virus with type 2 infection as a risk factor for HIV infection. JAMA 1988; 259:1048-1050.

230. Report of the U.S. Preventive Services Task Force. Screening for gonorrhea. In: Guide to Clinical Preventive Services. Health and Human Services, Prepublication copy, 1989, pp. 91-92.

231. Report of the U.S. Preventive Services Task Force. Screening for chlamydial infection. In: Guide to Clinical Preventive Services. Health and Human Services, Prepublication copy, 1989, pp. 99-101.

232. Centers for Disease Control. Chlamydia trachomatis infections: Policy guidelines for prevention and control. MMWR (Suppl 3) 1985;34.

233. Report of the U.S. Preventive Services Task Force. Screening for genital herpes simplex. In: Guide to Clinical Preventive Services. Health and Human Services, Prepublication copy, 1989, pp. 102-103.

234. Chuang TY, Su WPD, Perry HO, et al. Incidence and trend of herpes progenitals: A 15-year population study. Mayo Clin Proc 1983; 58:436-441.

235. Report of the U.S. Preventive Services Task Force. Screening for infection with human immunodeficiency virus. In: Guide to Clinical Preventive Services. Health and Human Services, Prepublication copy, 1989, pp. 93-98.

236. Report of the U.S. Preventive Services Task Force. Screening for hepatitis B. In: Guide to Clinical Preventive Services. Health and Human Services, Prepublication copy, 1989, pp. 82-84.

237. Centers for Disease Control. Syphilis and congenital syphilis, United States, 1985-1988. MMWR 1988; 37:486-9.

238. Clark EG, Danbolt N. The Oslo study of the natural course of untreated syphilis: An epidemiologic investigation based on a restudy of the Boeck-Bruusgaard material. Med Clin North Am 1964; 48:613-623.

239. National Institutes of Health. NIAID Study Group on Sexually Transmitted Diseases: 1980 status report. Summaries and panel recommendations. Washington, D.C.: Government Printing Office, 1981:215-264.

240. Cates W Jr. Epidemiology and control of sexually transmitted diseases: Strategic evolution. Infect Dis Clin North Am 1987; 1:1-23.

241. Hook EW, Holmes KK. Gonococcal infections. Ann Intern Med 1985; 102:229-43.

242. Westrom L. Effect of acute pelvic inflammatory disease on fertility. Am J Obstet Gynecol 1975; 121:707-713.

243. Guinan ME, Wolinsky SM, Reichman RC. Epidemiology of genital herpes simplex virus infection. Epidemiol Rev 1985; 7:127-46.

244. Corey L, Spear PG. Infections with herpes simplex viruses. N Engl J Med 1986; 314:749-757.

245. Centers for Disease Control. AIDS weekly surveillance report, United States. January 2, 1989.

246. Centers for Disease Control. Years of potential life lost before age 65 – United States, 1987. MMWR 1989; 38:27-29.

247. Curran JW, Jaffe HW, Hardy AM, et al. Epidemiology of HIV infection and AIDS in the United States. Science 1988; 239:610-616.

248. Immunization Practices Advisory Committee. Recommendations for protection against viral hepatitis. MMWR 1985; 34:313-335.

249. Handsfield HH, Jasman LL, Roberts PL, et al. Criteria for selective screening on Chlamydia trachomatis infection in women attending family clinics. JAMA 1986; 255:1730-1734.

250. Centers for Disease Control. Quarterly report to the Domestic Policy Council on the prevalence and rate of spread of HIV and AIDS in the United States. MMWR 1988; 37:223-226.

251. Centers for Disease Control. Changing patterns of groups at high risk for hepatitis B in the United States. MMWR 1988; 37:429-32,437.

252. Food and Drug Administration. Counseling patients about prevention. FDA Drug Bull 1987; Sept:17-19.

253. Centers for Disease Control. Condoms for prevention of sexually transmitted diseases. MMWR 1988; 37:7, 9.

254. Report of the U.S. Preventive Services Task Force. Screening for risk of low back injury . In: *Guide to Clinical Preventive Services*. Health and Human Services, Prepublication copy, 1989, pp. 164-166.

255. Cottonwood Hospital Medical Center. *Back School*. Hunter S, ed. Murray, UT: IHC Hospitals, Inc., 1989.

256. Frymoyer JW. Back pain and sciatica. N Engl J Med 1988; 318:219-300.

257. Frymoyer JW, Pope MH, Clements JH, et al. Risk factors in low-back pain: an Epidemiological survey. J Bone Joint Surg 1983; 65:213-218.

258. Svensson HO, Anderson GBJ. Low-back pain in 40- to 47-year old men: Work history and work environment factors. Spine 1983; 8:272-276.

259. Kelsey JL, Githens PB, O'Conner T, et al. Acute prolapsed lumbar intervertebral disc: an epidemiologic study with special reference to driving automobiles and cigarette smoking. Spine 1984; 9:608-613.

260. Biering-Sorensen F. Physical measurements as risk indicators for low-back trouble over a one year period. Spine 1984; 9:106-119.

261. Waddell, G. A new clinical model for the treatment of low-back pain. Spine 1987; 12:632-644.

262. Cady LD, Bischoff DP, O'Connell, Thomas PC, Allan JH. Strength and fitness and subsequent back injuries in fire fighters. J Occup Med 1979; 21:269.

263. Moffett JA, Chase SM, Portek I, Ennis JR. A controlled, prospective study to evaluate the effectiveness of back school in the relief of chronic low-back pain. Spine 1986; 11:120.

264. Sims-Willaims H, Jayson MIV, Young SMS, Baddeley H, Collins E. Controlled trial of mobilization and manipulation for patients with low-back pain in general practice. Br Med J 1978; 11:1338-1340.

265. Deyo, R.A. Conservative therapy for low-back pain. JAMA 1983; 250(8):1057.

266. Selby, D.K. Conservative care of nonspecific low-back pain. Ortho Clinics of N Amer 1982; 13:427-437.

267. Weber, Henrik, et al. Traction therapy in patients with herniated intervertebral discs. J Oslo City Hosp 1984; 34:61-70.

268. Thorsteinsson G, Stonnington HH, Stillwell GK, Elveback LR. The placebo effect of transcutaneous electrical stimulation. Pain 1978; 5:31-41.31-41.

269. Bennett, WI, Goldfinger SE, Johnson GT. *Your Good Health - How To Stay Well, and What To Do When You're Not*. Cambridge, MA: Harvard University Press, 1987.

270. Sehnert KW, Eisenberg H. *How To Be Your Own Doctor (Sometimes)*. New York, N.Y.: (Perigee Book) Putnam Publishing Group, 1985.

271. Tapley DF, Weiss RJ, Morris TQ, Subak-Sharpe GJ, Goetz DM. *The Columbia University College of Physicians and Surgeons Complete Home Medical Guide*. New York, N.Y.: Crown Publishers, Inc., 1985.

272. Vickery DM, Fries JF. *Take Care Of Yourself - A Consumer's Guide To Medical Care*. Reading, MA: Addison-Wesley Publishing Company, 1981.

273. Williams RR. Understanding genetic and environmental risk factors in susceptible persons. West J Med 1984; 141(6):799-806.

274. Williams RR, Hasstedt SJ, Wilson DE, Ash KO, Yanowitz FG, Reiber GE, Kuida H. Evidence that men with familial hypercholesterolemia can avoid early coronary death: An analysis of 77 gene carriers in 4 Utah pedigrees. JAMA 1986; 255:219-224.

275. Marmot MG, Syme SL, Kagen A, et al. Epidemiologic studies of coronary heart disease and stroke in Japanese men living in Japan, Hawaii and California. Am J Epidemiol 1975; 102:514-525.

276. Farney RJ, Walker JM. Diagnosis and treatment of obstructive sleep apnea syndrome: Update and newer techniques. Intermountain Sleep Disorders Center, LDS Hospital, SLC, UT, 84103.

277. Hauri P. Eleven rules for better sleep hygiene. In: *The Sleep Disorders*. Kalamazoo, MI: The Upjohn Company, 1982, pp. 22.

278. Report of the U.S. Preventive Services Task Force. Screening for diabetes mellitus. In: *Guide to Clinical Preventive Services*. Health and Human Services, Prepublication Copy, 1989, 64-70.

279. Harris MI. Prevalence of non-insulin-dependent diabetes and impaired glucose tolerance. In: National Diabetes Data Group. Diabetes in America: Diabetes Data Compiled 1984. Washington DC, Dept. of Health and Human Services, 1985, VI-I to VI-31 (Publication # DHHS [NIH] 85-1460).

280. Harati Y. Diabetic peripheral neuropathies. Ann Intern Med 1987; 107:546-559.

281. American Diabetes Association. Diabetes Facts and Figures. Alexandria, VA, 1986.

282. The Carter Center. Closing the gap: The problem of diabetes mellitus in the United States. Diabetes Care 1985; 8:391-406.

283. Burditt AF, Caird FI, Draper GJ. The natural history of diabetes retinopathy. QJ Med 1968; 37:303-317.

284. Nathan DM, Singer DE, Godine JE, et al. Retinopathy in older type II diabetes: Association with glucose control. Diabetes 1986; 35:797-801.

285. Davidson MB. The case for control in diabetes mellitus. West J Med 1978; 129:193-200.

286. West KM, Erdreich LJ, Stober JA. A detailed study of risk factors for retinopathy and nephropathy in diabetes. Diabetes 1980; 29:501-508.

287. Report of the U.S. Preventive Services Task Force. Screening for asymptomatic bacteriuria, hematuria, and proteinuria. In: *Guide to Clinical Preventive Services*. Health and Human Services, Prepublication Copy, 1989, 104-108.

288. Carter HB, Amberson JB, Bander NH, et al. Newer Diagnostic Techniques for Bladder Cancer. Urol Clin 1989; 14:763-769.

289. Evans DA, Brauner E, Warren JW, et al. Randomized Trial of Vigorous Antimicrobial Therapy of Bacteriuria in a Community Population. In: *Program and Abstracts of the Twenty-Seventh Inter-science Conference on Antimicrobial Agents and Chemotherapy*. New York: American Society of Microbiology, 1987:148

290. Boscia JA, Kobasa WD, Knight RA, et al. Therapy is no therapy for bacteriuria in elderly ambulatory non-hospitalized women. JAMA 1987; 257:1067-1071.

291. Sobel DS, Ferguson T. *The People's Book of Medical Tests*. New York: Summit Books, 1985, pp. 112.

292. Report of the U.S. Preventive Services Task Force. Screening for breast cancer. In: *Guide to Clinical Preventive Services.* Health and Human Services, Prepublication Copy, 1989, 26-31.

293. Report of the U.S. Preventive Services Task Force. Screening for tuberculosis. In: *Guide to Clinical Preventive Services.* Health and Human Services, Prepublication Copy, 1989, 85-87.

294. Comstock GW, Woolpert SF. Preventive Therapy. In: Kubica GP, Wayne LG eds. *The Mycobacteria: A Source Book.* Marcel Dekker, Inc., New York, 1984, pp. 1071-1081.

295. International Union Against Tuberculosis Committee on Prophylaxis. Efficacy of various durations of isoniazid preventive therapy for tuberculosis: Five years of follow-up in the IUAT trial. Bull WHO 1982; 60:555-564.

296. Stead WW, Teresa T, Harrison RW, et al. Benefit-risk consideration in preventive treatment for tuberculosis in elderly persons. Ann Intern Med 1987; 107:843-845.

297. Sobel DS, Ferguson T. *The People's Book of Medical Tests.* New York: Summit Books, 1985, pp. 133-135.

298. Dalsky GP, Personal communication. Dr. Dalsky is affiliated with the University of Connecticut Health Center, Osteoporosis Center and Exercise Research Laboratory, Farmington, Connecticut.

299. Report of the U.S. Preventive Services Task Force. Screening for postmenopausal osteoporosis. In: *Guide to Clinical Preventive Services.* Health and Human Services Prepublication Copy, 1989, 161-163.

300. Osteoporosis Center, University of Connecticut. *Boning Up On Osteoporosis.* National Osteoporosis Foundation, 1989.

301. Report of the U.S. Preventive Services Task Force. Estrogen prophylaxis. In: *Guide to Clinical Preventive Services.* Health and Human Services, Prepublication Copy, 1989, 255-257.

302. Jewish Hospital of St. Louis. Division of Bone and Mineral Diseases. "Checklist of Risk Factors for Developing Osteoporosis." The Bone Health Program.

303. National Institutes of Health. Consensus Conference: Osteoporosis. JAMA 1984; 252:799-802.

304. Iskrant AP, Smith RW Jr. Osteoporosis in women 45 and over related to subsequent fractures. Public Health Rep 1969; 84:33-38.

305. Ferris MH. Bone-mineral screening for osteoporosis. AJR 1987; 149:120-122.

306. Jensen JS, Baggar J. Long term special prognosis after hip fractures. Acta Ortho Scand 1982; 53:97-101.

307. Christiansen C, Riis BJ, Ridbro R. Prediction of rapid bone loss in postmenopausal women. Lancet 1987; 1:1105-1108.

308. Holbrook TL, Grazier K, Kelsey JL, et al. The frequency of occupance, impact, and cost of selected musculoskeletal conditions in the United States. Chicago, Ill.: American Academy of Orthopedic Surgeons, 1984.

309. National Center for Health Services Research and Health Care Technology Assessment. Single photon absorptiometry for measuring bone mineral density. Health Technology Assessment Report No. 7 Rockville, Md.: Department of Health and Human Services, 1986.

310. *Idem.* Dual photon absorptiometry for measuring bone mineral density. Health Technology assessment Report No. 6. Rockville, Md.: Department of Health and Human Services, 1986.

311. Wahner HW, Dunn WL, Riggs BL. Assessment of bone mineral. Part 1. J Nucl Med 1984; 25:1134-1141.

312. *Idem.* Assessment of bone mineral. Part 2. J Nucl Med 1984; 25:1241-1253.

313. Krolner B, Nielsen SP. Bone mineral content of the lumbar spine in normal and osteoporotic women: Cross sectional and longitudinal studies. Clin Sci 1982; 62:329-336.

314. Cann CE, Genant HK, Folb FO, et al. Quantitated computed tomography for prediction of vertebral fracture risk. Bone 1985; 6:1-7.

315. Wahner HW, Dunn WL, Brown ML, et al. Comparison of dual energy absorptiometry and dual photon absorptiometry for bone mineral measurements of the lumbar spine. Mayo Clin Proc 1988; 63:1075-1084.

316. Riggs BL, Wahner HW, Seeman E, et al. Changes in the bone mineral density of the proximal femur and spine with aging: differences between the postmenopausal and senile osteoporosis syndromes. J Clin Invest 1982; 70:716-723.

317. Jensen GF, Christiansen C, Boesen J, et al. Epidemiology of post-menopausal spinal and long bone fractures: A unifying approach to postmenopausal osteoporosis. Clin Orthoped 1982; 166:75-81.

318. Firoozina H, Golimbu C, Rafii M, et al. Quantitated computed tomography assessment of spinal trabecular bone. II. In osteoporotic women with and without vertebral fractures. J Comput Tomogr 1984; 8:99-103.

319. Wasnich RD, Ross PD, Heilburn LK, et al. Prediction of post-menopausal fracture risk with use of bone mineral measurements. Am J Obstet Gynecol 1985; 153:745-751.

320. Nilsson BE, Westlin NE. The bone mineral content in the forearm of women with Colles' fracture. Acta Orthop Scand 1974; 45:836-844.

321. Cummings S. Are patients with hip fractures more osteoporotic? Review of the evidence. Am J Med 1985; 78:487-494.

322. Melton W, Wahner HW, Richelson LS, et al. Osteoporosis and the risk of hip fracture. Am J Epidemiol 1986; 124:254-261.

323. Riggs BL, Wahner HW, Dunn WL, et al. Differential changes in bone mineral density of the appendicular and axial skeleton with aging. J Clin Invest 1981; 67:328-335.

324. Hui SL, Slemenda CW, Johnston CC Jr. Age and bone mass as predictors of fracture in a prospective study. J Clin Invest 1988; 81:1804-1809.

325. Hall FM, Davis MA, Baran DT. Bone mineral screening for osteoporosis. N Engl J Med 1987; 316:212-214.

326. Shapiro S, Kelly JP, Rosenberg L, et al. Risk of localized and widespread endometrial cancer in relation to recent and discontinued use of conjugated estrogens. N Engl J Med 1985; 313:969-972.

327. Antunes CMF, Stolley PD, Rosenshein NB, et al. Endometrial cancer and estrogen use: Report of a large case-control study. N Engl J Med 1979; 300:9-13.

328. Buring JE, Bain CJ, Ehrmann RL. Conjugated estrogen use and risk of endometrial cancer. Am J Epidemiol 1986; 124:434-441.

329. Spengler RF, Clarke EA, Woolever CA, et al. Exogenous estrogens and endometrial cancer: A cross sectional study and assessment of potential biases. Am J Epidemiol 1981; 114:497-506.

330. Cali RW. Estrogen replacement therapy–boon or bane? Postgrad Med 1984; 75:279-286.

331. Report of the U.S. Preventive Services Task Force. Nutritional counseling. In: *Guide to Clinical Preventive Services*. Health and Human Services, Prepublication Copy, 1989, 203-209.

332. Recker RR, Saville PD, Heaney RP. Effect of estrogen and calcium carbonate on bone loss in postmenopausal women. Ann Intern Med 1977; 87:649-655.

333. Ettinger B, Genant HK, Cann CE. Postmenopausal bone loss is prevented by treatment with low-dosage estrogen with calcium. Ann Intern Med 1987; 106:40-45.

334. Riis B, Thomsen K, Christiansen C. Does calcium supplementation prevent postmenopausal bone loss? A double-blind, controlled clinical study. N Engl J Med 1987; 316:173-177.

335. Nilas L, Christiansen C, Rodbro P. Calcium supplementation and postmenopausal bone loss. Br Med J 1984; 289:1103-1106.

336. Stevenson JC, Whitehead MI, Padwick M, et al. Dietary intake of calcium and postmenopausal bone loss. Br Med J 1988; 297:15-17.

337. Dalsky GP, Stocke KS, Ehsani AA, et al. Weight-bearing exercise training and lumbar bone mineral content in postmenopausal women. Ann Intern Med 1988; 108:824-828.

338. Dalsky GP. The role of exercise in the prevention of osteoporosis. Comp Ther 1989; 15:30-37.

339. Report of the U.S. Preventive Services Task Force. Aspirin prophylaxis. In: *Guide to Clinical Preventive Services*. Health and Human Services, Prepublication Copy, 1989, 258-260.

340. The Steering Committee of the Physicians' Health Study Research Group. Preliminary report: Findings from the aspirin component of the ongoing Physicians' Health Study. N Engl J Med 1988; 318:262-264.

341. Peto R, Gray R, Collins R, et al. Randomized trial of prophylactic daily aspirin in British male doctors. Br Med J 1988; 296:313-316.

342. American Heart Association. *Aspirin and Your Heart*. Dallas, TX: American Heart Association, 1989.

343. Report of the U.S. Preventive Services Task Force. Screening for hemoglobinopathies. In: *Guide to Clinical Preventive Services*. Health and Human Services, Prepublication Copy, 1989, 82-84.

344. Report of the U.S. Preventive Services Task Force. Screening for hepatitis B. In: *Guide to Clinical Preventive Services*. Health and Human Services, Prepublication Copy, 1989, 82-84.

345. Immunization Practices Advisory Committee. Recommendations for protection against viral hepatitis. MMWR 1985; 34:313-335.

346. Immunization Practices Advisory Committee. Update on hepatitis B prevention. MMWR 1987; 36:353-360,366.

347. Stevens CE, Toy PE, Tong MJ, et al. Perinatal hepatitis B virus transmission in the United States: Prevention by passive-active immunization. JAMA 1985; 253:1740-1745.

348. Beasley RP, Hwang LY. Epidemiology of hepatocellular carcinoma. In: Vyas, G.N., Dienstag, J.L., Hoofnagle, J.H., et al., eds. *Viral Hepatitis and Liver Disease*. Grune and Stratton, Orlando, Fla., 1984, pp. 209-224.

349. Beasley RP. Hepatitis B virus as the etiologic agent in hepatocellular carcinoma: epidemiologic considerations. Hepatology 1982; 2:21S-6S.

350. Beasley RP, Hwang LY, Lin CC, et al. Hepatocellular carcinoma and HBV: A prospective study of 27,707 men in Taiwan. Lancet 1981; 2:1129-1133.

351. Report of the U.S. Preventive Services Task Force. Adult immunizations. In: *Guide to Clinical Preventive Services*. Health and Human Services, Prepublication Copy, 1989, 246-250.

352. Report of the U.S. Preventive Services Task Force. Screening for rubella. In: *Guide to Clinical Preventive Services*. Health and Human Services, Prepublication Copy, 1989, 144-47.

353. Centers for Disease Control. Rubella and Congenital Rubella Syndrome –United States, 1985-1988. MMWR 1989;38:173-178.

354. *Idem*. Rubella and Congenital Rubella – United States, 1984-86. MMWR 1987; 36:664.

355. *Idem*. Rubella and Congenital Rubella Syndrome – New York City. MMWR 1986;35:770-779.

356. Report of the U.S. Preventive Services Task Force. Screening for cerebrovascular disease. In: *Guide to Clinical Preventive Services*. Health and Human Services, Prepublication Copy, 1989, 20-23.

357. Heyman A, Wilkinson WE, Heyden S, et al. Risk of stroke in asymptomatic persons with cervical arterial bruits: A population study in Evans County, Georgia. N Engl J Med 1980; 302:838-841.

358. Wolf PA, Kannel WB, Sorlie P, et al. Asymptomatic carotid bruit and risk of stroke: the Framingham study. JAMA 1981; 245:1442-1445.

359. Bogousslavsky J, Despland PA, Regli F. Asymptomatic tight stenosis of the internal carotid artery: Long-tern prognosis. Neurology 1986; 36:861-863.

360. Report of the U.S. Preventive Services Task Force. Screening for chlamydial infection. In: *Guide to Clinical Preventive Services*. Health and Human Services, Prepublication Copy, 1989, 99-100.

361. Centers for Disease Control. Chlamydia trachomatous infections: Policy guidelines for prevention and control. MMWR [Suppl 3], 1985, 34.

362. Report of the U.S. Preventive Services Task Force. Screening for gonorrhea. In: *Guide to Clinical Preventive Services*. Health and Human Services, Prepublication Copy, 1989, pp. 91-92.

363. Report of the U.S. Preventive Services Task Force. Screening for syphilis. In: *Guide to Clinical Preventive Services*. Health and Human Services, Prepublication Copy, 1989, pp. 89-90.

364. Report of the U.S. Preventive Services Task Force. Screening for infection with human immunodeficiency virus. In: *Guide to Clinical Preventive Services*. Health and Human Services, Prepublication Copy, 1989, 93-98.

365. Kovar MG, Harris MI, Hadden WC. The scope of diabetes in the United States population. Am J Public Health 1987; 77:1549-1550.

366. Centers for Disease Control. Trends in diabetes mellitus mortality. MMWR 1988; 37:769-773.

367. Centers for Disease Control. Changing patterns of groups at high risk for hepatitis B in the United States. MMWR 1988; 37:429-32,437.

368. Stevens CE, Beasley RP, Tsui J, et al. Vertical transmission of hepatitis B antigen in Taiwan. N Engl J Med 1975; 292:271-274.

369. Pollock ML, Wilmore JH. *Exercise in Health and Disease: Evaluation and Prescription for Prevention and Rehabilitation*. Philadelphia: W.B. Saunders Company, 1990, pp. 354-355.

370. Government of Canada: *Fitness and Amateur Sports: Canadian Standardized Test of Fitness (CSTF) Operations Manual*, 3rd ED. Ottawa, Minister of State, FAS 73-78, 1986.

371. Anderson KM, Wilson PWF, Odell PM, Kannel WB. An updated coronary risk profile: A statement for health professionals. Circulation 1991; 83(1):356-362.

372. Comments from Robert L. DuPont, Jr., the first White House Drug Czar.

373. Lavie CJ, Squires RW, Gau GT. Prevention of cardiovascular disease: Of what value are risk factor modification, exercise, fish consumption, and aspirin therapy? Postgrad Med 1987; 81(5):52-72.

374. Personal communication with Dr. Charles Smart, Director of the Early Detection Branch of the National Cancer Institute.

375. Mayo Clinic Health Letter, Second Opinion, Volume 9 (2), pp. 8.

376. *Coronary Prone Behavior.* Dembroski TM, Weiss SM, Shields JL, Haynes SG, Feinleib M, eds. Spinger-Verlag, New York, 1978.

377. American College of Sports Medicine. Guidelines for Exercise Testing and Prescription, (Ed 4). Philadelphia: Lea & Febiger, 1991.

378. Fletcher GF, Froelicher VF, Hartley H, Haskell WL, Pollock ML. Exercise Standards: A Statement for Health Professionals from the American Heart Association. Circulation 1990; 82(6):2286-2322.

379. Abbott Laboratories. *Coping With Your Circulatory Problems: Getting Back in Circulation.* Gray LT, Fahey VA (consultants). Printed in USA.

380. The American Medical Association. *Family Medical Guide,* J.R.M. Kunz, ed. Random House, NY, 1982, pp. 454.

381. Eddy DM, Editor. *Common Screening Tests.* Published by American College of Physicians, Phil, PA, 1991.

382. Hayward RSA, Steinberg EP, Ford DE, Roizen MF, Roach KW. Preventive care guidelines: 1991. Ann Int Med 1991; 114:758-783.

383. Eddy DM. Screening for breast cancer. Ann Int Med 1989; 111:389-399.

384. Garber AM, Sox HC, Littenberg B. Screening asymptomatic adults for cardiac risk factors: The serum cholesterol level. Ann Int Med 1989; 110:622-639.

385. Littenberg B, Garber AM, Sox HC. Screening for hypertension. Ann Int Med 1990; 112:192-202.

386. Singer DE, Samet JH, Cole CM, Nathan DM. Screening for diabetes mellitus. Ann Int Med 1988; 109:639-649.

387. Eddy DM. Screening for colorectal cancer. Ann Int Med 1990; (in press).

388. Eddy DM. Screening for cervical cancer. Ann Int Med 1990; 113:214-226.

389. Helfand M, Crapo LM. Screening for thyroid disease. Ann Int Med 1990; 112:840-849.

390. Sox HC, Garber AM, Littenberg B. The resting electrocardiogram as a screening test: A clinical analysis. Ann Int Med 1989; 111:489-502.

391. Sox HC, Littenberg B, Garber AM. The role of exercise testing in screening for coronary artery disease. Ann Int Med 1989; 110:456-469.

392. Melton LJ, Eddy DM. Screening for osteoporosis. Ann Int Med 1990; 112:516-528.

393. Fox HC Jr., Editor. *Common Diagnostic Tests, Use and Interpretation, First Edition.* Published by American College of Physicians, Phil, PA, 1987.

394. American Academy of Ophthalmology. Preferred Practice Pattern: Comprehensive Adult Eye Examination. San Francisco, CA: American Academy of Ophthalmology, 1989.

395. Sobel DS, Ferguson T. *The People's Book of Medical Tests.* New York: Summit Books, 1985, pp. 245-248.

INDEX

human immunodeficiency virus (HIV-AIDS), 135-137, 156, 167 (see also "AIDS")
    children, 136
    counseling, 137
hunger, 150
hyperkalemia, 224
hypertension: 69, 84-86
    family history, 148, 172
    pregnancy, 172
    white coat, 85
hyperthyroidism, 101
hypoglycemia, 223
hypokalemia, 224
hypothyroidism, 102

– I –

immigrants, 156
immunization, 121-122, 163
immunosuppressants, 121
immunoassay, 162
infectious diseases, 3
infertility, 110, 136
influenza: 121, 122, 164
    vaccine, 121, 122, 164
    high risk for, 121
injuries: 127-131, 161
    adult, 127-129
    childhood, 127-129
    eye, 128
    household, 127, 129
    low-back, 138-141
    motor vehicle, 127
    physical, 130
    prevention, 127-129, 157
    violent, 128-129, 130-131
insulin: 71, 72, 73
    insulin-dependent diabetes mellitus (IDDM), 152
    non-insulin-dependent diabetes mellitus (NIDDM), 152
insulin-dependent diabetes mellitus (IDDM), 152
intensity, exercise, 42, 44, 150
intercourse, 110
internist, 143
intestine:
    large, 89, 111, 154
insomnia, 101
intravenous (IV) drug users, 126, 135, 136, 137, 162, 167
Ipecac, 127
irradiation, 101, 102

– J –

jaundice, 172
job, 66
jogging, 41, 42, 45

joint, 40, 47, 53
juices, 72

– K –

ketone tests, 220
kidney: 119, 120
    cancer, 153
    disease, 85, 121, 152, 160
    stones, 224
knee-to-chest exercise, 54

– L –

ladders, 128
large intestine, 89, 111, 154
larynx, 125
laxatives, 62
lens prescription, 117
LDH (lactic dehydrogenase), 223
LDL-cholesterol, 105-108
lean body mass (LBM), 47, 73, 219
leg raises, 50
legumes: 59, 61
    dry beans, 209
    lentils, 209
    peas, 209
leisure/occupational time (LOT) program, 40, 41, 44
lethargy, 102
leukemia, 221
lifestyle counseling, 76, 77
lifestyle history (personal), 178-181
lipids, 69
lipoprotein: 105-108
    HDL, 107
    LDL, 105-108
liver: 120
    cancer, 136, 162
    cirrhosis, 121, 123, 162
    disease, 3, 136, 160, 172
liquor, 124
log: 195-200
    activity, 6, 195-200
    relaxation, 195-200
    "something for self," 195-200
    weight, 195-200
longevity, 69
low-back injury: 53, 138-141
    risk factors, 138
    prevention, 139-141
    treatment, 139
low-calorie diet, 70
lump, 93, 99, 102, 104, 112, 113
lunch, 61, 209
lung cancer, 58, 112, 115
lung disease, 3, 121
lunge, 51, 54
lupus, 157
lymph system, 96, 99, 100

– M –

malaria, 172
malignant melanoma, 92-97
mammogram: 111-113, 155
    diagnostic, 113
    two-view, 113
margarine, 60
marijuana, 124
Marxer, Dr. Webster L., iii
massage, 139
Mayo Clinic, 145
mean corpuscular hemoglobin (MCH), 221
mean corpuscular hemoglobin concentration (MCHC), 221
mean corpuscular volume (MCV), 221
measles, 172
measles-mumps-rubella (MMR) vaccine, 163
meat, 59, 61, 212
medical procedures (history of), 174,
medications, 126, 127, 128, 129, 130, 175
meditation technique, 65, 67-78
melanocyte, 96
memory, 102
menstrual cycle, 111-112, 113
mental health, 40
menopause: 157, 158
    postmenopause, 158
metabolic diseases, 69, 121, 152
metabolic rate, 70, 72
metabolism, brain, 149, 150
milk, 60, 72
minerals, 62
mole(s): 92-97
    skin cancer, 92-99
mononucleosis, 172
mono-unsaturated fat, 59
monthly health checks, 7, 75
motor vehicle, 118, 123, 128
motorcycles, 127, 129
mouth, 97, 103-104
multiple myeloma, 121
mumps, 172
murder, 130
muscle:
    osteoporosis, 158-159
    paralysis, 150
    resistance, 44, 47-52
    strengthening activities, 48-52, 159
    tenderness, 102
    wasting, 101
    weight training, 47-52
muscle strength, 40, 47-52, 128, 138
muscle strength tests, 47, 52, 201-203

Easy Gourmet Menus to Lower Your Fat Thermostat™

by Howard Gifford

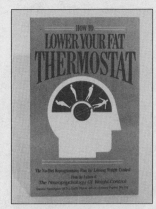

The latest from Chef Howard Gifford, author of *Gifford's Gourmet De-Lites*. Low-fat, gourmet cooking made easy. The 30 menus with over 150 irresistible recipes (including those presented by Chef Gifford on the popular Midday Show on KSL television, Salt Lake City, Utah) makes *Easy Gourmet Menus* a must for your cookbook library. Each easy to follow recipe gives the option of using his new, conveniently packaged spice mixes, or your own individual spices. Either way you'll be delighted with the taste of these wonderfully delicious meals.

How to Lower Your Fat Thermostat™

by Dennis W. Remington, M.D., A. Garth Fisher, Ph.D., Edward A. Parent, Ph.D.

Diets don't work and you know it! The less you eat, the more your body clings to its fat stores. This best-selling book contains the original program that teaches you to eat to lose weight. The *How to Lower Your Fat Thermostat* program is based on giving you plenty of nutrients and calories to convince the control centers in your brain to release excess fat stores. Your weight will come down naturally and comfortably, and stay at that lower level permanently.

Gifford's Spice Mixes

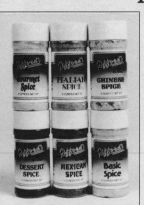

At the shake of a bottle, your cooking has just been made easier with the unique flavors created by Chef Gifford. Eliminate the cupboard full of spices that are seldom used and the time of mixing and measuring them. No more guess-work to create a desired taste. These new spice mixes are conveniently packaged with six inviting flavors: Gourmet Spice, Mexican Spice, Basic Spice, Italian Spice, Chinese Spice, and Dessert Spice. Use these spice mixes with the delicious recipes in the new book *Easy Gourmet Menus to Lower Your Fat Thermostat* or flavor your own meals with the desired spice mix. You'll be delighted by the results.

Recipes to Lower Your Fat Thermostat™

by La Rene Gaunt

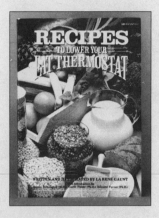

Companion cookbook to *How to Lower Your Fat Thermostat*. Once you understand the principles of the fat thermostat program, you will want to put them to work in your daily diet. Now you can with this full-color, beautifully illustrated cookbook. New ways to prepare more than 400 of your favorite recipes. Breakfast ideas. Soups and salads. Meats and vegetables. Wok food, potatoes, beans, and breads. Desserts and treats. All designed to please and satisfy while lowering your fat thermostat. It's Vitality House's most popular cookbook.

Gifford's Gourmet De-Lites

by Howard Gifford

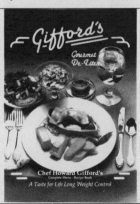

Vitality House is pleased to offer you an exciting work from a professional chef, Howard Gifford, whose meals have astonished guests at weight loss health resorts. Says Howard, "I love to create that which is pleasing both to the eye and the palate. Preparing healthy food is my medium! My tools? The common everyday household conveniences found in most American homes today. 'Simplicity' is my watchword. Become the creative gourmet cook you have always wanted to be! Learn what the magic of using just the right spices, extracts and natural juices can do for your foods! I'll also give you some helpful hints for shopping and organizing."

Acrylic Cookbook Holder

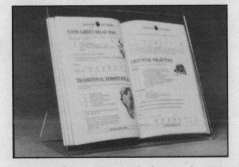

This acrylic cookbook holder is the perfect companion to your new cookbook. Desgined to hold any cookbook open without breaking the binding, it allows you to read recipes without distortion while protecting pages from splashes and spills.

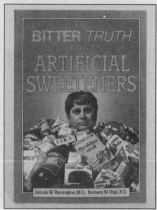

The Bitter Truth About Artificial Sweeteners

by Dennis W. Remington, M.D. and Barbara Higa, R.D.

Research proves that those people using artificial sweeteners tend to gain more weight. Not only do artificial sweeteners enchance the desire for sweets, they also cause many unpleasant side effects in addition to raising the Fat Thermostat. Learn the real truth about artificial sweeteners and sugars. Learn how they affect your health and weight and what you can do about them.

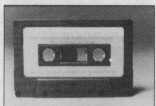

Five Roadblocks to Weight Loss

(Audiocassette)

If you have a serious weight problem that has failed to respond to the Fat Thermostat program, then you could be suffering from any of the five roadblocks to weight loss: food addictions, artificial sweeteners, food allergies, yeast overgrowth, and stress. Learn what these roadblocks are, what to do about them, and how the fat thermostat program relates to them . . . in an exclusive interview with Drs. Dennis Remington and Edward Parent.

Maintaining the Miracle

An Owner's Manual for the Human Body

by Ted D. Adams, Ph.D., A. Garth Fisher, Ph.D., Frank G. Yanowitz, M.D.

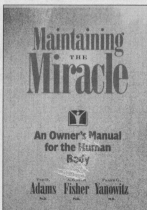

Your body is the most valuable possession you will ever own. Yet you may take better care of your car than you do your own body. In depth and up-to-date, this is the only book that tells you what to do and when to do it. You will thank yourself again and again for this invaluable help.

Desserts to Lower Your Fat Thermostat™

by Barbara Higa, R.D.

If you think you have to say goodbye to desserts, think again. At last there's a book that lets you have your cake and eat it too. *Desserts to Lower Your Fat Thermostat* is filled with what you thought you could never find: recipes for delicious desserts, snacks, and treats that are low in fat and free of sugar, salt and artificial sweeteners.

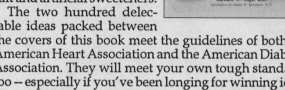
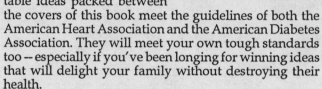

The two hundred delectable ideas packed between the covers of this book meet the guidelines of both the American Heart Association and the American Diabetes Association. They will meet your own tough standards too -- especially if you've been longing for winning ideas that will delight your family without destroying their health.

Back to Health: A Comprehensive Medical and Nutritional Yeast-Control Program

by Dennis W. Remington, M.D. and Barbara Higa, R.D.

New for the 1990's! With Expanded Physician Section!

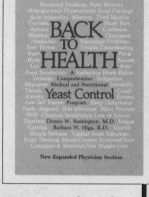

If you suffer from anxiety, depression, memory loss, heartburn or gas . . . if weight control is a constant battle . . . if you are tired, weak and sore all over . . . this book was written for you. While yeast occurs naturally in the body, when out of control it becomes the body's enemy, manifesting itself in dozens of symptoms. Getting yeast back under control can correct many conditions once considered chronic. More than 100 yeast-free recipes, plus special sections of weight control, hypoglycemia and PMS.

Pocket Progress Guide

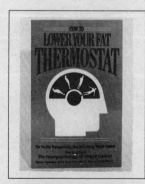

A pocket-sized summary of the fat thermostat program that includes food composition tables, daily records, and a progress summary for quick and easy reference.

The New Neuropsychology of Weight Control
(8 Audiocassettes and Study Guide)

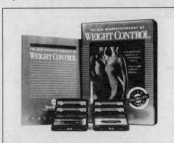

by Dennis W. Remington, M.D., A. Garth Fisher, Ph.D., Edward A. Parent, Ph.D., Barbara Higa, R.D.

More than a million people have purchased the most powerfully effective weight control program ever developed -- *The Neuropsychology of Weight Control*. Thousands of them have reported dramatic and permanent reductions in their weight.

The New Neuropsychology of Weight Control program is a scientifically-based weight-loss system that teaches you how your body works and shows you exactly what to do to change from a fat-storing to a fat-burning metabolism. Still included are the proven principles from the original program based on the best-selling book *How to Lower You Fat Thermostat*.

The New Neuropsychology of Weight Control program shows you how to set achievable weight loss goals and precisely what you need to do to reach them. You'll know how much weight you should lose and how long it will take. Included is a complete 12-week eating plan that provides daily menus, meal plans, tasty recipes, cooking instructions and eight shopping lists. You'll know exactly what to cook and how to cook it. And, you'll learn to create your own delicious meals that taste good while helping you to lose weight permanently.

The Will to Change
(Video Cassette)

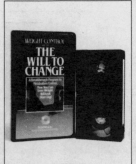

For some people, seeing is believing. While reviewing the key points of the program and the benefits of reaching your goal weight, this motivational video also features testimonials by people who have had dramatic success. In moments of doubt or discouragement, this video provides the needed support and encouragement.

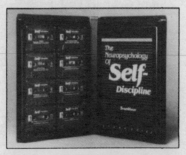

SyberVision's Neuropsychology of Self-Discipline
The Master Key to Success

There's one critical characteristic that makes the difference between success and failure: self-discipline. Without it, you can never hope to achieve your ambitions. With it, there's no goal you can't reach.

The Neuropsychology of Self-Discipline is a unique self-improvement pogram that allows you to instill a new and powerful self-mastery into your own mind and body. Armed with tools, insights, and skills of a highly disciplined achiever, you'll be able, perhaps for the first time in your life, to systematically pursue, and successfully realize, your most important goals.

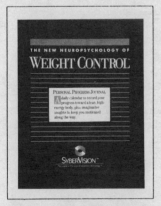

The Neuropsychology of Weight Control
Personal Progress Journal

This journal will be your six-month record of how well you're doing. By tracking your day-to-day progress you will ensure your long-term success.

QTY	CODE	DESCRIPTION	RETAIL	SUBTOTAL
	A	How To Lower Your Fat Thermostat	$ 9.95	
	B	Recipes To Lower Your Fat Thermostat	14.95	
	C	Acrylic Cookbook Holder	9.95	
	D	Neuropsychology of Weight Control (8 cassettes & guide)*	79.95	
	E	Back To Health (Yeast/Candida Guide)	10.95	
	F	Maintaining The Miracle	16.95	
	G	The Bitter Truth About Artificial Sweetners	9.95	
	H	Five Roadblocks To Weight Loss (Audiocassette)	7.95	
	I	Pocket Progress Guide	2.95	
	J	The Will To Change (Videocassette)	29.95	
	L	Neuropsychology of Self-Discipline (8 cassettes & guide)*	69.95	
	M	Personal Progress Journal (Sybervision weight program)	14.95	
	N	Desserts To Lower Your Fat Thermostat	12.95	
	O	Gifford's Gourmet De-Lites	12.95	
	P	Easy Gourmet Menus To Lower Your Fat Thermostat #	13.95	
	S	Gifford's Gourmet De-Lites Spice Mix Set #	20.95	
Shipping, 4th class book rate, $2.50 for the first item, $.50 each additional item.				+
For faster delivery, usually under five days, by UPS, add $1.50.				+
Canadian: $6.00 (U.S. dollars) for 1st item, $2.00 each additional item.				+
* Buy D or L and get 1 book free!		Utah residents add 6.25% sales tax.		+
# Buy P & S together and receive $5.00 off your order!			TOTAL	$

Prices subject to change without notice.

Name_____

Address_____

City_____ State_____ Zip_____

Day Phone_____

☐ Check   ☐ Money Order   -   Make payable to **Vitality House Publishing**
☐ MasterCard   ☐ VISA   ☐ American Express

Card No._____Expires_____

Signature_____

How did you hear about our products?   ☐ Friend   ☐ Book   ☐ Other _____

Mail to: 1675 No. Freedom Blvd. #11-C Provo, UT 84604 (801) 373-5100

Copyright© 1991 Vitality House International. Orders shipped upon receipt. Allow 2-3 weeks shipping.

EGM391   **To Order: Call Toll Free 1-800-637-0708 or FAX 801-373-5370**

Easy Gourmet Menus to Lower Your Fat Thermostat™
by Howard Gifford

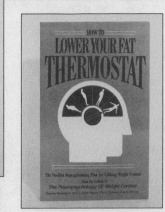

The latest from Chef Howard Gifford, author of *Gifford's Gourmet De-Lites.* Low-fat, gourmet cooking made easy. The 30 menus with over 150 irresistible recipes (including those presented by Chef Gifford on the popular Midday Show on KSL television, Salt Lake City, Utah) makes *Easy Gourmet Menus* a must for your cookbook library. Each easy to follow recipe gives the option of using his new, conveniently packaged spice mixes, or your own individual spices. Either way you'll be delighted with the taste of these wonderfully delicious meals.

How to Lower Your Fat Thermostat™
by Dennis W. Remington, M.D., A. Garth Fisher, Ph.D., Edward A. Parent, Ph.D.

Diets don't work and you know it! The less you eat, the more your body clings to its fat stores. This best-selling book contains the original program that teaches you to eat to lose weight. The *How to Lower Your Fat Thermostat* program is based on giving you plenty of nutrients and calories to convince the control centers in your brain to release excess fat stores. Your weight will come down naturally and comfortably, and stay at that lower level permanently.

Gifford's Spice Mixes

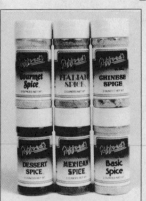

At the shake of a bottle, your cooking has just been made easier with the unique flavors created by Chef Gifford. Eliminate the cupboard full of spices that are seldom used and the time of mixing and measuring them. No more guess-work to create a desired taste. These new spice mixes are conveniently packaged with six inviting flavors: Gourmet Spice, Mexican Spice, Basic Spice, Italian Spice, Chinese Spice, and Dessert Spice. Use these spice mixes with the delicious recipes in the new book *Easy Gourmet Menus to Lower Your Fat Thermostat* or flavor your own meals with the desired spice mix. You'll be delighted by the results.

Recipes to Lower Your Fat Thermostat™
by La Rene Gaunt

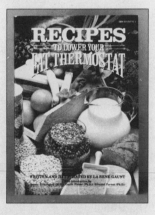

Companion cookbook to *How to Lower Your Fat Thermostat.* Once you understand the principles of the fat thermostat program, you will want to put them to work in your daily diet. Now you can with this full-color, beautifully illustrated cookbook. New ways to prepare more than 400 of your favorite recipes. Breakfast ideas. Soups and salads. Meats and vegetables. Wok food, potatoes, beans, and breads. Desserts and treats. All designed to please and satisfy while lowering your fat thermostat. It's Vitality House's most popular cookbook.

Gifford's Gourmet De-Lites
by Howard Gifford

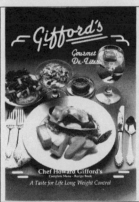

Vitality House is pleased to offer you an exciting work from a professional chef, Howard Gifford, whose meals have astonished guests at weight loss health resorts. Says Howard, "I love to create that which is pleasing both to the eye and the palate. Preparing healthy food is my medium! My tools? The common everyday household conveniences found in most American homes today. 'Simplicity' is my watchword. Become the creative gourmet cook you have always wanted to be! Learn what the magic of using just the right spices, extracts and natural juices can do for your foods! I'll also give you some helpful hints for shopping and organizing."

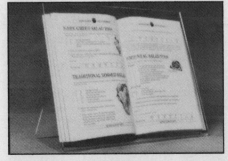

Acrylic Cookbook Holder
This acrylic cookbook holder is the perfect companion to your new cookbook. Desgined to hold any cookbook open without breaking the binding, it allows you to read recipes without distortion while protecting pages from splashes and spills.

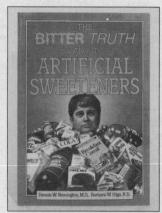

The Bitter Truth About Artificial Sweeteners

by Dennis W. Remington, M.D. and Barbara Higa, R.D.

Research proves that those people using artificial sweeteners tend to gain more weight. Not only do artificial sweeteners enchance the desire for sweets, they also cause many unpleasant side effects in addition to raising the Fat Thermostat. Learn the real truth about artificial sweeteners and sugars. Learn how they affect your health and weight and what you can do about them.

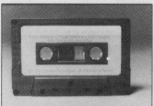

Five Roadblocks to Weight Loss

(Audiocassette)

If you have a serious weight problem that has failed to respond to the Fat Thermostat program, then you could be suffering from any of the five roadblocks to weight loss: food addictions, artificial sweeteners, food allergies, yeast overgrowth, and stress. Learn what these roadblocks are, what to do about them, and how the fat thermostat program relates to them . . . in an exclusive interview with Drs. Dennis Remington and Edward Parent.

Maintaining the Miracle

An Owner's Manual for the Human Body

by Ted D. Adams, Ph.D., A. Garth Fisher, Ph.D., Frank G. Yanowitz, M.D.

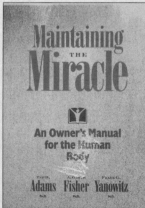

Your body is the most valuable possession you will ever own. Yet you may take better care of your car than you do your own body. In depth and up-to-date, this is the only book that tells you what to do and when to do it. You will thank yourself again and again for this invaluable help.

Desserts to Lower Your Fat Thermostat™

by Barbara Higa, R.D.

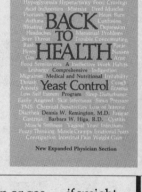

If you think you have to say goodbye to desserts, think again. At last there's a book that lets you have your cake and eat it too. *Desserts to Lower Your Fat Thermostat* is filled with what you thought you could never find: recipes for delicious desserts, snacks, and treats that are low in fat and free of sugar, salt and artificial sweeteners.

The two hundred delectable ideas packed between the covers of this book meet the guidelines of both the American Heart Association and the American Diabetes Association. They will meet your own tough standards too -- especially if you've been longing for winning ideas that will delight your family without destroying their health.

Back to Health: A Comprehensive Medical and Nutritional Yeast-Control Program

by Dennis W. Remington, M.D. and Barbara Higa, R.D.

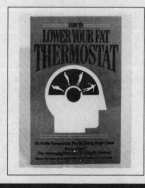

New for the 1990's! With Expanded Physician Section!

If you suffer from anxiety, depression, memory loss, heartburn or gas . . . if weight control is a constant battle . . . if you are tired, weak and sore all over . . . . this book was written for you. While yeast occurs naturally in the body, when out of control it becomes the body's enemy, manifesting itself in dozens of symptoms. Getting yeast back under control can correct many conditions once considered chronic. More than 100 yeast-free recipes, plus special sections of weight control, hypoglycemia and PMS.

Pocket Progress Guide

A pocket-sized summary of the fat thermostat program that includes food composition tables, daily records, and a progress summary for quick and easy reference.

The New Neuropsychology of Weight Control
(8 Audiocassettes and Study Guide)

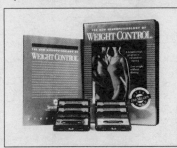

by Dennis W. Remington, M.D., A. Garth Fisher, Ph.D., Edward A. Parent, Ph.D., Barbara Higa, R.D.

More than a million people have purchased the most powerfully effective weight control program ever developed -- *The Neuropsychology of Weight Control*. Thousands of them have reported dramatic and permanent reductions in their weight.

The New Neuropsychology of Weight Control program is a scientifically-based weight-loss system that teaches you how your body works and shows you exactly what to do to change from a fat-storing to a fat-burning metabolism. Still included are the proven principles from the original program based on the best-selling book *How to Lower You Fat Thermostat*.

The New Neuropsychology of Weight Control program shows you how to set achievable weight loss goals and precisely what you need to do to reach them. You'll know how much weight you should lose and how long it will take. Included is a complete 12-week eating plan that provides daily menus, meal plans, tasty recipes, cooking instructions and eight shopping lists. You'll know exactly what to cook and how to cook it. And, you'll learn to create your own delicious meals that taste good while helping you to lose weight permanently.

The Will to Change
(Video Cassette)

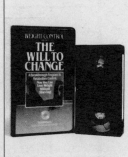

For some people, seeing is believing. While reviewing the key points of the program and the benefits of reaching your goal weight, this motivational video also features testimonials by people who have had dramatic success. In moments of doubt or discouragement, this video provides the needed support and encouragement.

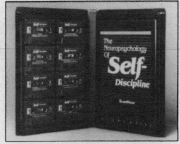

SyberVision's Neuropsychology of Self-Discipline
The Master Key to Success

There's one critical characteristic that makes the difference between success and failure: self-discipline. Without it, you can never hope to achieve your ambitions. With it, there's no goal you can't reach.

The Neuropsychology of Self-Discipline is a unique self-improvement pogram that allows you to instill a new and powerful self-mastery into your own mind and body. Armed with tools, insights, and skills of a highly disciplined achiever, you'll be able, perhaps for the first time in your life, to systematically pursue, and successfully realize, your most important goals.

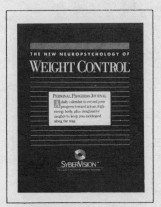

The Neuropsychology of Weight Control
Personal Progress Journal

This journal will be your six-month record of how well you're doing. By tracking your day-to-day progress you will ensure your long-term success.

QTY	CODE	DESCRIPTION	RETAIL	SUBTOTAL
	A	How To Lower Your Fat Thermostat	$ 9.95	
	B	Recipes To Lower Your Fat Thermostat	14.95	
	C	Acrylic Cookbook Holder	9.95	
	D	Neuropsychology of Weight Control (8 cassettes & guide)*	79.95	
	E	Back To Health (Yeast/Candida Guide)	10.95	
	F	Maintaining The Miracle	16.95	
	G	The Bitter Truth About Artificial Sweetners	9.95	
	H	Five Roadblocks To Weight Loss (Audiocassette)	7.95	
	I	Pocket Progress Guide	2.95	
	J	The Will To Change (Videocassette)	29.95	
	L	Neuropsychology of Self-Discipline (8 cassettes & guide)*	69.95	
	M	Personal Progress Journal (Sybervision weight program)	14.95	
	N	Desserts To Lower Your Fat Thermostat	12.95	
	O	Gifford's Gourmet De-Lites	12.95	
	P	Easy Gourmet Menus To Lower Your Fat Thermostat #	13.95	
	S	Gifford's Gourmet De-Lites Spice Mix Set #	20.95	
Shipping, 4th class book rate, $2.50 for the first item, $.50 each additional item.				+
For faster delivery, usually under five days, by UPS, add $1.50.				+
Canadian: $6.00 (U.S. dollars) for 1st item, $2.00 each additional item.				+
* Buy D or L and get 1 book free!		Utah residents add 6.25% sales tax.		+
# Buy P & S together and receive $5.00 off your order!			TOTAL	$

Prices subject to change without notice.

Name_____

Address_____

City_____ State_____ Zip_____

Day Phone_____

☐ Check   ☐ Money Order   -   Make payable to **Vitality House Publishing**
☐ MasterCard   ☐ VISA   ☐ American Express

Card No._____Expires_____

Signature_____

How did you hear about our products? ☐ Friend   ☐ Book   ☐ Other _____

Mail to: 1675 No. Freedom Blvd. #11-C Provo, UT 84604 (801) 373-5100

Copyright© 1991 Vitality House International. Orders shipped upon receipt. Allow 2-3 weeks shipping.

EGM391   **To Order: Call Toll Free 1-800-637-0708 or FAX 801-373-5370**